Textbook on
Novel Drug
Delivery System

As Per PCI Regulation for B Pharm and M Pharm Students

Textbook on
Novel Drug Delivery System

As Per PCI Regulation for B Pharm and M Pharm Students

Md Rafiul Haque
B Pharm M Pharm PhD
Associate Professor, HOD
HIMT College of Pharmacy
Greater Noida (UP)

Swati Mittal
B Pharm M Pharm
Assistant Professor
HIMT College of Pharmacy
Greater Noida (UP)

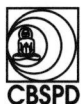

CBSPD

CBS Publishers & Distributors Pvt Ltd

New Delhi • Bengaluru • Chennai • Kochi • Kolkata • Lucknow • Mumbai
Gujarat • Hyderabad • Jharkhand • Nagpur • Patna • Pune • Uttarakhand

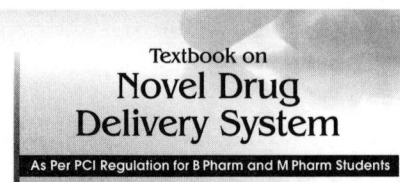

Textbook on
**Novel Drug
Delivery System**

As Per PCI Regulation for B Pharm and M Pharm Students

ISBN: 978-93-87964-88-4

Copyright © Authors and Publisher

First Edition: 2021

Reprint: 2023, 2024, **2026**

Published by Satish Kumar Jain and produced by Varun Jain for

CBS Publishers & Distributors Pvt Ltd

4819/XI Prahlad Street, 24 Ansari Road, Daryaganj, New Delhi 110 002, India
Ph: 011-23289259, 23266838

Website: www.cbspd.com

e-mail: delhi@cbspd.com; cbspubs@airtelmail.in.

Corporate Office: 204 FIE, Industrial Area, Patparganj, Delhi 110 092
Ph: 011-4934 4934 Fax: 011-4934 4935 e-mail: publishing@cbspd.com; publicity@cbspd.com

Branches

- **Bengaluru:** Seema House 2975, 17th Cross, K.R. Road, Banasankari 2nd Stage, Bengaluru 560 070 Karnataka, India
  Ph: +91-80-26771678/79 Fax: +91-80-26771680 e-mail: bangalore@cbspd.com
- **Chennai:** 18/8B, Subbarayan Street, Shenoy Nagar, Chennai 600 030, Tamil Nadu, India
  Ph: +91-44-42032115, 26681266 e-mail: chennai@cbspd.com
- **Kochi:** 42/1325, 1326, Power House Road, Opp KSEB, Power House, Ernakulam, Kochi, 682 018, Kerala, India
  Ph: +91-484-4059061-65,67 Fax: +91-484-4059065 e-mail: kochi@cbspd.com
- **Kolkata:** 147, Hind Ceramics Compound, 1st Floor, Nilgunj Road, Belghoria, Kolkata 700 056 West Bengal, India
  Ph: +91-33-25633055/56 e-mail: kolkata@cbspd.com
- **Lucknow:** Basement, Khushnuma Complex, 7-Meerabai Marg (behind Jawahar Bhawan) Lucknow 226 001, UP, India
  Ph: +91-522-4000032 e-mail: tiwari.lucknow@cbspd.com
- **Mumbai:** PWD Shed, Gala no. 25/26, Ramchandra Bhatt Marg, Next to JJ Hospital Gate no. 2, Opp. Union Bank of India, Noorbaug, Mumbai 400 009, Maharashtra, India
  Ph: +91-22-66661880/89 e-mail: mumbai@cbspd.com

Representatives

- Hyderabad • Jharkhand • Nagpur • Patna • Pune • Uttarakhand

For trade terms please contact: customercare@cbspd.com
For general enquiries please contact: info@cbspd.com

Printed at: Glorious Printers, Delhi, India

Preface

It is an enormous pleasure to familiarize the first edition of *Textbook on Novel Drug Delivery System* for B Pharm and M Pharm students.

It is well-known that diversified dosage form and delivery system have been developed to provide the precaution and well-being of society. It is essential to introduce these novel dosage forms with their applicability. This book will help the reader to flawless and updated such novel system in the discipline of pharmaceutical science.

Novel drug delivery system has received abundant consideration from the past 3–4 decades with an intention of treating illness in more scientific way rather than adopting a common policy for all types of diseases. This methodology makes use of changes in the physicochemical nature of the drug and to make maximum use of the administered drug for therapeutic benefit and minimizing undesirable and toxic effect.

In this book, we have discussed a number of drug delivery systems. Those are of macro- and micro-types. These systems are developed using advancement in conventional formulation technologies. Much talked and researched systems include controlled, transdermal, implantable, targeted, ocular, protein–peptide and vaccine drug delivery systems.

We have tried our best to understand the subject matter in an easy style and in a comprehensive manner. The subject matter is liberally illustrated with a number of clear and labelled diagrams. We sincerely feel that this book will fulfill the requirement of the students as well as teachers. While preparing this book, several standard reference books and textbooks have been consulted. Emphasis has been laid on famishing maximum information required for students in a simple and lucid language.

We are extremely thankful to staff members of CBS Publishers & Distributors Pvt Ltd, New Delhi for their full efforts in bringing out this edition.

We shall gratefully accept constructive suggestions from the teachers as well as students for upgrading this book.

Md Rafiul Haque
Swati Mittal

Contents

List of Abbreviations

API—active pharmaceutical ingredient
APC—antigen presenting cell
BCS—biopharmaceutical classification system
BMS—bare-metal stents
BBB—blood–brain barrier
CR—controlled release
CMC—carboxymethyl cellulose
CMC—critical micelle concentration
CGM—continuous glucose monitoring
CTL—cytotoxic T cell
CNT—carbon nanotubes
CHP—cholesteryl pollutant
COPD—chronic obstructive pulmonary disease
CRDDS—controlled release drug delivery system
Dex-HEMA—dextran hydroxyethyl methacrylate
DNA—deoxyribonucleic acid
DPI—dry powder inhaler
EPR—enhanced permeability retention
EDTA—ethylenediamine tetraacetic acid
FDA—food and drug administration
FDDS—floating drug delivery system
GRDDS—gastroretentive drug delivery system
GI—gastrointestinal
GRT—Gastric residence time
GET—Gastric emptying time
GIT—gastrointestinal tract
HBS—hydrodynamically balanced system
HFA—hydrofluoroalkane
HPC—Hydroxypropyl cellulose
HPMC—Hydroxypropyl methylcellulose
IR—immediate release
IM—intramuscularly
IV—intravenous
IUD—intrauterine devices
IVR—intravaginal ring
LDPE—low-density polyethene
LH—luteinizing hormone
MTC—minimum toxic concentration
MEC—minimum effective concentration

MDI—metered-dose inhaler
MHC—major histocompatibility complex
NP—nanoparticle
OROS—osmotic-controlled release oral delivery system
PEG—polyethylene glycol
PVA—polyvinyl alcohol
PVC—polyvinyl chloride
PMMA—poly (methyl methacrylate)
PEVA—poly (ethylene-vinyl acetate)
PVP—polyvinyl pyrrolidone
RE—release efficiency
RNA—ribonucleic acid
RSVE—reconstituted Sendai virus envelopes
SR—sustain release
SC—subcutaneous
TDDS—transdermal drug delivery system
TEM—transmission electron microscope
TNF—tumour necrosis factor
TSA—Trichostatin A
UVA—ultraviolet A
UVB—ultraviolet B
VCM—vinyl C monomer

Controlled Drug Delivery Systems and Polymers

CONTROLLED DRUG DELIVERY SYSTEMS

Introduction

The term, controlled drug delivery (CDD), is used to obtain specific release rates or locally targeting of active ingredients. CDD system is the one which delivers the drug at a predetermined rate, locally or systematically for a specified period of time. Drug delivery system can be a controlled release drug delivery system where there is predictive control over the release pattern, and subsequent tissue or blood levels may be achieved. Administration of drug in conventional dosage form needs large dose, frequent administration and lacks extended duration, with chances of toxicity. CDD system has been introduced to overcome the drawback of fluctuating drug levels associated with conventional dosage forms. While in CDD devices, there is efficient consumption of drug, desired extended duration with very low chances of toxicity, facilitating enhanced complication of patient, leading to better management of therapeutics. The efficacious use of drug influences cost factor, economy of therapy and adverse effect. Thus, control release formulation (CRF) involves a minimization of the amount of drug that is needed and a reduction of possible side effects. Generally concerning oral CRF, the gastrointestinal (GI) tract is of great importance to consider since it is the location of the drug release and from which the drug will be further transported to the target location. The pH value varies throughout the GIT and does also vary depending on fasting or fed condition. The pH value varies between 1 and 5.5 in the upper part while it is between 5.5 and 7 in the lower part. The different pH values of the different parts need to be considered when selecting the soft material to be designed to dissolve in the upper GI tract.

For the preparation of CRF, both natural and synthetic polymers are used. Natural polymers are various types of modified cellulose and cellulose derivatives. They are commonly used due to their susceptibility to chemical modification offering possibilities for material design. Although two cellulose derivatives have the same backbone, substitution groups can be added, resulting in one cellulose derivative becoming hydrophobic while another can become hydrophilic. To manufacture such type of the formulations is to raise the pharmaceutical efficiency for the patient, all involved materials require to fulfill the requirements for being human-body friendly. Hence, free from toxicity and not being harmful either before or after degradation.

Many different types of CDD system exist for the treatment of different pathological conditions. In these systems, *in vivo* performance is usually affected by the composition of the formulation along with manufacturing procedures. Apart from drug, such systems are usually manufactured by using polymer alone or combinations of polymers, waxy materials, and supplementary functional excipients. For the achievement of controlled drug release system, many approaches and technologies are available. Thus, it seems that the controlled delivery should be the goal for all products.

Terminology

Controlled release formulation: CDD or modified release delivery systems may be defined as the delivery of a regular supply of the active ingredient by continuously releasing for a certain period of time. An ideal CCD system is the one which delivers the active ingredient at a predetermined rate, locally or systematically, for a specific period of time.

Repeat action preparation (RAP): A dose of the drug (bioactive moiety) initially is released instantly after administration, which is generally equivalent to a single dose of the conventional drug formulation. After a definite period of time, a second single dose is released. In some preparation, one-third single dose is released after a definite time has elapsed, following the second dose. It provides the convenience supplying of additional dose or doses without the need of re-administration.

Extended release formulation (ERF): ERF is usually designed to reduce dose frequency and maintain relatively constant blood plasma drug concentration. This helps avoid the adverse effects associated with high concentration.

Delayed release preparation (DRP): The drug is released at a delay time after administration. The delayed action is obtained by the incorporation of a special coat, such as enteric coating. The purposes of such preparations are to reduce side effects related to the drug presence in the stomach, protect the active ingredient from degradation in the highly acidic pH of the gastric fluid.

Site-specific targeting: These systems refer to targeting of a bioactive molecule directly to a certain biological site. In such condition, the target is adjacent to or in the diseased organ or tissue.

Receptor targeting: These systems refer to targeting of a drug not indirectly to a certain biological location. In such condition, the target is the particular receptor for a drug within organ or tissue. Site-specific targeting and receptor targeting systems satisfy the spatial aspect of drug delivery and are also considered to be CDD systems.

Rationale of CDD System

The main objective for CDD is to modify the pharmacokinetics and pharmacodynamics of bioactive moiety by using novel drug delivery systems or by altering the molecular structure or physiological parameters inherent in a selected route of administration. Thus, optimal design of controlled release systems requires a thorough understanding of the pharmacokinetics and pharmacodynamics of drugs. However, when doses are not administered properly, the resulting drug action is less than optimum drug therapy. For example, if doses are given too frequently, minimum toxic concentration (MTC) of bioactive moiety may be reached with toxic side effects resulting. Extended release tablets and capsules are normally taken only once or twice daily compared with

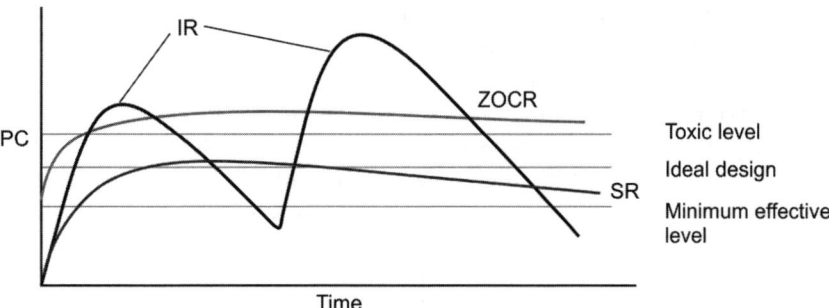

Fig. 1.1: Characteristic representation of plasma concentrations (PC) of a conventional immediate release (IR) dosage form, a sustained release (SR) dosage form and an idealized zero-order controlled release (ZOCR) dosage form (in combination with a start-up dose)

counterpart conventional forms that may need to be taken three to four times daily to achieve the same therapeutic effect. Typically, ERF gives an instant release of drug which then is followed by the gradual and continual release of additional amounts of drug to maintain this effect over a predetermined period of time (Fig. 1.1).

Advantages of Controlled Drug Therapy

- This delivery system improves the patient fulfillment especially with long-term treatments for chronic diseases.
- Conventional dosage form produces fluctuation in bioavailability. These fluctuations depend on the pharmacokinetics within the body like absorption, distribution, metabolism and excretion. Controlled release eliminates this type of fluctuation in bioavailability.
- Lessening in dose and dosing frequencies.
- Maintenance of required drug concentration in plasma thus eliminates the failure of drug therapy and improves the efficacy of treatments.
- An appropriate delivery system for drugs which is having a short biological half-life (3–4 hours) and drug rapidly eradicates from the body.

Disadvantages of Controlled Drug Therapy

- Dumping is a major disadvantage of control release DDS, which refers to the rapid release of a relatively large quantity of drug from controlled release formulations. This phenomenon becomes hazardous with potent drugs.
- Poor *in vivo* and *in vitro* correlation.
- Not easy to optimize the accurate dose and dosing interval.
- Patient variability affects the release rate like GI emptying rate, residential time, fasting or non-fasting conditions, etc.

Properties of Drug Candidate for Controlled Drug Delivery System

Physiological Properties

1. **Aqueous solubility:** Most of the active pharmaceutical ingredients (API) are weakly acidic or basic in nature that affect the H_2O solubility of API. Weak water-soluble drugs are difficult to design the CRF. High aqueous solubility drugs show burst

release followed by a rapid increment in blood plasma drug concentration. Such types of drugs are a good candidate for CRDDS. The pH depends on solubility also creates a problem in formulating CRDDS.

2. **Partition coefficient (P-value):** P-value denotes the fraction of the bioactive moiety into oil and aqueous phase that is a significant factor that affects the passive diffusion of the bioactive moiety across the biological membrane. The bioactive moiety is having high or low P-value not suitable for control release (CR), it should be appropriate to dissolve in both phases.

3. **Drug pKa:** pKa is the factor that determined the ionization of bioactive moiety at physiological pH in GIT. Generally, the high ionized bioactive moiety is poor candidate for CRDDS. The absorption of the unionized drug occurs rapidly as compared to ionized drugs from the biological membranes. The pKa ranges for acidic drug, pH is 3 to 5 and for a basic drug, pH is 7 to 11.

4. **Drug stability:** Bioactive moieties that are stable in acid/base, enzymatic degradation, and other gastric fluids are good candidates for CRDDS. If drug degraded in the stomach and small intestine, it is not suitable for CRF because it will decrease bioavailability of concerned drug.

5. **Molecular weight and molecular size:** The molecular weight and molecular size are two most significant factors which affect the molecular diffusibility across a biological membrane. The molecular size less than 400D is easily diffusible but greater than 400D generates problem in drug diffusion.

6. **Protein binding:** The drug–protein complex acts as a reservoir in plasma for the bioactive moiety. Bioactive moieties showing high plasma protein binding are not a good candidate for CRDDS because the protein binding increases the biological half-life. So, there is no need to sustain the drug release.

Biological Factors

1. **Absorption:** Uniformity in rate and extent of absorption is a significant factor in formulating the CRDDS. However, the rate-limiting step is drug released from the dosage form. The absorption rate should be faster than release rate to prevent the dose dumping. The various factors like aqueous solubility, acid hydrolysis affect the absorption of drugs.

2. **Biological half-life (t½):** Normally, the drug is having short half-life needed frequent dosing and suitable candidate for controlled release system. A drug with long half-life needed dosing after a long-time interval. Ideally, the drugs having half-life 2–3 hours are a suitable candidate for CRDDS. Drugs have half-life more than 7–8 hours are not used for CR system.

3. **Dose size:** The CRDDS formulated to eliminate the repetitive dosing, so it should contain the large dose than conventional dosage form. But the dose used in conventional dosage form provides an indication of the dose to be used in CRDDS. The volume of sustained dose must be as large as it comes under acceptance criteria.

4. **Therapeutic window:** The drugs with narrow therapeutic index are not good for CRDDS. If the delivery system failed to CR, it would cause dose dumping and ultimate toxicity.

5. **Absorption window:** The bioactive moieties which show absorption from the specific segment in GI tract are not a good candidate for CRDDS. Drugs which absorbed throughout the GIT are suitable candidates for CR.

6. **Patient physiology:** The physiological conditions of the patient like gastric emptying rate, residential time, and GI diseases influence the release of the drug from the dosage form directly or indirectly.

Approaches to Design CR Formulations

Based on the release mechanism, these are classified as follows:
1. Diffusion-controlled products
2. Dissolution-controlled products
3. Erosion products
4. Osmotic pump systems
5. Ion exchange resins

Diffusion-Controlled Products

In such a system, there is water-insoluble polymer which controls the flow of water and the subsequent release of dissolved bioactive moiety from the dosage form. Diffusion occurs when a drug passes through the polymer that forms the CR device. The diffusion may occur through pores in the polymer matrix or by passing between polymer chains (Fig. 1.2). These are broadly divided into two groups:
a. Reservoir devices
b. Matrix devices

The basic mechanisms of drug release from these two systems are basically different.

a. **Reservoir devices:** In such system, a water insoluble polymeric material encases a core of drug. Drug will partition into the membrane and exchange with the fluid surrounding the particles or tablet. The bioactive agent is released to the surrounding environment by diffusion process through the rate limiting membrane. In these reservoir systems, the drug (bioactive moiety) delivery rate remains fairly constant.

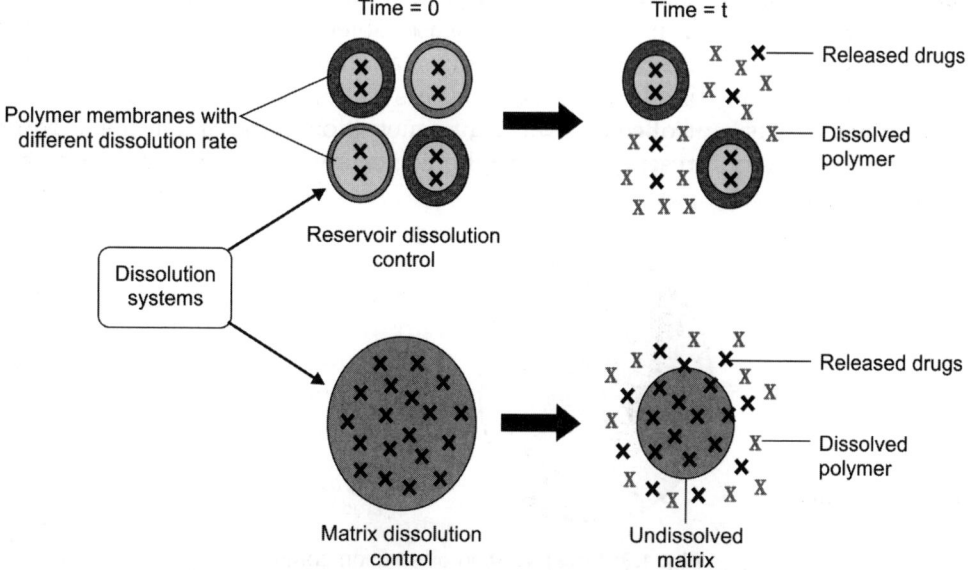

Fig. 1.2: Diffusion-controlled system

b. **Matrix devices:** In such matrix devices, the drug or bioactive molecule is dispersed in polymer matrix to form a homogeneous system known as a matrix system. Diffusion occurs when the bioactive molecule passes from the polymer matrix into the external environment. As the release continues, its rate normally decreases with such type of system, since the bioactive molecule has a progressively longer distance to travel and, therefore, needs a longer diffusion time to release.

Dissolution-Controlled Products

In such products, the rate of dissolution of the drug or bioactive molecule is controlled by slowly soluble polymers or by microencapsulation. Once the coating is dissolved, the bioactive molecule becomes available for dissolution. By varying the thicknesses of the coat and its composition, the rate of bioactive molecule release may be controlled. Some formulations contain a fraction of the total dose as an immediate release component to give a pulse dose soon after administration. The pellet dosage forms of diffusion- or dissolution-controlled products may be encapsulated or prepared as a tablet. Dissolution-controlled products can be subdivided into two groups:

a. Encapsulation dissolution control
b. Matrix dissolution control

a. **Encapsulation dissolution control:** These systems involve coating of individual particles or granules of drug or bioactive molecule with a slow dissolving material. The coated particles may be compressed directly into tablets or placed in capsules. The rate of dissolution of the drug or bioactive moiety (and thereby availability for absorption) is controlled by microencapsulation. Once the coating is dissolved, the bioactive molecule becomes available for dissolution. By changing the thicknesses of the coat and its composition, the rate of drug release may be controlled. Such type of products should not be chewed as the coating may be damaged. One of the major advantages of encapsulated pelleted products is that the onset of absorption is less sensitive to stomach emptying. The entrance of the pellets into the small intestine (where the majority of drug absorption occurs) is generally more uniform than with non-disintegrating sustained-release tablet preparations (Fig. 1.3).

b. **Matrix dissolution control:** In such system, an alternative approach is to compress the drug with a slow dissolving carrier. In this system, the rate of drug or bioactive molecule release is controlled by the rate of penetration of the dissolution fluid into the matrix, porosity, presence of hydrophobic additives and the wet capability of system and surface of particle (Fig. 1.4).

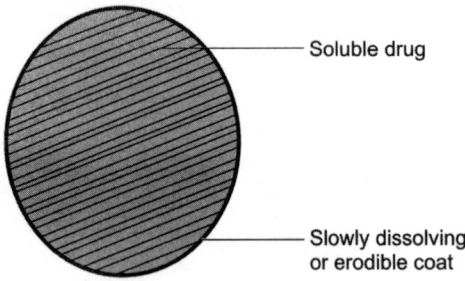

Soluble drug

Slowly dissolving or erodible coat

Fig. 1.3: Encapsulation dissolution control

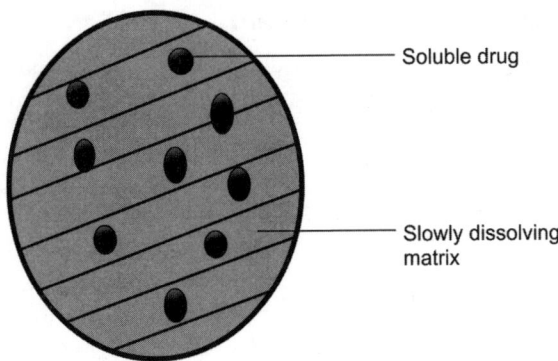

Fig. 1.4: Matrix dissolution control

Erosion Products

In such type of system, drugs or bioactive agents are mixed with biodegradable polymers. Such materials degrade within the body as a result of natural biological processes and drug release occurs at fixed rate. Many biodegradable polymers are designed to degrade as a result of hydrolysis of the polymer chains into biologically acceptable and progressively smaller compounds. The release of drug from such products is controlled by the erosion rate of a carrier matrix. The rate of release is determined by the rate of erosion.

Osmotic Pump Systems

The osmotic pump is like a reservoir device but contains an osmotic agent (e.g. the active agent in salt form) which acts to imbibe water from the surrounding medium via a semipermeable membrane. A pressure is generated within the device which forces the active agent out of the device via an orifice (of a size designed to minimize solute diffusion, whilst preventing the build-up of a hydrostatic pressure head which has the effect of decreasing the osmotic pressure and altering the dimensions {volume} of the device). The advantage of such type of product is that the fixed release is unchanged by the environment of the gastrointestinal tract and relies simply on the passage of water into the dosage form. The rate of release may be modified by changing the osmotic agent and the size of the hole.

Ion Exchange Resins

A drug–resin complex for extended release is known and is successfully used commercially. The drug is bound to the resin and released by exchanging with suitable charged ions in contact with the ion exchange groups. Such a technique is applicable to certain drugs which have particular characteristics in terms of their relative affinity for the polymers being used.

Types of CR Preparation

On the basis of technical sophistication, controlled drug delivery system may be grouped into three major classes.

1. Rate-Programmed Drug Delivery System

This drug delivery system is that from which the drug release has been programmed at specific rate profiles. They are further subdivided into following subclasses.

a. Dissolution drug delivery system
  - Slow dissolution rate of the drug
  - Slow dissolution rate of the reservoir membrane or matrix

b. Diffusion drug delivery system
  - Porous matrix-controlled system
  - Porous membrane-controlled system

c. Erosion drug delivery system
  - Surface erosion
  - Bulk erosion

d. Dissolution, diffusion and/or erosion drug delivery system
  - Reservoir system (membrane rectal drug delivery system)
  - Matrix system (monolithic drug delivery system)
  - Hybrid system (membrane cum matrix drug delivery system)

2. Stimuli-Activated Drug Delivery System

a. Activation by physical process
b. Activation by chemical process
c. Activation by biological system

3. Site-Targeted Drug Delivery System

a. Polymeric carriers for drug targeting
b. Albumin as carrier for drug targeting
c. Lipoprotein as carrier for drug targeting
d. Liposomes as carrier for drug targeting

Liquid-Sustained Release Systems

The development of liquid oral-sustained release formulations is gained much interest currently. Such preparations eradicate the problems associated with the solid dosage forms while maintaining the advantages and convenience of sustained release drug delivery. Alternative strategies are adopted to develop such systems. One of the techniques examined the use of suspended microspheres which are incorporated as a dispersed phase in a suspension. Another strategy studied the use of ion exchange resins or employing sparingly soluble salts to prepare oral sustained release suspensions. The use of *in situ* gelling systems gives other promising alternative with most of the reported investigations employing the sol to gel phase transition of alginate solution after addition of polyvalent cations as calcium. A suspension is reported to form a gel when comes in contact with simulated gastric fluid. In recent study, a liquid-sustained release formulation for eradication of *Helicobacter pylori* is developed in presence of alginate solution. In such study, the *in situ* gelation is obtained by separate oral administration of calcium solution which is taken immediately after administration of sodium alginate solution. Shortly after this, it is attempted to prepare systems containing sodium alginate combined with calcium. Such systems retained the fluidity in the bottle but undergo immediate gelation on coming into contact with gastric or simulated gastric acidity. To inhibit the interaction of calcium with alginate in the bottle, calcium ions are sequestered with sodium citrate. This complex breaks immediately in strong acidity librating free calcium which can interact with alginate lead to spontaneous gelation. The optimal quantities of calcium chloride and sodium citrate that maintain fluidity of the preparation before administration but gel spontaneously after contact with simulated gastric fluid (pH 1.2) are determined. It should be noted that such type of gel is pH sensitive and breaks in presence of intestinal pH. Accordingly, the release pattern will depend on the gastric emptying rate which is highly changeable. Such a problem draws the attention to new *in situ* gelling system with a stronger gel structure that can keep up the sustained release pattern after gastric emptying. The gel structure of alginate-based systems is enhanced by combination with chitosan. This combination is employed in development of controlled release particulate and other solid drug delivery systems. The synergism between chitosan and alginate is due to the electrostatic interactions between carboxyl groups of alginate and amino groups ($-NH_2$) of chitosan and existence of interactive Coulomb forces. Such effects increase the gel strength. This drug is selected as it has high water solubility and short half-life.

Preparation of In Situ Gelling Systems

In situ gelling liquid formulations consisting of increasing concentrations of sodium alginate is prepared in absence and presence of chitosan. Sodium alginate is added to ultrapure water containing 0.45% w/v sodium citrate and 0.15% w/v calcium chloride and 0.6% w/v dextromethorphan hydrobromide. Such mixtures are heated to 60°C while stirring. Stirring is continued at ambient temperature until cooling to less than 40°C. For chitosan-containing systems, amount of chitosan is levigated gradually with the lead to alginate solution under continuous stirring using a mortar and pestle to produce homogenous dispersion.

Evaluation

This type of study is conducted to assess the gel forming property of the tested formulation. The formulation (10 ml) is packed into cellulose bag. This is immersed in 0.1 N HCl (100 ml) and maintained at 37°C for 24 hours. The fluid content of the cellulose bag is separated from the gel by sieving through a 355 μm sieve for 30 seconds. The weight of the gel remaining on the sieve is determined.

Determination of In Vitro Drug Release

The method of assessment of drug release from enteric-coated systems is adopted (USP 24). In addition, the study is further extended to monitor drug release at pH 7.4. The release experiments employed a USP dissolution apparatus (Model: UDT-804, LOGAN Inst. USA) with a paddle stirrer being maintained at 50 rpm. The release medium is 500 ml of simulated gastric fluid without enzymes (0.1 N HCl, pH 1.2) and the temperature is maintained at 37 ± 0.2°C. The test preparation (10 ml) is loaded into a petri dish (2.7 cm, internal diameter) before immersion into the dissolution vessel containing release medium without much disturbance. Samples (5 ml) are collected at predetermined time intervals (5, 15, 30, 60, 90 and 120 minutes, respectively). Fresh release medium is added to replenish for each sample. The samples are filtered through 0.45 μm filter, immediately after collection and the filtrate is analyzed for drug content using the HPLC method. After the last sample (2 hours), the pH of the release medium is adjusted to 6.8 to simulate the intestinal pH (USP 24). This is achieved by addition of 200 ml of 0.3 M dibasic sodium phosphate and 25 ml of 1 N sodium hydroxide. Sampling is then continued for another 4 hours at the end of which the medium is adjusted to 7.4 using 1N NaOH and sampling is continued for another 2 hours. These samples are treated as before. The cumulative amounts of the drug released (expressed as % of the total drug added) are plotted as a function of time to produce the drug release profiles. The release efficiency is calculated from the area under the release curve at time t (determined using the non-linear trapezoidal rule) and expressed as a % of the area of the rectangle describe by 100% release in the same time. The results are compared to the release data of the marketed formulation (Delsym® suspension). In addition, the release data for each phase are fitted to different kinetic models to determine the release kinetics. This includes fitting the data to zero order, first order and Higuchi diffusion system. Each study is conducted in triplicate.

Pharmacokinetic Design for DDS

The objective of drug therapy is to maximize the desired pharmacological response while minimizing drug toxicity. The goal of CR or SR formulations is to minimize the ratio of maximum to minimum plasma drug concentrations (C_{max}/C_{min}) at steady-state; this depends on the dosing interval and the terminal half-life ($t\frac{1}{2}$) of the drug. However, this is true for drugs that decline monoexponentially in plasma or for drugs that do not distribute extensively in tissues. For drugs with a distinct distribution phase (drugs that distribute extensively in tissues), plasma concentrations during the terminal phase would be very much lower than those during the early distribution phase. The use of the terminal $t\frac{1}{2}$ of these drugs (those with distinct distribution phase) as a guide for multiple dosing could result in large C_{max}/C_{min} ratios and in unsuccessful drug therapy, if the C_{max}/C_{min} ratio exceeds the therapeutic index (TI), which is defined as the ratio of effective and safe plasma concentrations to concentrations eliciting unwanted toxic effects. For drugs with narrow TI values and those that decline multi-exponentially in plasma, it is necessary to identify the $t\frac{1}{2}$ of a particular phase of the log concentration-time profile as a guide for multiple-dosing calculations. The $t\frac{1}{2}$ value that is used as the guide for multiple-dosing therapy should be the multiple-dosing $t\frac{1}{2}$ ($t\frac{1}{2}$, md). This $t\frac{1}{2}$ value is the one that most significantly affects drug concentrations after multiple dosing. In general, the terminal or distribution $t\frac{1}{2}$ should be used as the $t\frac{1}{2}$, md for drugs with shallow or steep distribution phases, respectively. However, it should be emphasized that the use of the distribution $t\frac{1}{2}$ as the $t\frac{1}{2}$, md would result in extensive accumulation of drug in the body. The $t\frac{1}{2}$, md should also be chosen based on the site(s) of action related to the pharmacologic and toxic effects of the drug. For example, if the site of action is located in deep tissue compartments of the body, the terminal $t\frac{1}{2}$ used should be the $t\frac{1}{2}$, md. To minimize the C_{max}/C_{min} ratio, the, md has to be longer than τ. For drugs with $t_{1/2}$, md values less than r, a smaller C_{max}/C_{min} ratio can be achieved by controlling the rate of drug release (and absorption) from the formulation. If a formulation can be developed with a release rate much slower than the quotient of $t\frac{1}{2}$, md, the $t\frac{1}{2}$ of a drug after administration of the SR or CR formulation will reflect the rate of release of drug from the formulation (flip-flop) and a smaller C_{max}/C_{min} ratio can, therefore, be achieved. The first step in the development of CR or SR formulations, therefore, is to determine, if a CR or SR formulation is even necessary. This can be determined by comparing the C_{max}/C_{min} ratio to the therapeutic index of the drug. However, this criterion requires that a relationship be known between the effect of the drug (pharmacologic and toxic) and plasma concentrations. If there is no such relationship, other considerations can be reviewed. For example, one can consider whether the pharmacologic or toxic effects of the drug are a function of drug input rate or a function of the maximum plasma concentrations attained.

In the simplest release pattern called zero-order release (Fig. 1.5). In zero-order release, the delivery rate remains constant. The release rate from these devices is given as,

$$dMt/dt = k$$

where, k is constant, t is time and Mt representing the mass of active agent released.

The release rate is directly proportional to the amount of active ingredient loaded in device (Fig. 1.6). Mathematically, this may be represented as:

$$dMt/dt = k (Mo–Mt)$$

where, Mo = mass of active moiety in the device

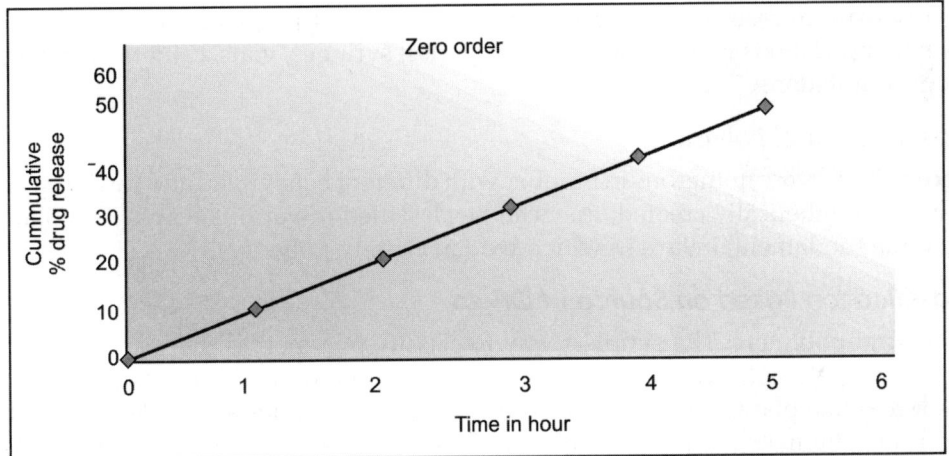

Fig. 1.5: Zero-order release of a drug from CR formulation

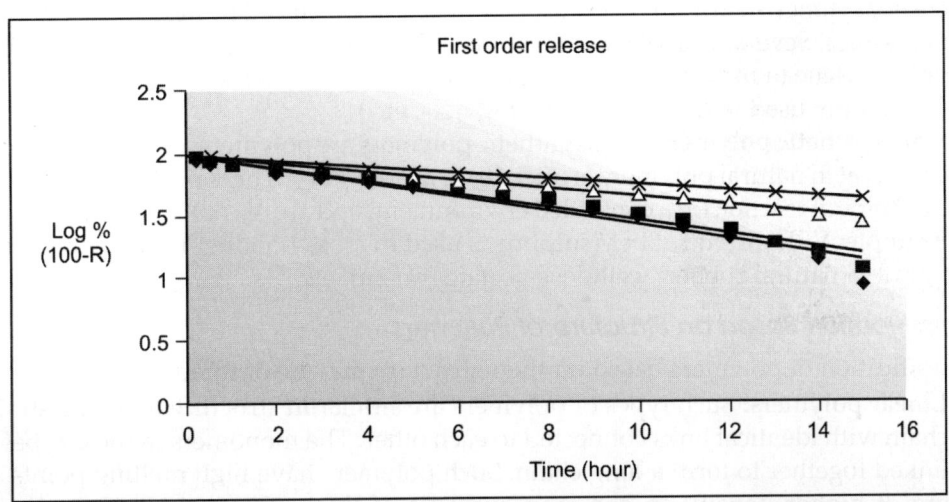

Fig. 1.6: First-order release of a drug from CR formulation

This indicates that the release rates decline exponentially with time and with depletion of active ingredient the release rate approaches zero.

POLYMERS

Introduction

Polymer is long chain organic molecule assembled from several smaller molecules called monomers. Natural-based and synthetic polymers have found their way into the pharmaceutical and biomedical industries and their applications are growing at a fast pace. Polymers may be applied in drug delivery systems, as scaffolds for tissue engineering and repair, and as novel biomaterials. Polymer is becoming increasingly significant in the field of drug delivery. The pharmaceutical utilization of polymers varies from their use as binders in tablets to viscosity and flow controlling agents in liquids, suspensions and emulsions. Polymers may be used as film coatings to mask the unpleasant taste of a drug or bioactive molecule, to enhance drug stability, and to modify drug release characteristics. In pharmaceutical preparations also, they have several applications in manufacturing of bottles, syringes, vials, catheters, and also in drug formulations.

Classification of Polymers

Since polymers are numerous in number with different behaviours and can be naturally found or synthetically created, they can be classified in various ways. The following are some fundamental ways in which we can classify polymers.

Classification Based on Source of Origin

1. **Natural polymers:** The simplest way to classify polymers is their source of origin. Natural polymers are polymers which occur in nature and are existing in natural sources like plants and animals. Some common examples are proteins (which are found in humans and animals alike), cellulose and starch (which are found in plants) or rubber (which we harvest from the latex of a tropical plant).
2. **Synthetic polymers:** Synthetic polymers are polymers which humans can artificially create/synthesize in a lab. These are commercially produced by industries for human necessities. Several commonly produced polymers which we utilize day-to-day are polyethylene (a mass-produced plastic which we use in packaging) or nylon fibres (commonly used in our clothes, fishing nets, etc.)
3. **Semisynthetic polymers:** Semisynthetic polymers are polymers achieved by making changing in natural polymers artificially in a laboratory. These polymers synthesize by chemical reaction (in a controlled environment) and are of commercial importance. Example: Vulcanized rubber (sulphur is used in cross-bonding the polymer chains found in natural rubber), cellulose acetate (rayon), etc.

Classification Based on Structure of Polymers

Classification of polymers based on their structure may be of three types:
1. **Linear polymers:** Such types of polymers are similar in structure to a long straight chain with identical links connected to each other. The monomers in these types are linked together to form a long chain. Such polymers have high melting points and are of higher density. A common example of this polymer is PVC (polyvinyl chloride). This type of polymer is largely used for making electric cables and pipes.

2. **Branch chain polymers:** The structure of such polymers is like branches originating at random points from a single linear chain. Monomers unite together to form a long straight chain with some branched chains of different lengths. As a result of such branches, the polymers are not closely packed together. They are of low density having low MP. Low-density polyethene (LDPE) used in plastic bags and general-purpose container is a very common example.
3. **Cross-linked or network polymers:** In such type of polymers, monomers are joined together to form a three-dimensional network. The monomers having strong covalent bonds as they are composed of bifunctional and trifunctional in nature. Such polymers are hard and brittle, e.g. melamine, bakelite (used in electrical insulators), etc.

Classification Based on Mode of Polymerization

Polymerization is a process by which monomer molecules are reacted each other in a chemical reaction to form a polymer chain, which is a three-dimensional network. On the basis of type of polymerization, polymers may be classified as:

1. **Addition polymers:** Such types of polymers are generally formed by the repeated addition of monomer molecules. The polymer is formed by polymerization of monomers with double or triple bonds such as unsaturated hydrocarbon compounds. Note, in such process, there is no removal of small molecules like H_2O or alcohol (–OH), etc. (no byproduct of the process). They always have their empirical formulas same as their monomers, e.g. ethene ($CH_2 = CH_2$) to polyethene $- (CH_2 - CH_2) \, n^-$.
2. **Condensation polymers:** Such polymers are formed by the combination of monomers, with the removal of small molecules like H_2O or alcohol (–OH), etc. The monomers in such types of condensation reactions are bifunctional or trifunctional in nature. A very common example is the polymerization of hexamethylenediamine and adipic acid to give nylon-66, where molecules of water are removed in the process.

Classification Based on Molecular Forces

Intramolecular forces are those forces that join atoms together within a molecule. In polymers, strong covalent bonds link atoms to each other in individual polymer molecules. Intermolecular forces (between the molecules) attract polymer molecules towards each other. The properties exhibited by solid materials like polymers depend largely on the strength of the forces between these molecules. Using this, polymers may be classified into four types:

1. **Elastomers:** These are rubber-like solid polymers, which are elastic in nature. Elastic basically mean that the polymer can be easily stretched by applying a little force. The very common example of this can be seen in rubber bands (or hair bands). Applying a few stresses elongates the band. The polymer chains are held by the weakest intermolecular forces, hence allowing the polymer to be stretched. But removing that stress results in the rubber band taking up its original form. This happens as cross-links between the polymer chain which help it in retracting to its original position, and taking its original form. Car tyres are made of vulcanized rubber. This is when introduce sulphur to cross-bond the polymer chains.
2. **Thermoplastics:** Thermoplastic polymers are those long-chain polymers in which intermolecule forces (van der Waals forces) unite the polymer chains together. Such

polymers become softened after heating (thick fluid like) and hardened when they are allowed to cool down, forming a hard mass. They do not have cross-bond and can easily be shaped by heating and using moulds. A very common example is polystyrene or PVC (which is used in making pipes).

3. **Thermosetting:** Thermosetting plastics are those polymers which are semi-fluid in nature with low molecular masses. When heated, they start cross-linking between polymer chains, hence becoming hard and infusible. They form a three-dimensional structure on the application of heat. This reaction is irreversible in nature. The most common example of a thermosetting polymer is that of Bakelite, which is used in preparing electrical insulation.

4. **Fibres:** These are a class of polymers which are thread-like in nature, and can easily be woven. They have strong intermolecular forces between the chains giving them less elasticity and high tensile strength. The intermolecular forces may be hydrogen bonds or dipole-dipole interaction. Fibres have sharp and high melting points (MP). A very common example is that of nylon-66, which is used in carpets and apparels.

Above are the very general ways to classify polymers. Another category of polymers is that of biopolymers. Biopolymers are those polymers which are obtained from living organisms. They are very biodegradable and have a very well-defined structure. Many biomolecules like carbohydrates and proteins are a part of the category.

Characteristics of an Ideal Polymer

- It should be inert and compatible with the environment.
- It should be non-toxic.
- It should be easily administered.
- It should be easy and inexpensive to fabricate.
- It should have good mechanical strength.
- Low density
- Poor temperature resistance
- It can be produced transparent or in different colours.
- Low coefficient of friction
- Good mould ability

Properties of Polymers

Physical Properties

- As chain length and cross-linking increases, the tensile strength of the polymer increases.
- Polymers do not melt; they change state from crystalline to semicrystalline.

Chemical Properties

- Compared to conventional molecules with different side molecules, the polymer is enabled with hydrogen bonding and ionic bonding resulting in better cross-linking strength.
- Dipole-dipole bonding side chains enable the polymer for high flexibility.
- Polymers with van der Waals forces linking chains are known to be weak, but give the polymer a low melting point.

Optical Properties

Due to their ability to change their refractive index with temperature as in the case of PMMA and HEMA: MMA, they are used in lasers for applications in spectroscopy and analytical applications.

Advantages of Polymers

- Cheap to make
- Many uses because of their different properties
- Provide jobs in firms which make the polymer and the product.
- Some polymers can be recycled, melted down and made into something else which saves valuable natural resources.
- If polymers are used instead of wood, fewer trees will have to be cut down.

Disadvantages of Polymers

- People do not like to live near polymer-producing industrial works.
- Some people think plastic products look cheap compared with natural materials.
- Made from oil, a non-renewable resource.
- Most plastics are not biodegradable, so there is a problem of how to get rid of them.
- Landfill sites are ugly.
- Give off toxic fumes when they burn.
- Sorting types of polymers for recycling can be expensive.

Applications of Polymers for Controlled Drug Delivery

Over the past four decades, an interest has developed in the design and formulation of dosage forms that control the subsequent release of drug from the dosage form into the surrounding biological fluids. This rate process effectively controls the therapeutic properties of the medicinal agent. Vital to the development of these systems is role of pharmaceutical polymers. In light of the current and continuing importance of this category of drug delivery system provides a concise range of designs of CRDDS and the contribution/significance of polymers to their function.

Reservoir Systems

In such type of systems, the drug having core is separated from the biological fluids by a water insoluble polymeric coat or layer, depending on the geometry of the drug delivery system. Examples of polymers that are commonly used as the polymeric coats/layers include ethyl cellulose, poly (ethylene-vinyl acetate), silicone and various acrylate copolymers. A diagrammatic representation of the design and operation of a reservoir system is presented in Figure 1.7.

Drug release from these systems occurs in a number of steps, initially involving the partitioning of the drug into the polymeric coat/layer.

The Ocusert System

The delivery of therapeutic agents to the eye for the treatment of disorders of the eye (e.g. glaucoma) using conventional drug delivery systems, e.g. drops, ointments, is an inefficient process. These are primarily due to the rapid clearance of drugs from the surface of the eye due to blinking and tear flow. One method by which the efficiency of ocular drug delivery may be improved is through the use of polymeric implants

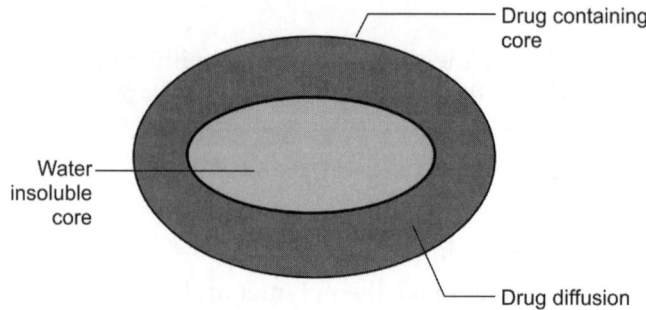

Fig. 1.7: Diagrammatic representation of the design and operation of a reservoir-controlled release system

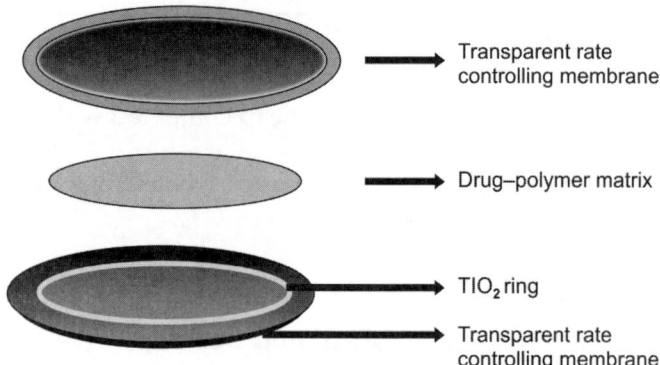

Fig. 1.8: Ellipsoidal shaped Ocusert

that are implanted under the lower cul-de-sac of the eye. The Ocusert represents one such example that has been designed to release either 20 μg h⁻¹ or 40 μg h⁻¹ of a therapeutic agent (pilocarpine) for a 7-day period following implantation. In design terms, the Ocusert is an ellipsoidal-shaped implant that is composed of several layers, diagrammatic representations of which are shown in Figure 1.8.

In this system, pilocarpine is dispersed within an alginic acid matrix which is sandwiched between two layers each composed of poly (ethylene-co-vinyl acetate). These layers act as the rate controlling membranes. The fourth layer is composed of an opaque, annular ring that is housed beneath the rate controlling layer and, as both the rate controlling membranes and the drug-containing matrix are transparent, the function of this ring is to offer visibility of the device following instillation. Drug release from this delivery system occurs by diffusion.

The Progestasert System

A second example of a reservoir CDDS is the Progestasert intrauterine device (IUD), a medicated implant that is used for contraceptive purposes. In the 1960s, IUDs emerged as an available method of contraception that prevented implantation of the ovum due to the mechanical effects of the device on the uterine endometrium. It is accepted that to achieve greater contraceptive efficiency, larger IUDs should be used, as these offer greater coverage of the endometrium. However, patients using these larger IUDs will be more prone to side effects including bleeding, cramps and possibly expulsion. One method by which the contraceptive efficacy of these devices may be improved whilst lowering the incidence of side effects is to use the IUD to locally deliver contraceptive agents to the endometrium at a defined rate for a prolonged period. Local delivery of progesterone is advantageous for a number of reasons. Most noticeably, the drug is rapidly metabolized oral administration and, therefore, requires frequent oral administration of high doses of this drug.

Reservoir-Designed Transdermal Patches

One-third example of the use of reservoir systems for controlled drug delivery may be observed in the transdermal delivery of therapeutic agents. Transdermal drug delivery involves the diffusion of the drug through the skin and ultimately absorption into the systemic circulation. One of the anatomical purposes of the skin is to protect the body from the ingress of possibly dangerous chemicals and, therefore, it is little surprise that only a limited number of therapeutic agents possess the appropriate physicochemical properties to traverse this anatomical barrier. There are three main anatomical barriers that therapeutic agents must partition into and diffuse through prior to possible absorption into the systemic circulation, namely the stratum corneum (a keratinized layer at the outermost region of the skin), the viable epidermis and the dermis, into which the microcirculation may be found (Fig. 1.9).

Matrix Systems

In this matrix designed drug delivery systems, the drug or bioactive moiety is homogeneously dispersed, either at the molecular scale or as solid particles, within a polymeric medium. In comparison to reservoir systems, the manufacture of matrix designed drug delivery systems is more straight forward and may be performed using a number of different approaches. Examples of these include:
- Mixing of a polymer with the drug or bioactive particles followed by direct compression into tablets.
- Incorporation of a drug into a polymer by polymerization of a drug-monomer mixture or by hydrogel swelling within a drug solution.
- Dissolving the drug and polymer in an appropriate solvent followed by solvent removal.
- Curing the polymer in the presence of dissolved/dispersed drug.

Swelling-Controlled Release Systems

In the previous sections, the release of therapeutic agents from reservoir and matrix designs was described. Whilst the designs of these systems differ, it is assumed that

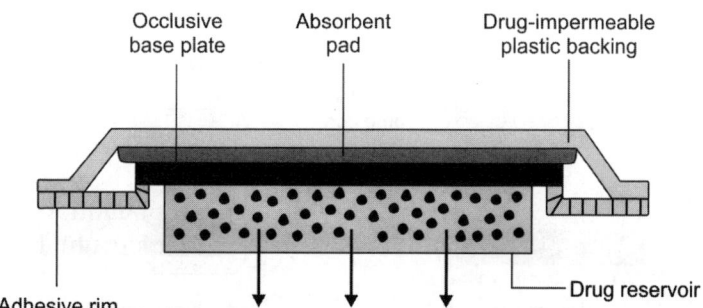

Fig. 1.9: Cross-section view of matrix diffusion controlled transdermal drug delivery system showing major structural components

the shape and dimensions of the devices do not change during the course of drug release. This is due to the hydrophobic nature of the polymers used in the formulation of these systems. Hence, in the reservoir systems, the thickness of the coating remains constant whereas in matrix systems there is a defined thickness of the device (e.g. slab, cylinder, sphere) over which diffusion occurs. As a result, in the equations that describe drug release, the thickness of the system/membrane is defined. However, in many drug delivery systems, the dimensions of the dosage form will change during the course of drug release due to swelling of the polymer matrix. Although the mechanism for drug release is diffusion.

Biodegradable Systems

Biodegradable systems are those in which a therapeutic agent has been incorporated into a matrix that is composed of a biodegradable polymer, i.e. a polymer that will undergo controlled degradation within a biological environment. As a result, following implantation, the molecular weight of the polymer matrix will be reduced due to hydrolysis of crosslinks or hydrolysis of the main polymer chain, and in doing so the previously insoluble polymer matrix will be rendered soluble in the biological fluids thereby facilitating elimination. There are several examples of biodegradable polymers that have been examined for controlled release applications. These include poly (lactic acid), poly (glycolic acid) and their copolymers, poly (ε-caprolactone), poly (ortho esters) and polyanhydrides.

Osmotically Controlled Drug Delivery Systems

In these systems, the difference between the osmotic pressure within a formulation and the surrounding biological fluids is used as the driving force for drug release. The first osmotic systems were developed by the Alza Corporation in the 1970s and since that time, both the number and types of designs of these systems have increased. The basic design of the OROS system, one of the original elementary osmotic pumps (Fig. 1.10).

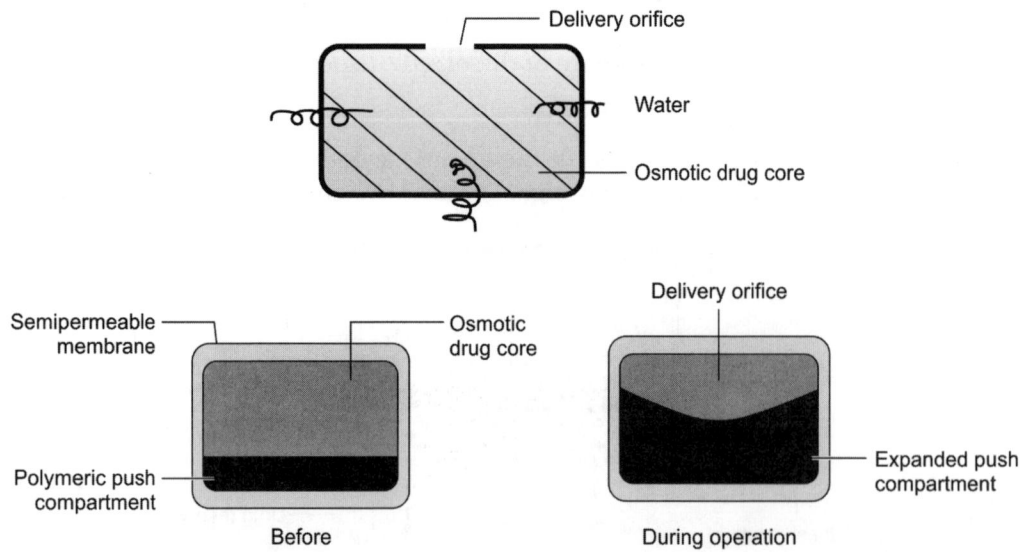

Fig. 1.10: The basic design of the OROS system

Stimulus Responsive Drug Release

Up to this section, the discussion of drug release is primarily concerned with systems from which drug release is facilitated by simple diffusion. Osmotically controlled systems and the use of biodegradable polymers offer possibilities for the enhancement of drug release through ancillary processes, namely osmotic pressure and polymer degradation. However, another aspect of great interest in drug delivery is the ability to engineer dosage forms to release the drug on demand following the application of an appropriate stimulus, e.g. drug release at a specific location within the gastrointestinal tract.

Polymer-Drug Conjugates

Polymer-drug conjugates offer an exciting strategy for the improved delivery of therapeutic agents, both in terms of the provision of controlled release but also for the improved targeting of the therapeutic agent to a particular site. As the title suggests, polymer-drug conjugates are composed of a drug that is covalently bound to a polymer, which may be either hydrophilic or hydrophobic.

QUESTIONS

A. Short Answer Type Questions

1. Describe properties of drug candidates for controlled drug delivery system.
2. Discuss about biological properties of drugs appropriate to controlled release formulations.
3. Write a short note on pharmacokinetic design for drug delivery system.
4. Mention the application of polymers.
5. Write about physicochemical properties of drugs related to controlled release formulations.
6. Write a short note on controlled release preparation and their formulations.
7. Define polymers and classify them.
8. What are the characteristics for ideal polymers?

B. Long Answer Type Questions

1. Write different approaches for design-controlled release formulation.
2. Mention advantages and disadvantages of polymers in detail.
3. Discuss on physicochemical and biological properties of drugs relevant to controlled release formulations.
4. Describe in detail about controlled drug delivery systems and their importance.
5. What are the advantages and disadvantages for controlled release drug formulation?
6. Define site specific and receptor targeting. Discuss about rationale for controlled release drug formulation.
7. Give the different properties and application of polymers comprehensively.

Microencapsulation, Mucosal and Implantable Drug Delivery Systems

MICROENCAPSULATION

Introduction

Microencapsulation (ME) is a process by which very small droplets or particles of solid or liquid material are coated or surrounded with a continuous film of polymeric material. It is mainly bioencapsulation or entrapment of a bioactive ingredient (e.g. from DNA to whole cell or cluster of cells) normally to improve its performance or enhance its shelf life. ME provides the means of altering liquids to solids and changing of colloidal and surface properties. It also providing environmental protection and controlling the release qualities or availability of coated materials and several of these properties can be accomplished by macropackaging techniques. But, the unique property of ME is the smallness of the surrounded particles and their subsequent use and adaptation to a large variety of dosage forms and not has been technically possible (Fig. 2.1).

The terminology used to describe microparticulate formulations can sometimes be inconsistent and confusing to readers unfamiliar with the field. Basically, the word "microparticle" refers to a particle with a diameter of 1–1000 µm, irrespective of the precise interior or exterior structure. Within the broad category of microparticles, "microspheres" specifically refer to spherical microparticles and the subcategory of "microcapsules" applies to microparticles which have a core surrounded by a material which is distinctly different from that of the core. The core may be liquid, solid or even gas (Fig. 2.2).

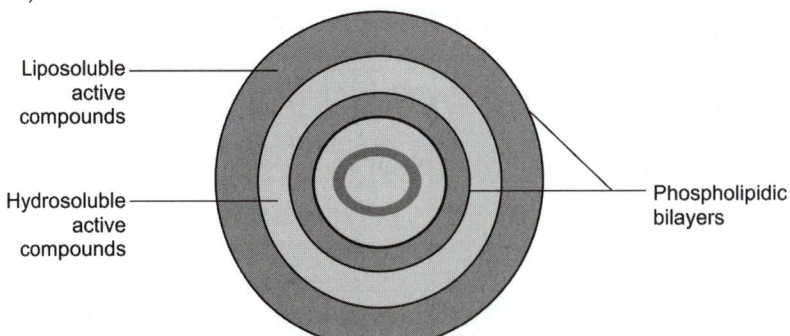

Fig. 2.1: The diagram of ME

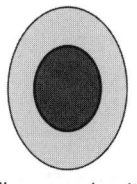 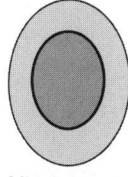 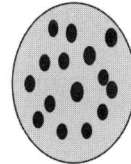 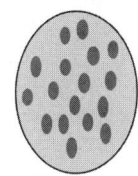 

| Microcapsule with solid core | Microcapsule with non-solid core | Microcapsule with solid microdomain or nanodomains | Microcapsule with non-solid microdomain or nanodomains | Microcapsule with molecular mix of matrix and encansulated agent |

Single domain of active agent   Molecular mix of matrix and active agent

Fig. 2.2: Different structures of microcapsules and microspheres

Reasons for Microencapsulation

- The primary reason for microencapsulation is found to be either for sustained or prolonged drug release.
- This technique has been widely used for masking taste and odour of many drugs to improve patient compliance.
- This technique can be used for converting liquid drugs in a free-flowing powder.
- The drugs, which are sensitive to oxygen, moisture or light can be stabilized by microencapsulation.
- Incompatibility among the drugs can be prevented by microencapsulation.
- Vaporization of many volatile drugs, e.g. methyl salicylate and mint oil can be prevented by microencapsulation.
- Many drugs have been microencapsulated to reduce toxicity and GI irritation including ferrous sulphate and potassium chloride.
- Alteration in site of absorption can also be achieved by microencapsulation.
- Toxic chemicals such as insecticides may be microencapsulated to reduce the possibility of sensitization of factorial person.
- It is reported that microencapsulated vitamin A palmitate enhances stability.

Importance of Microencapsulation

- It protects core material from environment (e.g. protection of vitamins from oxidation).
- It prevents evaporation of core material which is volatile in nature.
- For preparation of handy formulations from sticky core materials.
- Separating reactive core material from other chemicals.
- For preparing controlled release capsules that slowly release core material (active agent) from shell of the capsule.
- Taste masking of drugs.
- For reducing irritant effects of gastric irritants.

Advantages of Microencapsulation

- An effective protection of the encapsulated active agent against (e.g. enzymatic) degradation.
- Control the release rate of the incorporated drug over periods of hours to months.

- An easy administration (compared to alternative parenteral controlled release dosage forms, such as macro-sized implants).
- Desired, preprogrammed drug release profiles can be provided which match the therapeutic needs of the patient.

Disadvantages of Microencapsulation

- Microencapsulation techniques are of high cost.
- This causes reduction in shelf life of hygroscopic drugs.
- Different dosage forms like tablets, capsules, lozenges cannot be encapsulated by single microencapsulation process.
- Coating may not be uniform; this can affect release pattern of a drug in the body.

Microspheres (MS)/Microcapsules (MC)

Microspheres are multi-particulate drug delivery systems. They are prepared to obtain prolonged or controlled drug delivery to improve bioavailability and stability. It also helps in targeting the drug to specific site at a predetermined rate. MS/MC is made from polymeric waxy or other protective materials such as natural, semisynthetic and synthetic polymers. MS are characteristically free flowing powders having particle size ranging from 1–1000 μm consisting of proteins or synthetic polymers. The range of techniques for the preparation of MS provides multiple options to control as drug administration aspects and to enhance the therapeutic efficacy of a given drug. These drug delivery systems offer various different advantages compared to conventional dosage form. It includes improve in efficacy; reduce the toxicity and improve in patient compliance and convenience. Such drug delivery systems generally use macromolecules as carriers for the drugs.

Ideal Characteristics of Microspheres

- Ability to control the release rate for a predefined period of time.
- Higher concentrations of the drug can be given for serve as depot.
- Stability of the preparation after synthesis with a clinically acceptable shelf life.
- Controlled particle size and dispersion of the drug in aqueous solvent for parenterals.
- Biocompatibility with a controllable biodegradability.

Materials used for the preparation of microspheres:

1. Synthetic polymers
2. Natural polymers.

Synthetic polymers:

- *Non-biodegradable polymers:* Polymethylmethacrylate (PMMA), acrolein, glycidyl methacrylate, epoxy polymers
- *Biodegradable polymers:* Lactides, their glycolides and their copolymers, poly (alkyl cyanoacrylate), polyanhydrides

Natural polymers: These are obtained from different sources like proteins, carbohydrates and chemically modified carbohydrates.

- *Proteins:* Albumin, gelatin and collagen
- *Carbohydrates:* Agarose, carrageenan, chitosan, starch,
- *Chemically modified carbohydrates:* Poly (acryl) dextran, poly (acryl) starch

Types of Microspheres

1. **Bioadhesive microspheres:** These types of MS show a prolonged residence time at the site of application. It causes intimate contact with the absorption site and produces better therapeutic action.
2. **Magnetic microspheres:** They are supramolecular particles that circulate through capillaries without producing embolic occlusion (<4 μm). But they are sufficiently susceptible (ferromagnetic) to be captured in microvessels and dragged into the adjacent tissues by magnetic field of 0.5–0.8 tesla.
3. **Floating microspheres:** It is gastroretentive floating microspheres. They are low-density systems that have sufficient buoyancy to float over gastric contents and remain in stomach for prolonged period without affecting any gastric emptying rate and the drug is released slowly at the desired rate.
4. **Radioactive microspheres:** They deliver high radiation dose to the targeted areas without damaging the normal surrounding tissues and inject to the arteries that lead to tumour of interest. The different types of radioactive microspheres are α emitters, β emitters and γ emitters.
5. **Biodegradable polymeric microspheres:** They contain biodegradable polymers which prolong the residence time when contact with mucous membrane due to its high degree of swelling property with aqueous medium, resulting gel formation. The rate and extent of drug release is controlled by concentration of polymer.
6. **Synthetic polymeric microspheres:** They are made up of synthetic polymers. They are used as bulking agent, fillers, embolic particles, drug delivery vehicles, etc.

Techniques to Manufacture Microcapsules

Physical methods:

1. *Pan coating:* This process is widely used in the pharma industry. It is the oldest industrial method for forming small, coated particles or tablets. The particles are tumbled in a pan.
2. *Centrifugal extrusion:* Liquids are encapsulated by a rotating head containing concentric nozzles. A jet of core liquid is surrounded by a sheath of wall solution or melt in the process.
3. *Vibrational nozzle:* Matrix-encapsulation or core-shell encapsulation or micro-granulation can be done using a laminar flow through a nozzle and an additional vibration of the nozzle or the liquid. The vibration in resonance with the Rayleigh instability leads to very uniform droplets. The liquid can consist of any liquids with limited viscosities (0–10,000 mPa-s; e.g. solutions, emulsions, suspensions, melts, etc). The solidification can be achieved according to the used gelation system with an external (additional binder system, e.g. in a slurry) or an internal gelation (e.g. Sol-gel processing, melt). This process works very well for generating droplets between 20 and 10,000 μm (0.79–393.70 mils). The units are organized in industries and research mostly with capacities of 1–20,000 kg per hour (2–44,000 lb/h) at working temperatures of 20–1,500°C. Heads are available vary from one up to several hundred thousand nozzles.
4. *Spray drying:* Spray drying technique applies when an active material is suspended or dissolved in a melt or polymer solution and resulting trapped in the dried particle. The major advantages are the ability to handle labile materials due to short contact time in the dryer. In modern spray dryers, the viscosity of the solutions can be

spray as high as 300 mPa-s. Applying this technique along with the use of supercritical CO_2, sensitive materials like proteins can be encapsulated.

Physicochemical methods:

1. *Ionotropic gelation:* It takes places when units of uric acid in alginate polymer chain crosslink with multivalent cations. These may contain iron, calcium, zinc and aluminium.

2. *Coacervation-phase separation:* It consists of three steps carried out under continuous agitation.

   a. *Formation of three immiscible chemical phases:* Core material phase, liquid manufacturing vehicle phase, and coating material phase.

   b. *Deposition of coating material:* Core material is dispersed in the coating polymer solution and coating polymer material coated around core. Deposition of liquid polymer coating around core by polymer adsorbed at the interface formed between vehicle phase and core material.

   c. *Hardening of coating:* Coating material is immiscible in vehicle phase and is made rigid. This is done by cross-linking, thermal, or dissolution techniques.

Chemical methods:

1. *Interfacial polycondensation:* There are two reactants in a polycondensation meet at an interface in interfacial polycondensation, which react rapidly. This method is based on the classical Schotten-Baumann reaction between an acid chloride and a compound containing an active hydrogen atom such as an amine or alcohol, etc. Thin flexible walls form rapidly at the interface under the right conditions. A pesticide solution and a diacid chloride are emulsified in H_2O and an aqueous solution containing an amine and a polyfunctional isocyanate is added. Base is added to neutralize the acid formed during the reaction and condensed polymer walls form instantaneously at the interface of the emulsion droplets.

2. *Interfacial cross-linking:* It is derived from interfacial polycondensation. It is developed to avoid the use of toxic diamines for the application of pharmaceutical or cosmetic. In this method, the tiny bifunctional monomer containing active hydrogen atoms is replaced by a biosourced polymer, like a protein. When the reaction is carried out at the interface of an emulsion, the acid chloride reacts with the various different functional groups of the protein, result in the formation of a membrane. The method is very versatile. The properties of the microcapsules (size, porosity, degradability, mechanical resistance, etc.) can be customized.

3. *In situ polymerization:* In a few microencapsulation processes, the direct polymerization of a single monomer is performed on the particle surface. In one process, e.g. cellulose fibres are encapsulated in polyethylene at the same time as immersed in dry toluene. Usual deposition rates are about 0.5 µm/min. Coating thickness ranges 0.2–75 µm (0.0079–2.9528 mils). The coating is uniform, even over sharp projections. Protein microcapsules are biocompatible and biodegradable. The presence of the protein backbone renders the membrane more resistant and elastic than those obtained by interfacial polycondensation.

4. *Matrix polymerization:* In various processes, a core material is imbedded in a polymeric matrix during formation of the particles. An example of this type is spray drying, in which the particle is formed by evaporation of the solvent from the matrix material. On the other hand, the solidification of the matrix also can be caused by a chemical change.

Microparticles (MP)

They are formed by shedding or blebbing of cell membrane upon injury. These particles contain microvesicles, exosomes, and apoptotic bodies and cellular contents. These small particles also contain RNA, DNA and miRNA and they range from 0.05–3 µm in diameter. Normally, these particles are present at a low concentration in the circulation. Under pathological conditions and an injury, these particles are released into the circulation. There is a growing interest in utilizing these microparticles as biomarkers of specific organ or cell injuries. Hence, they reflect the cellular origin for different organ systems. The pathology and identifying these markers allow one to predict their origin and the pathological or injury process. However, these particles can be released or fused with endothelial cells, and can trigger a variety of systemic responses. Thus, their role as biomarkers and also in inducing pathobiological processes away from their site of origin is of great significance. As far as predicting lung injury is concern, it is reported that circulating microparticles from smokers can provide insight into the ongoing lung injury. It is reported that microparticles contain tissue factor which, upon its release, can induce thrombogenic effects on the vasculature. Acute lung injury leads to increased microparticles in the circulation. Sputum microparticles have been reported to have proinflammatory effects. Various different types of flow cytometry-based techniques are available to isolate them from blood plasma and characterize their properties.

Microencapsulation Process

1. Encapsulant (material) preparation
2. Core preparation and incorporation
3. Core dispersion and homogenization
4. Particle/droplet formation
5. Matrix/shell hardening or stabilization

Applications

Some of the applications of microencapsulation can be mentioned in detail as given below.

- Prolonged release dosage forms: The microencapsulated drug can be given as microencapsulation is perhaps most useful for the preparation of capsules or tablets, or parenteral dosage forms.
- Microencapsulation can be used to prepare enteric-coated dosage forms, so that the medicament will be selectively absorbed in the intestine rather than the stomach.
- It can be used to mask the taste of bitter drugs.
- From the mechanical point of view, microencapsulation has been used to aid in the addition of oily medicines to tableted dosage forms. This has been used to overcome problems inherent in producing tablets from otherwise tacky granulations and in direct compression to tablets.
- It has been used to protect drugs from environmental hazards such as humidity, light, oxygen or heat. Microencapsulation does not yet provide a perfect barrier for materials, which degrade in the presence of air (oxygen), moisture or heat, however, a great degree of protection against these elements can be provided.
- The separations of incompatible substances, e.g. pharmaceutical eutectics, have been achieved by encapsulation.

- Microencapsulation can be used to decrease the volatility. An encapsulated volatile substance can be stored for longer times without considerable evaporation.
- Microencapsulation has also been used to decrease potential danger of handling of toxic or noxious substances. The toxicity occurred due to handling of herbicides, insecticides, fumigants, and pesticides has been advantageously reduced after microencapsulation.
- The hygroscopic properties of many core materials may be reduced by microencapsulation.
- Many drugs have been microencapsulated to reduce gastric irritation.
- Microencapsulation method has also been proposed to prepare intrauterine contraceptive device.
- In the fabrication of multilayered tablet formulations for controlled release of medicament contained in medial layers of tableted particles.

Bioadhesion/Mucoadhesion

The word bioadhesion can be defined as the state in which two materials, at least one biological in nature, are held together for an extended period of time by interfacial forces. In biological systems, bioadhesion can be categorized into three types:

- **Type 1:** Adhesion between two biological phases, e.g. platelet aggregation and wound healing.
- **Type 2:** Adhesion of a biological phase to a synthetic substrate, e.g. cell adhesion to culture dishes and biofilm formation on prosthetic devices and inserts.
- **Type 3:** Adhesion of a synthetic material to a biological substrate, e.g. adhesion of synthetic hydrogels to soft tissues and adhesion of sealants to dental enamel.

For drug delivery purposes, the term bioadhesion implies attachment of a drug carrier system to a specified biological site. The biological surface can be the mucus coat or epithelial tissue on the surface of a tissue. If adhesive attachment is with a mucus coat, the phenomenon is referred to as mucoadhesion. Leung and Robinson described mucoadhesion as the interaction between a mucin surface and a synthetic or natural polymer. Bioadhesion should not be confused with mucoadhesion. In bioadhesion, the polymer is attached to the biological membrane, but if the substrate is mucus membrane, the term mucoadhesion is used.

Mechanism of Bioadhesion

The mechanisms responsible in the formation of bioadhesive bonds are not fully known. However, most researches have explained bioadhesion bond formation as a three-step process.

- **Step 1:** Wetting and swelling of polymer (the contact stage)
- **Step 2:** Interpretation between the polymer chains and mucosal membrane.
- **Step 3:** Formation of chemical bond between the entangled chains (both known as consolidation stage).

Step 1: When the polymer spreads over the surface of biological substrate or mucosal membrane, the wetting and swelling step occurs that develops an intimate contact with the substrate. By the help of the surface tension and forces that exist at the site of adsorption or contact, bioadhesives are able to adhere to or bond with biological tissues. Swellings of polymers occur because the components within the polymers have an affinity for H_2O (Fig. 2.3).

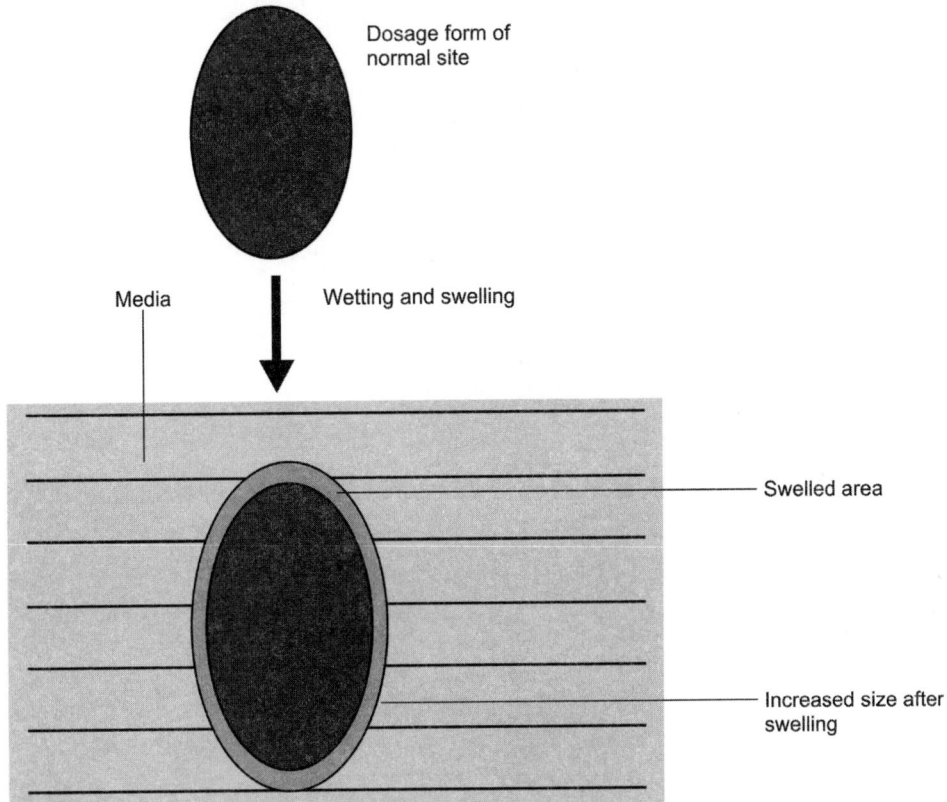

Fig. 2.3: Wetting and swelling of polymer interpenetration

Step 2: The surface of mucosal membranes consists of high molecular weight polymers known as glycoproteins. Interdiffusion and interpenetration occur between the chains of mucoadhesive polymers and the mucus gel network creating a great area of contact. The strength of the bond depends on the degree of penetration between the two polymer groups. In order to produce strong adhesive bonds, one polymer group must be soluble in the other and both polymer types must be of similar chemical structure (Fig. 2.4).

Step 3: Entanglement and configuration of weak chemical bonds as well as secondary bonds between the polymer chains mucin molecule. The types of bonding formed between the chains include primary bonds such as covalent bonds and weaker secondary interactions such as hydrogen bonds and van der Waals interactions. Both primary and secondary bonds are developed in the manufacture of bioadhesive formulations in which strong adhesions between polymers are formed (Fig. 2.5).

Theories of Mucoadhesion

Various theories exist to give explanation at least some of the experimental observations made during the bioadhesion process. Unfortunately, each theoretical model can only describe a limited number of the diverse range of interactions that constitute the bioadhesive bond. However, four major theories can be distinguished.

1. **Electronic theory:** Electronic theory is based on the idea that both mucoadhesive and biological materials possess opposing electrical charges. Therefore, when both

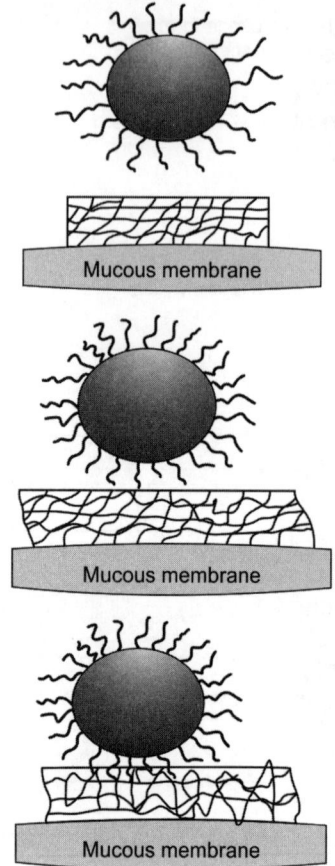

Fig. 2.4: Interdiffusion and interpenetration of polymer and mucus

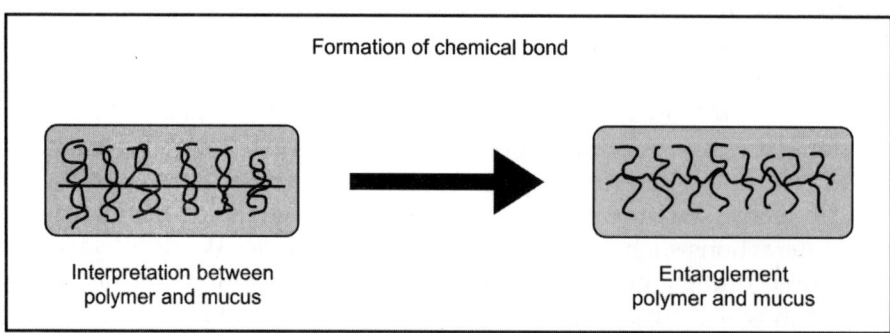

Fig. 2.5: Entanglement of polymer and mucus by chemical bonds

materials come into contact, they transfer electrons resulting in building of a double electronic layer at the interface, where the attractive forces within this electronic double layer find outs the mucoadhesive.

2. **Adsorption theory:** In accordance with the adsorption theory, the mucoadhesive device adheres to the mucus by secondary chemical interactions, such as in hydrogen bonds and van der Waals, electrostatic attraction or hydrophobic interactions.

Example, hydrogen bonds are the prevalent interfacial forces in polymers containing carboxyl groups. Such forces are considered the most vital in the adhesive interaction phenomenon because, although they are individually weak, a large number of interactions can result in an intense global adhesion.

3. **Wetting theory:** The wetting theory applies to liquid systems which present affinity to the surface that spread over it. This affinity can be observed by using measuring techniques such as the contact angle. The common rule states that the lower the contact angle, the greater the affinity. The contact angle must be equal or near to zero to provide adequate spread ability (Fig. 2.6).

The spread ability coefficient (S_{AB}) can be calculated from the difference between the surface energies γb and γa and the interfacial energy γab, as indicated in equation.

$$S_{AB} = \gamma b - \gamma a - \gamma ab$$

The greater the individual surface energy of mucus and device in relation to the interfacial energy, the greater the adhesion work, W_A, i.e. the greater the energy required to separate the two phases.

$$W_A = \gamma a + \gamma b - \gamma ab$$

4. **Diffusion theory:** Diffusion theory expresses the interpenetration of both polymer and mucin chains to a sufficient depth to create a semipermanent adhesive bond. It is generally believed that the adhesion force increases with the degree of penetration of the polymer chains. This penetration rate mainly depends on the diffusion coefficient, flexibility and nature of the mucoadhesive chains, mobility and contact time (Fig. 2.7).

5. **Fracture theory:** This is perhaps the most common used theory in studies on the mechanical measurement of mucoadhesion. It analyses the force needed to separate two surfaces after adhesion is established (Fig. 2.8). This force, S_m, is normally calculated in tests of resistance to rupture by the ratio of the maximal detachment force, F_m, and the total surface area, A_o involved in the adhesive interaction.

$$S_m = F_m / A_o$$

6. **Mechanical theory:** Mechanical theory is believed that adhesion to be due to the filling of the irregularities on a rough surface by a mucoadhesive liquid. Moreover, such roughness enhances the interfacial area available to interactions thereby aiding

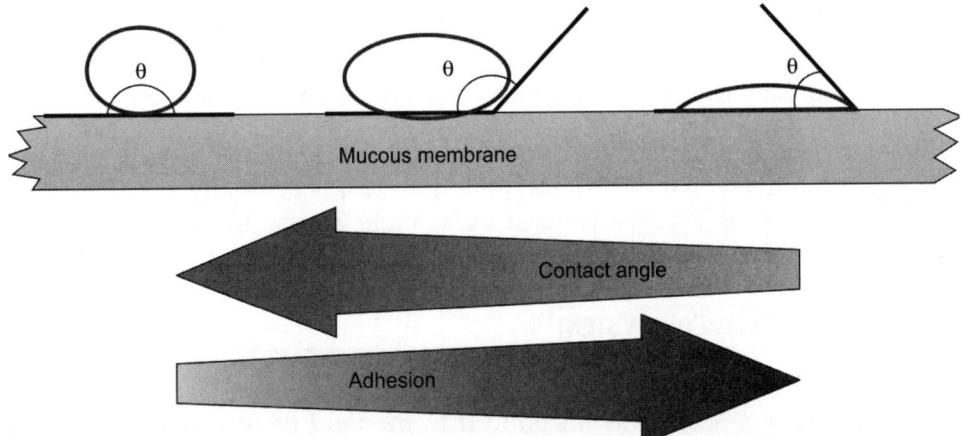

Fig. 2.6: Influence of contact angle between device and mucous membrane on bioadhesion (schematic)

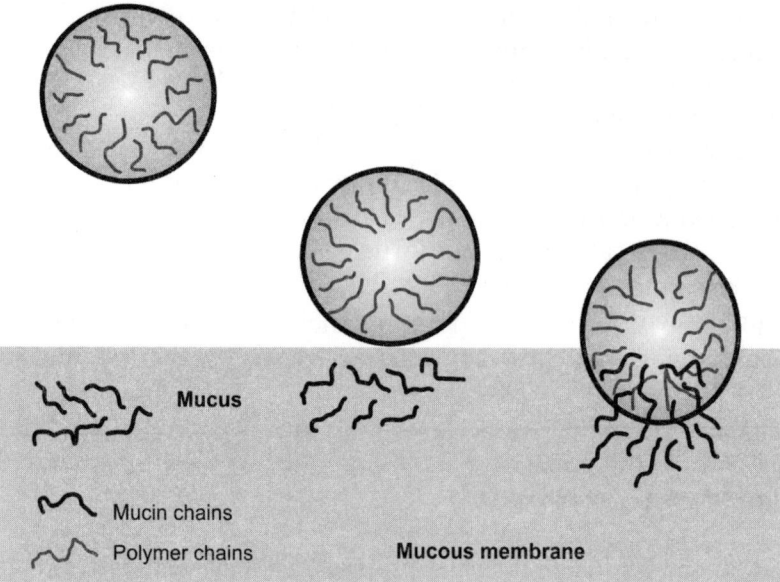

Fig. 2.7: Secondary interactions resulting from interdiffusion of polymer chains of bioadhesive device and of mucus

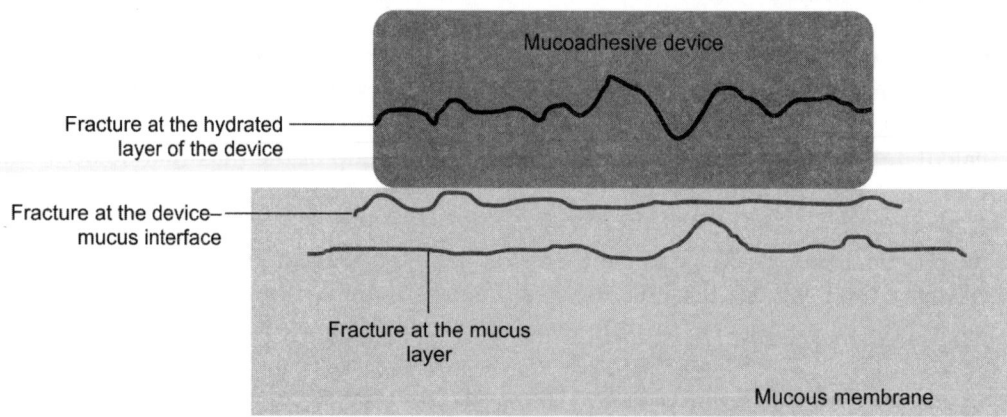

Fig. 2.8: Regions where the mucoadhesive bonds rupture can occur

dissipating energy and can be considered the most significant phenomenon of the process. It is unlikely that the mucoadhesion process is generally same for all cases and, therefore, it cannot be expressed by a single theory. In fact, all theories are relevant to identify the significant process variables.

MUCOSAL DRUG DELIVERY SYSTEM

Introduction

The mucoadhesion concept was introduced in the field of controlled release drug delivery systems in the early 1980. Thereafter, several researchers have focused on the investigations of the phenomena of mucoadhesive hydrogels with the mucus. For drug delivery purpose, the term bioadhesion implies attachment of a drug carrier system to a specific biological site. The biological site can be epithelial tissue. If adhesive attachment is to a mucus coat, the phenomenon is termed to as mucoadhesion. That's why a bacterial attachment is to tissue surfaces, and mucoadhesion can be modeled after the adherence of mucus on epithelial tissue. Mucoadhesion is the relatively novel and emerging conception in drug delivery and it keeps the delivery system adhering to the mucous membrane. By this characterization, the mucosal routes for drug delivery are:

- Buccal delivery system
- Oral delivery system
- Vaginal delivery system
- Rectal delivery system
- Nasal delivery system
- Ocular delivery system

Advantages of Mucoadhesive Drug Delivery Systems

- Prolongs the residence time of the dosage form at the site of absorption, therefore, increases the bioavailability.
- Excellent accessibility, rapid onset of action.
- Fast absorption because of huge blood supply and good blood flow rates.
- Drug is defended from degradation in the acidic media in the GIT.
- Improved patient compliance.

Disadvantages of Mucoadhesive Drug Delivery Systems

- Occurrence of local ulcerous effects due to prolonged contact of the drug containing ulcerogenic property.
- One of the most important restrictions in the development of oral mucosal delivery is the lack of a good model for *in vitro* screening to identify drugs suitable for such administration.
- Patient acceptability in terms to taste and irritancy.
- Eating and drinking is prohibited.

Transmucosal Permeability

The transcellular and paracellular routes are involved in drug permeation across the epithelial membrane. Normally, skin and gastrointestinal mucosa viewed as lipodal barriers, so partition coefficient and molecular size are very important for diffusion. Recent study shows that the absorption of drug increases as the lipophilicity of drug increases in the mucosa. It is studied that ionic and lipid-soluble compounds rapidly absorbed thorough rat rectal mucosa. The correlation between the rectal absorption and their partition coefficient shows the rectal mucosa as a lipoidal barrier. It is investigated that human nasal mucosa using propranolol of difference lipophilicity suggests that most lipophilic drug absorbed highest but several other works show the presence of aqueous pores along with lipoidal pores. In the similar way, the study on rabbit vaginal barrier suggests that there is no absence of both the pathways lipoidal and aqueous pores. It is studied that vaginal absorption of straight long chain alkanoic acids in rabbits revealed that permeability coefficient increases as the length of alkyl chain increase but does not correlate linearly with their partition coefficient, indicating neither purely lipophilic nor pure hydrophilic nature (Fig. 2.9).

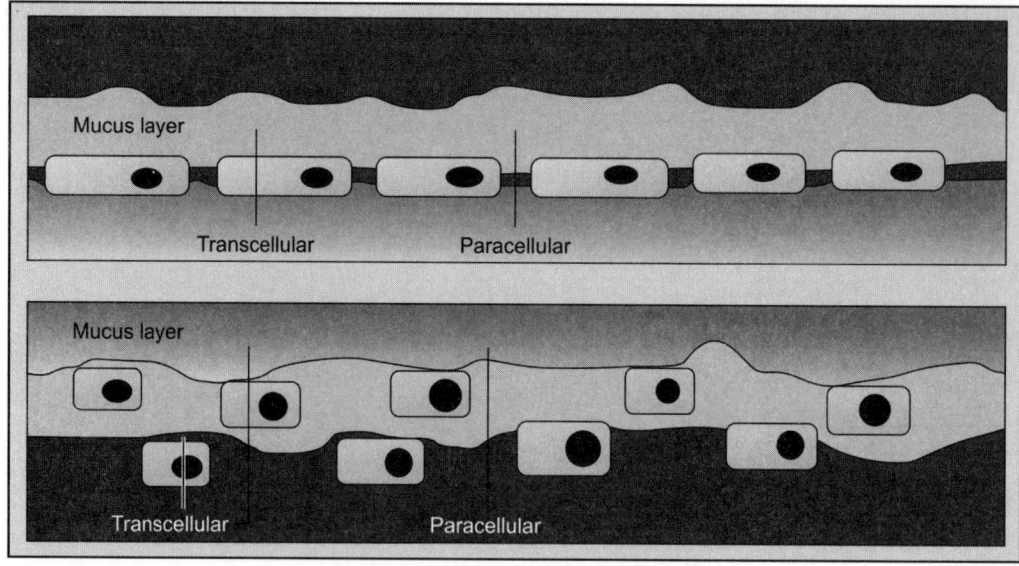

Fig. 2.9: Transmucosal permeability

Factors to be considered in the transmucosal permeability are:
- Lipophilicity of drug
- Salivary secretion
- pH of saliva
- Binding to oral mucosa
- Oral epithelium thickness

Formulation Considerations of Buccal Delivery Systems
- Buccal bioadhesive tablets
- Buccal bioadhesive semisolid dosage forms
- Buccal bioadhesive patches and films
- Buccal bioadhesive powder dosage forms

Buccal Bioadhesive Tablets

Buccal bioadhesive tablets are dry dosage forms that are to be moistened before to placing in contact with buccal mucosa. Double and multilayered tablets are already prepared using bioadhesive polymers and excipients. The two buccal bioadhesive tablets, commercially available in United Kingdom, are 'Bucastem' and 'Suscard buccaP'.

Buccal Bioadhesive Semisolid Dosage Forms

Buccal bioadhesive semisolid dosage form containing finally powdered natural or synthetic polymer dispersed in a polyethylene or in aqueous solution, e.g. Arabase.21.

Buccal Bioadhesive Patches and Films

Buccal bioadhesive patches containing two polylaminates or multilayered thin film round or oval as containing basically of bioadhesive polymeric layer and impermeable backing layer to provide unidirectional flow of drug across buccal mucosa. Buccal bioadhesive films are prepared by incorporating the drug in alcohol solution of bioadhesive polymer.

1. Isosorbide dinitrate in the form of unidirectional erodible buccal film is developed and characterized for improving bioavailability.
2. Buccal film of salbutamol sulphate and terbutaline sulphate for the treatment of asthma.
3. Buccoadhesive film of clindamycin used for pyorrhoea treatment.

Buccal Bioadhesive Powder Dosage Forms

Buccal bioadhesive powder dosage forms are a mixture of bioadhesive polymers and the drug or bioactive moiety. These are sprayed onto the buccal mucosa.

Example, buccal tablet or buccal film of nifedipine.

Advantages

- Bypasses gastrointestinal tract and hepatic portal system, thus increasing the bioavailability of orally administered drugs.
- Improved patient compliance due to the removal of associated pain with injections.
- A relatively rapid onset of action may be obtained relative to the oral route and the formulation can be eliminated, if therapy is needed to be discontinued.
- Increased ease of drug administration.
- The buccal mucosa is well vascularized and drugs can be rapidly absorbed into the venous system underneath the oral mucosa.
- Transmucosal delivery shows fewer variables between patients, resulting in lower intersubject variability as compared to transdermal patches.
- The large contact surface of the oral cavity contributes to rapid and extensive drug absorption.
- Drugs, which show not good bioavailability via the oral route can be administered conveniently.

Disadvantages

- Drugs with bulky dose are difficult to be administered.
- Drugs which are not stable at buccal pH cannot be administered.
- If formulation contains antimicrobial agents, it affects the natural microbes in the buccal cavity.
- Low permeability of the buccal membrane specifically when compared to the sublingual membrane.
- Drugs which irritate oral mucosa or have bitter taste, or cause allergic reactions, discolouration of teeth cannot be formulated.
- Swallowing of saliva may also potentially lead to the loss of dissolved or suspended drug.

Basic Components of Buccal Bioadhesive Drug Delivery System

The basic components of buccal bioadhesive drug delivery system are:

- Drug substance
- Bioadhesive polymers
- Backing membrane
- Penetration enhancers
- Adhesives

Drug Substance

Prior preparing buccoadhesive drug delivery systems, one has to decide whether the intended, action is for rapid release/prolonged release and for local/systemic effect. The drug should have following characteristics.

1. The conventional single dose of the drug should be small. The drugs having biological half-life between 2 and 8 hours are good agent for controlled drug delivery.
2. T_{max} of the drug shows wider-fluctuations or higher values when given orally.
3. The drug absorption should be passive when administered orally.

Bioadhesive Polymers

The first step in the development of buccoadhesive dosage forms is the selection and characterization of selective bioadhesive polymers in the formulation. Bioadhesive polymers play a major role in buccoadhesive drug delivery systems of drugs. Polymers or bioactive moiety are also used in matrix devices in which the drug is embedded in the polymer matrix, which controls the duration of release of drugs. An ideal polymer for buccoadhesive drug delivery systems should have following characteristics.

1. It should be inert and compatible with the environment.
2. The polymer and its degradation products must be non-toxic absorbable from the mucus layer.
3. It must adhere quickly to moist tissue surface and should possess some site specificity.
4. The polymer must not decay on storage or during the shelf life of the dosage form.
5. The polymer must be easily available in the market and economical.

Criteria followed in polymer selection

- It should form a strong non-covalent bond with the mucin/epithelial surface.
- It must have high molecular weight and narrow distribution.
- It should be compatible with the biological membrane.

The polymers that are generally used as bioadhesive in pharmaceutical applications are:

   a. *Natural polymers:* Gelatin, sodium alginate.
   b. *Synthetic and semisynthetic polymers:* PVA, PEG, HPMC, PVP, carbomers, etc.

Backing Membrane

Backing membrane plays a key role in the attachment of bioadhesive devices to the mucous membrane. The materials used as backing membrane must be inert, and impermeable to the drug and penetration enhancer. The commonly used materials in backing membrane include carbopol, HPMC, HPC, CMC, magnesium stearate, polycarbophil, etc.

Penetration Enhancers

Penetration enhancers are used in buccoadhesive formulations to improve the release of the drug. They help the systemic delivery of the drug by allowing the drug to penetrate more readily into the viable tissues.

- Nasal route
- Ocular route
- Vaginal route
- Gastrointestinal route

IMPLANTABLE DRUG DELIVERY SYSTEMS (IDDS)

Introduction

Implantable devices are known upon to serve various functions, from vascular stents that preserve blood flow to electrostimulation devices that regulate heart rhythm or block spurious signals in the brain, to orthopaedic devices that mechanically support the spine or restore range of motion of knees and hip. For over a decade, there has been a raising convergence between implantable devices and drug therapies, containing devices that deliver drugs as a primary of action. Implants are meant for implantation in the body subcutaneous or intramuscular tissue by a minor surgical incision or injected through a large bore needle. Implants are developed with a view to supply continuous release of the drug into the blood.

Stream over long periods of time without the repeated insertion of needles.

Advantages

- **Convenience:** Effective concentration of drug in the bloodstream can be maintained for an extremely long time by techniques such as continuous intravenous infusion or repeated injections. Implantation treatment allows patients to get medication outside the hospital setting with marginal medical observation.
- **Compliance:** By decreasing the frequency of drug administration over the entire period of treatment improves patient compliance. Patient can forget to take a medicine, but drug delivery from an implant is not generally dependent of patient input.
- **Stability:** Implants are environmentally stable. They should not breakdown under the influence of physical factors such as heat, light, air and moisture. It must be stable and safe and have good mechanical strength.
- **Improved drug delivery:** The drug (active ingredients) is distributed locally or in systemic circulation with least interfering by metabolic or biological barriers. For example, the bioactive moiety bypassed the GIT and the liver. The bypassing effect is favourable to bioactive compounds, which are either easily inactivated or absorbed poorly in the GIT and/or the liver before systemic distribution.
- **Controlled release:** Implants are available which deliver bioactive moiety by zero order-controlled release kinetics. In order that dosing frequency is reduced, and patient compliance is increased. It leads to raising effectiveness and reduces side effects.
- **Flexibility:** In the choice of materials, methods of manufacture, degree of drug loading, drug release rate, etc., considerable flexibility is probable. From a regulatory perspective, it is regarded as a new product and can lengthen the market protection of the bioactive moiety.

Disadvantages

- **Invasive:** To initiate therapy, either a major or a minor surgical procedure is needed. Appropriate surgical personnel are required for this, and may be time-consuming. This causes some scar formation at the site of implantation and surgery-related complications in a few patients. Uncomfortable feeling for the patient wearing such type of device.

- **Danger of device failure:** There is no associated danger with this treatment that the device may for some reason fail to work properly. This again needs surgical involvement to correct.
- **Termination:** Osmotic pumps and non-biodegradable polymeric implants are also surgically recovered at the last time of therapy. Even though surgical recovery is not needed in biodegradable polymeric implants. Its on-going biodegradation makes it difficult to end drug delivery, or to maintain the correct dose at the end of its lifetime.
- **Limited to potent drugs:** In order to minimize patient's discomfort, the size of an implant is generally kept small. Therefore, most of the implants have a limited loading capacity so that only for potent medicines such as hormones may be appropriate for delivery by implantable devices.
- **Biocompatibility issues:** Concerns over body reactions to foreign matters regularly increase the issues of biocompatibility and safety of an implant.
- **Possibility of adverse reactions:** A high concentration of the drug (bioactive moiety) delivered by an implantable device at the implantation site may create adverse reactions.

Ideal Properties of Implants

1. Biostable
2. Biocompatible
3. Easily removable
4. Non-toxic and non-carcinogenic
5. Minimum surface area and smooth texture
6. Rate-controlled release of the drug

Classification of Implantable Drug Delivery Systems (IDDS)

Classification of IDDS is very difficult, given that there are many exceptions and hybrids that may be listed under multiple categories. However, drug implants can be generally subdivided into active and passive systems. Passive systems can be further classified into non-degradable and degradable implants, which typically have no moving parts or mechanisms. Active systems employ some energy-dependent method for providing a positive driving force to change drug release and these energy sources may be as diverse as osmotic pressure gradients or electromechanical drives.

Passive Implants

Passive implants tend to be relatively simple, homogenous and singular devices, typically consisting of the simple packaging of drugs in a biocompatible material or matrix. By definition, they do not contain any moving parts and depend on a passive, diffusion-mediated phenomenon to change drug release. Delivery kinetics is partially tunable by the selection of bioactive moiety, its concentration, overall implant external appearance, matrix material and surface properties.

Non-degradable implantable drug delivery systems: While membrane-enclosed reservoirs and matrix-controlled systems are by far the most common, many other variants of non-degradable implants are commercially available. The matrix materials used in all these systems are typically polymers, with a documented history of both pre-clinical and clinical assessments. Commonly used polymers include elastomers such as silicones and acrylates, urethanes, and their copolymers within the polymeric matrices forming most passive monolithic implants; the drug is typically dispersed homogeneously throughout the matrix material. Alternatively, reservoir-type systems are characterized by a compact drug core, surrounded by a permeable non-degradable membrane, the thickness and permeability which regulate the diffusion of the drug into the body.

Biodegradable implants: To overcome the drawbacks of non-biodegradable implants, biodegradable systems, based on polymers such as polylactic acid (PLA), polylactic-co-glycolic acid (PLGA), polycaprolactone (PCL) or their block copolymer variants with other polymers are developed. A most important advantage of biodegradable systems is that the biocompatible polymers used for fabricating these delivery systems are eventually broken down into safe metabolites and absorbed or excreted by the body. Labile bonds that are prone to degradation by hydrolysis or enzymes, such as amide, ester and anhydride bonds, are characteristic of the backbone of biodegradable polymers. Complete degradation of the implant post-drug release makes surgical removal of the implant after the conclusion of therapy unnecessary, thereby decreasing potential complications with explanation and increasing patient acceptance and compliance.

Dynamic Implants

Dynamic implant systems harness a positive driving force to enable and control drug release. As a result, these are typically able to change drug doses and delivery rates much more precisely than passive systems. However, this comes at a higher cost, both in terms of complexity and actual device price.

Implantable pump systems: External control of dosing is a requirement for many bioactive moieties, a feature that is not easy to obtain when using biodegradable or non-degradable delivery systems. Pump systems are used to provide the higher precision and remote control needed in these situations. Additionally, they offer various advantages, such as evasion of the GI tract, avoidance of repeated injections, and improved release rates (faster than diffusion-limited systems). With advances in microelectronics since 1970s, remote control over delivery rates or integration of implantable sensors to generate feedback-controlled drug delivery is now feasible. Implantable pumps mainly use osmosis, propellant-driven fluids, or electromechanical drives to generate pressure gradients and facilitate controlled bioactive moiety release as described below.

Osmotic pumps: Osmotic pumps have found wide acceptability among all active IDDS. The first osmotic pump was devised by Australian pharmacologists, Rose and Nelson, who developed an implantable osmotic pump in 1955, termed as Rose and Nelson osmotic pump. Higuchi and Leeper made a few alterations to this design and introduced it to the pharmaceutical world in the year 1973. In the same year, a dispensing device with means of filling, containing a powdered agent capable of creating osmotic pressure, was also designed.

Propellant infusion pumps: While osmotic pumps offer a higher level of control and zero-order release, compared to biodegradable systems, the volume of bioactive moiety that they can release limits them. To counter this deficit, an alternative design uses propellant gas instead of an osmotic agent to create a constant positive pressure for zero-order release. The use of a compressible medium, such as gas, permits for a larger volume of bioactive moiety to be stored and released.

Electromechanical systems: While osmotic and propellant-driven constant pressure pumps work well for low volumes of medication, this may be a severe limitation for certain chronic diseases requiring daily infusion of medication, precluding their use over long time spans. In such cases, it may be necessary to consider larger implants, wherein the storage capacity of the pump may be replenished from time to time, while the pumping mechanisms stay implanted. By necessity, this implies the use of electrically powered mechanical pumps, typically with moving parts and advanced control systems.

Mechanisms

1. **Diffusion controlled:** Reservoir type of system consists of a core of bioactive moiety surrounded by a polymer and diffusion of the drug across the polymer layer is the rate-limiting step. Zero-order release kinetic easily obtained. In matrix type systems, zero-order release rate can be obtained by compensating for the increased diffusional distance with an increasing area of the drug.
2. **Chemically controlled:** The drug is distributed uniformly throughout the bioerodible polymer, which erodes and reduces in geometry with time to allow the drug release. Zero-order kinetics can be obtained, if the surface area remains unchanged with time.
3. **Swelling controlled:** In this type of system, the release rate is equal to the product of surface area and a rate constant corresponding to rate of advance of boundary separating the outer shell from central core.
4. **Osmotically controlled:** The system in the form of matrix where the core is surrounded by semipermeable film utilizes osmotic pressure as driving force for delivery of drugs.
5. **Magnetically controlled:** This type of system consists of drug and small magnetic beads uniformly dispersed within a polymer matrix. In contact with aqueous media, drug is generally released in diffusion-controlled manner.

Implantable Drug Delivery Devices (IDDD)

1. **Transdermal patches:** Transdermal patches usually have hollow microneedles made of a biocompatible polymer through which the drug is delivered below the skin. Transdermal patches have many advantages compared with other systems of drug delivery the drugs are not degraded in the GIT, they are painless, and they deliver a constant dosage without the need for patient's compliance.
2. **Polymer implants:** Polymer implants are biodegradable polymers loaded with the bioactive molecules. The polymer degrades when it comes in interaction with body fluids and in the process releases bioactive molecules. The rate of degradation of the polymer and hence the bioactive molecule release can be optimized by modifying the properties of the polymers. The polymer materials which are most extensively used for these applications include, but are not restricted to, polyglycolic acid (PGA), polylactic acid (PLA), polyurethane and the combinations of these in different proportions.
3. **Bioadhesives:** They are substances which form bonds with biological surfaces. The most common substances which are used as bioadehsives are polymer hydrogels.
4. **Microencapsulation:** Microencapsulation refers to the method of covering the bioactive molecule with a material which will prolong the time before the drug is release. There are variety of methods in which microencapsulation is prepared. Some of them are use of polymer microspheres, liposomes, nanoparticles, etc.

Applications

IDDS is being used in the areas of women's health, chronic diseases (including lifestyle diseases), oncology, pain management, and neurology.

Women's Health

In the area of women's health, IDDS plays a key role, especially in field of contraception. A modern version of the Norplant, known Jadelle, is recently marketed by Bayer pharmaceuticals. Pfizer has developed a silicone intravaginal ring (IVR), marketed under the brand name Estring and it is designed to treat symptoms associated with menopause and releases 2 mg of oestradiol for 90 days. The Nuvaring IVR from Merck offers combined delivery of 120 µg of etonogestrel and 15 µg of ethinyl oestradiol per day over a 3-week period. Nexplanon is a new version of the Implanon implant also from Merck that is capable of delivering 68 mg of etonogestrel for up to 3 years. Similar to Norplant and Implanon, Nexplanon also has a cylindrical rod shape for subcutaneous implantation in the arm.

Chronic Diseases

In all clinical use scenarios, IDDS perhaps find their best applicability in the treatment of chronic diseases. As such, devices for an extensive variety of clinical applications against chronic illnesses are developed, as described further:

- *Cardiovascular disease:* DES is the best example of IDDS for vascular disease treatment. DES is developed to specifically address the problems of restenosis encountered with bare-metal stents (BMS), and typically consist of a BMS, coated with a polymer which gradually releases a drug to inhibit cell proliferation that causes restenosis.
- *Cancer:* The major challenge in anticancer therapy is to develop IDDS to deliver chemotherapeutic bioactive molecules safely and effectively without side effects. Therefore, IDDS has a great potential to deliver chemotherapeutic drugs in a more effective and safe manner.
- *Diabetes:* Diabetes, a condition already at the level of global epidemic affecting 371 million patients, is a chronic disease state where implantable systems have the potential to transform the current standard of both diagnosis and treatment. On the diagnostic end, continuous glucose monitoring (CGM) may be achieved by SC implanted sensors for blood glucose measurement. Sensors like Medtronic's Enlite, Dexcom's G4 Platinum, and Glysen's ICGMTM are already available commercially. However, these are mostly restricted to a sensing function without subsequent insulin deliver.
- *Ocular therapy:* Various different implantable systems are evaluated to provide prolonged ocular delivery. These include implantable silicone devices, membrane-controlled devices and implantable infusion systems. A good example of the membrane-controlled system is the Ocusert device.
- *Pain management:* Chronic pain is a particularly challenging disease state, because of the need for repeated dosage, morbidity and mortality from overdosing, and the high risk for addiction to oral and parenteral medications. Data from the CDC between 1999 and 2010 show a reported rise in deaths from prescription pain drug over doses of 400% among women and a 265% in men (CDC, 2013). IDDS, therefore, offers some unique and potent solutions for managing chronic pain.

Infectious Diseases (Tuberculosis)

A fundamental problem in the treatment of tuberculosis (TB) is the long duration of therapy and side effects of drugs, which can hamper patient lifestyle and induce patient non-compliance, treatment failure, and development of drug resistant strains. In this context, IDDSs are a promising approach for the development of more effective and more compliant DDSs for TB treatment.

Neurology and Central Nervous System Health

Schizophrenia is a mental health condition wherein approximately 50% of patients under treatment are non-compliant. For such patients, systems capable of controlled and sustained delivery antipsychotics are of great value. One such system available commercially is the subcutaneous Med Launch Implant Program developed by Endo pharmaceuticals, for delivery of risperidone. Braeburn is the commercialization partner for this technology as well, similar to the Probuphine device mentioned earlier.

QUESTIONS

A. Short Answer Type Questions

1. Give importance of microencapsulation.
2. Briefly describe transmucosal permeability.
3. Write applications of microencapsulation.
4. Define implantable drug delivery system and classify them.
5. Give the reason for necessities of microencapsulation.
6. What are the materials used for the preparation of microsphere?
7. Briefly discuss the types of microsphere.
8. Discuss the mechanism of bioadhesion.
9. What are the basic components used for buccal drug delivery system?
10. Mention different devices for implantable drug delivery.
11. Give different methods for microencapsulation processes used in drug delivery system.

B. Long Answer Type Questions

1. Discuss in detail about implantable drug delivery systems.
2. What are the formulations considered for buccal drug delivery systems?
3. What is microencapsulation? Give its advantages and disadvantages.
4. Discuss the techniques used to manufacture microcapsules.
5. Write in detail about theories of mucoadhesion.
6. What do you mean by buccal drug delivery system? Give its advantages.
7. Discuss the mechanism for implantable drug delivery system.
8. Give the various applications for implantable drug delivery system.

Transdermal, Gastroretentive and Nasopulmonary Drug Delivery Systems

TRANSDERMAL DRUG DELIVERY SYSTEM (TDDS)

Introduction

Human skin (integument) acts as a protective barrier towards the external environment. It is a well-fabricated structure makes one-way channelization. Skin allows internal body fluids like sweat to come out but prevents entry of any external foreign matters. Skin's outermost obstruction, the stratum corneum, acts as a shield in such a way that it prevents aridity caused by water lost from the body. This barrier also furnishes a strong resistance towards absorption, either intentional or accidental, of chemicals that get in touch with the outer surface. However, the last two decades have witnessed the progress in the transdermal delivery of therapeutic agents initiated by pharmaceutical scientists. So, what type of challenges would scientists be faced? What examinations would they be done on the skin to explore its potential as a route for systemic transport of therapeutic agents? Significant conclusions have been drawn from critical analysis, that is, firstly skin offers a wide and freely reachable surface for drug transport. Secondly, in comparison to other routes, transdermal applications are relatively non-invasive, entailing effortless techniques like sticking of a patch, e.g. Band-Aid. Third, patient compatibility is easily achieved. Fourth, another fruitful alternative for patient compliance is that any transdermal application can be voluntarily removed or discontinued at any point in time; no other formulation approach provides this freedom. Although delivery of therapeutic agents through the integument is confined to reasonably only a small number of therapeutic agents, it has proved to be a significant market victory in comparison to added "controlled release" tools. At current, transdermal systems have an annual market of around two billion worldwide.

Advantages

Transdermal delivery of therapeutic agents offers some important advantages, which are as follows:
- Problems like significant pre-systemic metabolism are avoided.
- Prevention of degradation of the drug in the gastrointestinal tract or liver.
- The decrease of variations in inter-/intra-subjects: It is mainly realistic in the case where the release of preparation from the transdermal patch is a bit slow in contrast to the passage of the drug from the outermost keratinized layer of integument.

- As per basic concept of pharmacokinetics, drug volumes can be retained within the therapeutic window for a considerably long time.
- In relevance to the previous point, the duration of the action, i.e. area under the curve of the drug following single administration, can be absolute and accordingly, the frequency of dosing can be minimized.
- Enhanced compatibility and acceptance from patients towards drug treatment.
- The curative application might be stopped (by a simple detachment of patch) at any point of time on the occurrence of any kind of difficulties.

Disadvantages

- TDDS cannot deliver ionic drugs.
- TDDS cannot achieve high drug levels in blood/plasma.
- This type of drug delivery system cannot develop for drugs of large molecular size.
- Such drug delivery system cannot deliver drugs in a pulsatile fashion.
- This system cannot develop, if drug or formulation causes irritation to skin.

Limitation of such type of drug delivery system (TDDS) can be overcome to some extent by novel approaches such as iontophoresis, electroporation and ultrasound.

Basic Components of TDDS

1. Polymer matrix or matrices
2. The drug
3. Permeation enhancers
4. Other excipients

Polymer Matrix

The polymer controls the release of the drug from device. Potential useful polymers for transdermal devices are:

a. **Natural polymers:** Cellulose derivatives, shellac, waxes, zein, gelatin, proteins, gums and their derivatives, natural rubber, starch, etc.
b. **Synthetic elastomers:** Polybutadiene, hydrin rubber, polysiloxane, silicone rubber, butyl rubber, styrene-butadiene rubber, neoprene, nitrile, acrylonitrile, etc.
c. **Synthetic polymers:** Polyvinyl alcohol, polyacrylate, polyvinyl chloride, polyethylene, polypropylene, polyamide, polyurea, polyvinyl pyrrolidone, polymethylmethacrylate, epoxy, etc.

Drug

For successfully developing TDDS, the drug should be selected with great care. The following are some of the desirable physicochemical properties of a drug for transdermal delivery.

Physicochemical properties

- The drug must have a molecular weight less than approximately 1000 Daltons.
- The drug should have affinity for both lipophilic and hydrophilic phases. Extreme partitioning characteristics are not favourable to successful drug delivery via the integument.
- The drug must have low melting point.
- Along with above such properties, the drug should be potent, having short half-life and be non-irritating.

Permeation Enhancers

These are compounds which promote integument permeability by altering the skin as a barrier to the flux of a desired penetrate. These may easily be classified under the following main headlines:

a. **Solvents:** Such compounds enhance penetration possibly by swallowing the polar pathway and/or by fluidizing lipids such as water, alcohols—methanol and ethanol; alkyl methyl sulfoxides, dimethyl sulfoxide, alkyl homologs of methyl sulfoxide, dimethyl acetamide and dimethyl formamide; 2 pyrrolidone, N-methyl, 2-purrolidone; laurocapram (Azone), miscellaneous solvents—propylene glycol, glycerol, silicone fluids, isopropyl palmitate.

b. **Surfactants:** Such compounds are proposed to increase polar pathway transport, especially of hydrophilic drugs. The ability of a surfactant to change penetration is a function of the polar head group and the hydrocarbon chain length.

   • *Anionic surfactants:* Dioctyl sulphosuccinate, decodecyl-methyl sulphoxide, sodium lauryl sulphate, etc.

   • *Non-ionic surfactants:* Pluronic F127, Pluronic F68, etc.

   • *Bile salts:* Sodium taurocholate, sodium deoxycholate, sodium tauroglycocholate.

   • *Binary system:* Such systems actually open up the heterogeneous multilaminate pathway as well as the continuous pathways, e.g. propylene glycol and 1, 4-butane diol-linoleic acid.

c. **Miscellaneous chemicals:** These chemicals are urea, a hydrating and keratolytic agent; N,N-dimethyl-m-toluamide; calcium thioglycolate; anticholinergic agents. Some possible permeation enhancers have recently been described but the present data on their effectiveness sparse. These are di-*o*-methyl-β-cyclodextrin eucalyptol and soyabean casein.

Other Excipients

a. **Adhesives:** The fastening of all transdermal devices to the integument has so far been done by using a pressure sensitive adhesive which can be positioned on the face of the device and in the back of the device and extending peripherally. Both adhesive systems should fulfill the following criteria.

   • Should adhere to the integument aggressively, should be easily removed.

   • Should not leave an unwashable residue on the integument.

   • Should not irritate or sensitize the integument.

The adhesive system should also fulfill the following important criteria;

   • Physical and chemical compatibility with the drug, excipients and enhancers of the device of which it is a part.

   • Permeation of drug should not be affected.

   • The delivery of simple or blended permeation enhancers should not be affected.

b. **Backing membrane:** Backing membranes are flexible and they afford a good bond to the drug reservoir, prevent drug from leaving the dosage form through the top, and accept printing. It is impermeable substance that protects the product during use on the integument, e.g. metallic plastic laminate, plastic backing with absorbent pad and occlusive base plate (aluminium foil), adhesive foam pad (flexible polyurethane) with occlusive base plate (aluminium foil disc), etc.

Ideal Drug Candidates for Transdermal Delivery

An ideal drug candidate must follow a few eligibility criteria and conditions as
- It should have an optimal partition coefficient, i.e. Log P value (water-octanol) between 1 and 4.
- It must have low melting point, i.e. 200°C and shelf life must be up to 2 years.
- The half-life of the drug must be less than 10 h.
- It should not fabricate any local irritation or sensitization.
- It should have high potency, i.e. daily dose should be low (20 mg/day) and a low molecular weight (500 Daltons).
- It should have skin permeability coefficient greater than $>0.5 \times 10^{-3}$ cm/h.
- It should also have potential performance characteristics towards both hydrophilic and lipophilic phases.
- Excessive division characteristic is not favourable for successful delivery via the integument. A diagram view of selection criteria is presented in Fig. 3.1.

Drug Penetration Through Skin

In percutaneous permeation process, a drug molecule may pass through the epidermis itself or may get diffuse through shunts, particularly those offered by the relatively widely distributed hair follicles and eccrine glands. In the initial transient diffusion stage, drug molecules may penetrate the integument along the hair follicles or sweat ducts and then absorbed through the follicular epithelium and the sebaceous glands. When a steady state is achieved the diffusion through the intact stratum corneum becomes the primary pathway for transdermal permeation (Fig. 3.2).

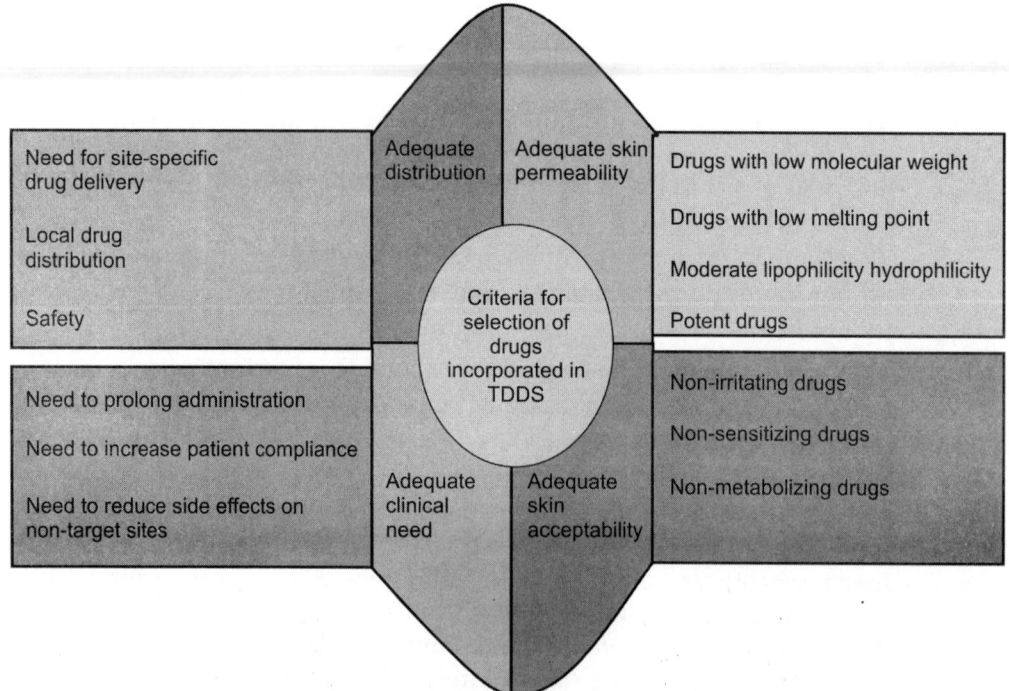

Fig. 3.1: Criteria for selection of drugs incorporated in TDDS

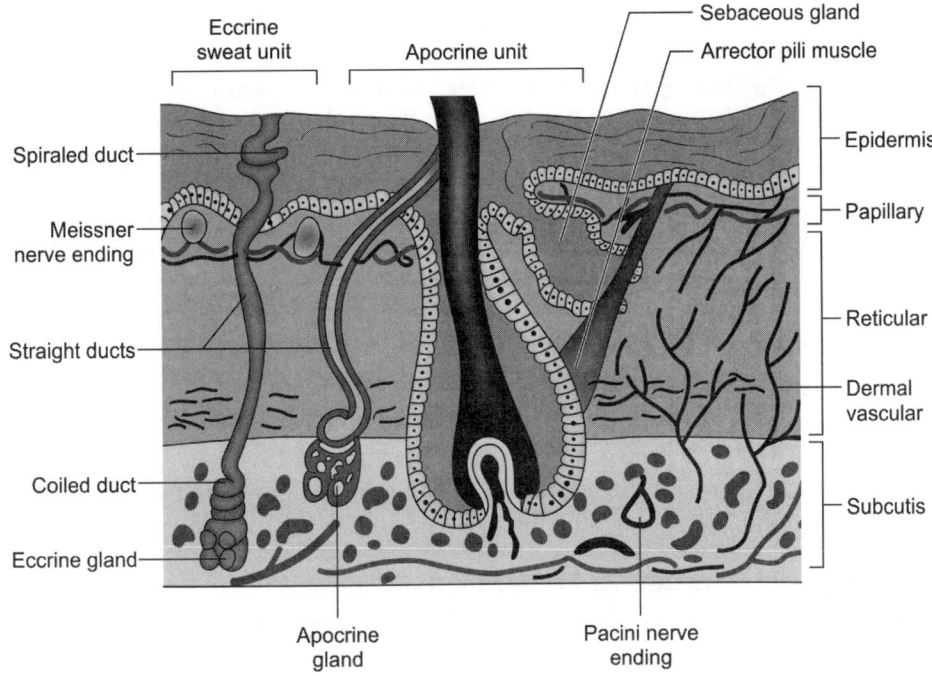

Fig. 3.2: Possible macroroutes for drug penetration

Possible macroroutes for drug penetration

1. Intact horny layer   2. Hair follicles   3. Eccrine glands

For any molecules applied to the skin, two main routes of skin permeation can be defined:

1. Transepidermal route   2. Transfollicular route

Transepidermal Route

In transepidermal transport, drug molecules cross the intact horny layer. Two potential microroutes of entry exist, the transcellular (or intracellular) and the intercellular pathway as shown in Fig. 3.3.

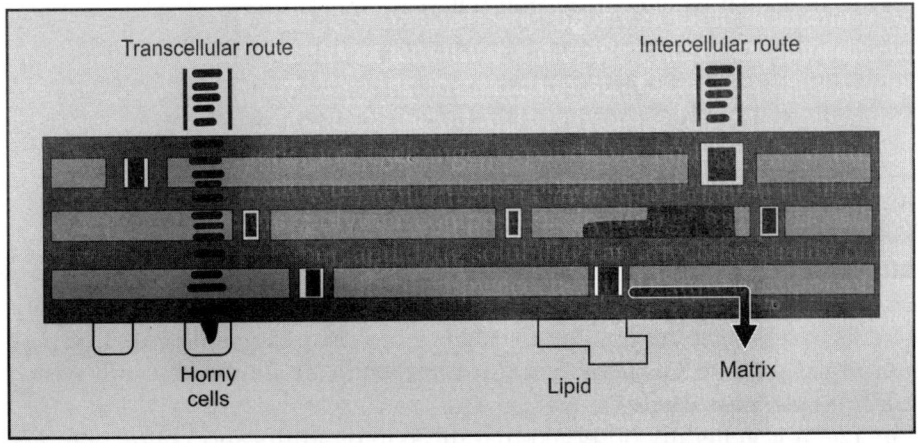

Fig. 3.3: Schematic representation of transepidermal route

Both polar and non-polar substances diffuse via transcellular and intercellular routes by various different mechanisms. The polar molecules primarily diffuse through the polar pathway consisting of "bound water" within the hydrated stratum corneum while the non-polar molecules dissolve and diffuse through the non-aqueous lipid matrix of the stratum corneum. Thus, the principal pathway taken by a penetrate is decided mainly by the partition coefficient (log K). Water-philic drugs (active moiety molecule) partition preferentially into the intracellular domains, whereas lipophilic permeants (octanol/water log K >2) traverse the stratum corneum via the intercellular route. Most of the molecules pass through the stratum corneum by both routes.

Transfollicular Route (Shunt Pathway)

These routes comprise transport through the sweat glands and the hair follicles with their associated sebaceous glands. Although this route offers high permeability, they are considered to be of minor significance because of their relatively small area, approximately 0.1% area of the total skin. These routes seem to be most significant for ions and large polar molecules which hardly permeate through the stratum corneum.

Basic Principle of Transdermal Permeation

Transdermal permeation is mainly based on passive diffusion. Integument is the most intensive and readily accessible organ of the body as only a fraction of millimeter of tissue separates its surface from the underlying capillary network. The release of an active ingredient from a preparation applied to the skin surface and its transport to the systemic circulation is a multistep process, which includes:

1. Flow of drug to the rate-controlling membrane.
2. Dissolution within and release from the preparation.
3. Sorption through stratum corneum and penetration by viable epidermis.
4. Uptake of drug through capillary network in the dermal papillary layer.
5. Effect on the target body parts (organ).
6. Partitioning into the outermost layer of integument, the stratum corneum.
7. Diffusion by the stratum corneum, principally through a lipidic intercellular pathway.

Properties that influence transdermal delivery

- Release of the medicament from the vehicle
- Penetration through the skin barrier
- Activation of the pharmacological response

Factors Affecting Transdermal Permeation

Biological Factors

1. **Skin conditions:** The intact integument itself acts as barrier but many agents like acids, alkali cross the barrier cells and penetrate through the integument, many solvents open the complex dense structure of horny layer solvents like methanol, chloroform remove lipid fraction, forming artificial shunts through which drug molecules can pass easily.
2. **Skin age:** It is generally observed that the skin of adults and young ones are more permeable than the older ones but there is no dramatic difference. A child shows

toxic effects because of the larger surface area per unit body weight. Thus, potent steroids, boric acid, hexachlorophene produces severe side effects.

3. **Blood supply:** Changes in peripheral circulation may affect transdermal absorption.
4. **Regional skin site:** Thickness of integument, nature of stratum corneum and density of appendages vary site-to-site. These factors affect considerably penetration.
5. **Skin metabolism:** Skin metabolizes hormones, steroids, chemical carcinogens and some drugs. So, skin metabolism determines efficacy of drug permeated through the integuments.
6. **Species differences:** The integument thickness, density of appendages and formation of keratin in integument vary species-to-species, therefore, affect the penetration.

Physicochemical Factors

1. **Skin hydration:** In contact with H_2O, the permeability of integuments increases considerably. Hydration is one of the most significant factors which increases the permeation of skin. Therefore, use of humectants (moistening agent) is done in transdermal delivery.
2. **Temperature and pH:** The permeation of drug increases 10-fold with temperature variation. The diffusion coefficient decreases as temperature drops. Weak acids and weak bases dissociate depending on the pH and pKa or pKb values. The proportion of unionized drug find outs the drug concentration in integument. Thus, temperature and pH are very important factors for affecting drug penetration.
3. **Diffusion coefficient:** Penetration of drug depends on the diffusion coefficient of drug. At a fixed temperature, the diffusion coefficient of drug depends on the properties of drug, diffusion medium and interaction between them.
4. **Drug concentration:** Normally, the flux is proportional to the concentration gradient across the barrier and concentration gradient will be greater, if the concentration of drug will be more across the barrier.
5. **Partition coefficient:** The most favourable partition coefficient (K) is required for good action. Drugs with high K are not ready to leave the lipid portion of integument. Also, drugs with low K will not be permeated.
6. **Molecular size and shape:** Drug absorption is inversely associated to molecular weight; small molecule penetrates faster than large ones.

Environmental Factors

1. **Sunlight:** The walls of blood vessels become thinner due to sunlight leading to bruising with only minor trauma in sun-exposed areas. The most common noticeable sun-induced pigment change is a freckle or solar lentigo.
2. **Cold season:** Normally result in itchy, dry skin, skin responds by increasing oil production to compensate for the weather's drying effects. A good moisturizer will help relieve symptoms of dry skin. Also, drinking lots of H_2O can keep skin hydrated and looking radiant.
3. **Air pollution:** Dust may obstruct pores and increase bacteria on the face and surface of integument, which may lead to acne or spots. These affect drug delivery through the skin. Invisible or gaseous chemical air pollutants may interfere with skin's natural protection system, breaking down the natural skin's oils that normally trap moisture in integument and keep it supple.

4. **Effect of heat on transdermal patch:** Heat induces high absorption of transdermally delivered drugs. Patient should be advised to avoid exposing the patch application site to external heat sources, like heated water bags, hot H_2O bottles. Even high body temperature may also raise the transdermally delivered drugs. In this case, the patch should be eliminated immediately. Transdermal drug patches are stored in their original packing and keep in a cool, dry place until they are ready to use.

GASTRORETENTIVE DRUG DELIVERY SYSTEMS (GRDDS)

Oral drug delivery systems have dominated other drug delivery systems for human administration due to their various different advantages including:
- Ease of administration
- Flexibility in formulation
- Cost-effectiveness
- Easy storage and transport
- High patient compliance.

However, oral drug delivery systems face various challenges such as:
- Low bioavailability due to the heterogeneity of the gastrointestinal system
- pH of the commensal flora
- Gastric retention time of the dosage form
- Surface area and enzymatic activity.

Conventional drug delivery systems may not overcome the problems imposed by the GI tract such as incomplete release of drugs, reduce in dose effectiveness and frequent dose requirement. Due to the failure of conventional drug delivery systems to retain drugs in the stomach may lead to the development of GRDDS. This system offers several advantages such as prolonged gastric residence time of dosage forms in the stomach up to several hours, enhanced therapeutic efficacy of drugs through improving drug absorption and suitability for targeted delivery in the stomach. Additionally, GRDDS can enhance the controlled delivery of drugs by continuously releasing the drug for an extended period at the desired rate and to the desired absorption site until the active chemical substances is completely released from the dosage form. GRDDS is reasonable for drugs that have low absorption in the lower part of the GI tract, are unstable and poorly soluble at alkaline pH, have a short half-life, and reveal local activity at the upper part of the intestine for eradication of *Helicobacter pylori.* Various formulation strategies are used to design successful controlled release GRDDS including superporous hydrogel, bio-/mucoadhesive, raft-forming, magnetic, ion-exchange, expandable, and low- and high-density systems. Various preparation-related factors—polymer types such as non-ionic, cationic, and anionic polymers, polymer composition in dosage form, viscosity grade, molecular weight of the polymer, and drug solubility can affect the quality of the gastroretentive dosage form. Additionally, the physicochemical nature of excipients plays a significant role in various GRDDS. For instance, excipient's density and composition of effervescent agents are critical factors in effervescent floating systems. In a superporous hydrogel system, high swelling excipients such as sodium carboxymethyl cellulose and crospovidone are needed to form a superporous hydrogel. Similarly process variables can also influence the quality of the gastroretentive dosage form, as the density of a tablet can be changed by the compression pressure during tableting.

Advantages of GRDDS

- The bioavailability of therapeutic agents can be significantly enhanced especially for those which get metabolized in the upper GIT by this gastroretentive drug delivery approach in comparison to the administration of non-gastroretentive drug delivery. There are various factors associated to absorption and transit of the drug in the gastrointestinal tract (GIT) that act concomitantly to influence the magnitude of drug absorption.
- For drugs with relatively short t½, sustained release may result in a flip-flop pharmacokinetics and also enable reduced frequency of dosing with improved patient compliance.
- They also have an advantage over their conventional system as it can be used to overcome the adversities of the gastric retention time as well as the gastric emptying time. As this system is expected to remain buoyant on the gastric fluid without affecting the intrinsic rate of employing because their bulk density is lower than that of the gastric fluids.
- Gastroretentive drug delivery can produce prolong and sustain release of medicines from dosage forms which avail local therapy in the stomach and small intestine. Hence, they are useful in the treatment of disorders associated with stomach and small intestine.
- The controlled, slow delivery of medicine form gastroretentive dosage form provides sufficient local action at the diseased site, thus minimizing or eliminating systemic exposure of drugs. This site-specific drug delivery minimizes undesirable side effects.
- Gastroretentive dosage forms minimize the fluctuation of drug concentrations and effects. Therefore, concentration-dependent adverse effects that are related to peak concentrations may present. This feature is of special importance for medicine with a narrow therapeutic index.
- Gastroretentive drug delivery can minimize the counter-activity of the body leading to greater drug efficiency.
- Decrease of fluctuation in drug concentration makes it easy to obtain improved selectivity in receptor activation.
- The sustained mode of drug release from gastroretentive doses form enables extension of the time over a critical concentration and thus enhances the therapeutic effects and betters the chemical outcomes.

Disadvantages of Gastroretentive Drug Delivery System

- Gastroretentive drug delivery system requires high fluid level in stomach to float and work efficiently.
- Not feasible for those drugs that have solubility of stability problem in GIT.
- In patient with achlorhydria can be questionable in case of swellable system.
- The mucus on the wall of the stomach is in a state of constant renewal, resulting in unpredictable adherence.
- Retention of high-density system in the antrum part under the migrating waves of the stomach is questionable.
- Unsuitable for the drugs with limited acid solubility, e.g. phenytoin.
- Unsuitable for the drugs that are unstable in acidic environment, e.g. erythromycin.
- Unsuitable for the drugs that irritate or cause gastric lesions on slow release, e.g. aspirin and NSAIDs.
- Unsuitable for the drugs that are absorbed selectively in colon, e.g. corticosteroids.

Potential Drug Candidates for Gastroretentive Drug Delivery Systems

- Drugs that have narrow absorption window in GI tract (e.g. L-DOPA, furosemide, p-aminobenzoic acid, riboflavin).
- Drugs which are locally active in the stomach (e.g. misoprostol, antacids).
- Drugs which are not stable in the intestinal or colonic environment (e.g. ranitidine, captopril, HCl, metronidazole).
- Drugs that disturb normal colonic microbes (e.g. antibiotics used for the removal of *Helicobacter pylori*, such as tetracycline, amoxicillin, clarithromycin).
- Drugs that show low solubility at high pH values (e.g. chlordiazepoxide, diazepam, verapamil).

Approaches to Prolong Gastric Residence Time of Drug Delivery System

Several devices such as mucoadhesive, high-density, swelling, and floating systems are developed to increase gastric residence time of a dosage form. Physiological features of the upper gastrointestinal tract pose a considerable challenge to develop such systems.

Floating Systems

Floating drug delivery system (FDDS) is one of the important drug delivery systems that floats immediately upon contact with gastric fluids present promising approaches for enhancing drug bioavailability with absorption windows in the upper small intestine. FDDS have less bulk density than gastric fluids and so remain buoyant in the stomach without affecting gastric emptying rate for a prolonged period of time and the drug is released slowly as a desired rate from the system. After drug releasing, the residual system is emptied from the stomach. These result in an enhanced GRT and a better control of the fluctuation in plasma drug concentration. However, besides a minimal gastric content required allowing the proper achievement of the buoyancy retention principle, a minimal level of floating force is also needed to keep the dosage form reliably buoyant on the surface of the meal. The main requirements for FDDS are:

- It should release contents slowly to serve as a reservoir.
- It must maintain specific gravity lower than gastric contents ($1.004 - 1.01$ g/cm^3).
- It must form a cohesive gel barrier.

The inherent low density may be provided through the entrapment of air (e.g. hollow chambers) or by the incorporation of low-density materials (e.g. fatty materials or oils, or foam powder). The good floating behaviour of this system could be successfully combined with accurate control of the resulting drug release patterns. The single-unit floating dosage forms are related with problems such as sticking together or being obstructed in the GI tract, which may produce gastric irritation. However, multiple-unit floating systems can be an attractive alternative since they have been shown to reduce inter- and intra-subject availabilities in drug absorption as well as to lower the possibility of dose dumping. Based on the mechanism of buoyancy, two distinctly different technologies, i.e. non-effervescent and effervescent systems have been utilized in the development of FDDS.

a. **Effervescent systems:** These systems utilize gas (CO_2) producing agents (e.g. sodium bicarbonate, citric acid or tartaric acid) to obtain floatability. After oral administration in the GI tract, CO_2 is liberated from these drug delivery systems, which reduces the density of the system and making it float on the gastric fluid. The optimum stoichiometric ratio of citric acid and sodium bicarbonate for gas production is reported to be 0.76:1. The buoyancy may be obtained also by using matrices prepared with swellable polymers like methocel, hydroxypropyl methylcellulose (HPMC), chitosan. An alternative is the incorporation of the matrix-containing portion of liquid, which produces gas that evaporates at body temperature. These effervescent systems further can be classified as gas-generating systems and volatile liquid/vacuum systems.

1. *Gas-generating systems:*
   - *Intragastric single-layered floating tablets* (Fig. 3.4): These are prepared by intimately mixing the CO_2 generating components and drug candidates within tablet matrix. These have lower bulk density than the gastric content and, therefore, obtain buoyancy in the stomach unflattering the gastric emptying rate for a prolonged period of time. The drug is released from the matrix tablet in a sustained manner at a controlled rate. After completion of the drug release, the residual system is to be expelled from the stomach.
   - *Intragastric bilayered floating tablets:* Intragastric bilayered floating tablets can be compressed that contains the gas generating mechanism in one hydrocolloid containing sustained release layer and immediate release layer. It is shown in Fig. 3.5.
   - *Multiple-unit type of floating pills:* A multiple-unit type of floating pill, which produces CO_2 gas, is developed. It is shown in Fig. 3.6.

   The system containing sustained release pills as seeds surrounded by double layers. The inner layer is an effervescent layer consists of tartaric acid and sodium bicarbonate. The outer layer is a swellable membrane layer. Moreover, the effervescent layer is divided into two sublayers to avoid direct contact between these two gas-generating agents. Sodium bicarbonate is contained

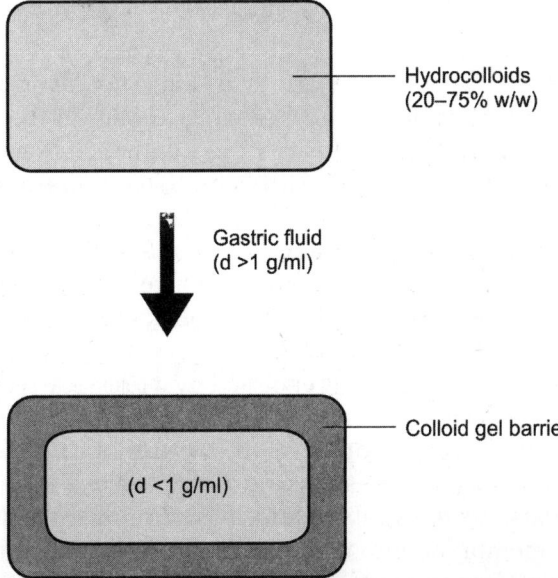

Hydrocolloids
(20–75% w/w)

Gastric fluid
(d >1 g/ml)

Colloid gel barrier

(d <1 g/ml)

Fig. 3.4: Intragastric single-layered floating tablet

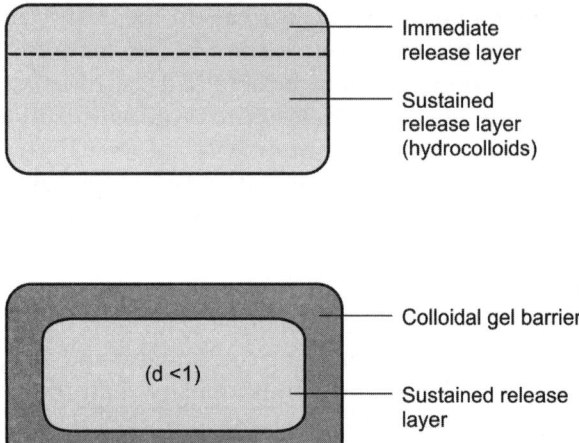

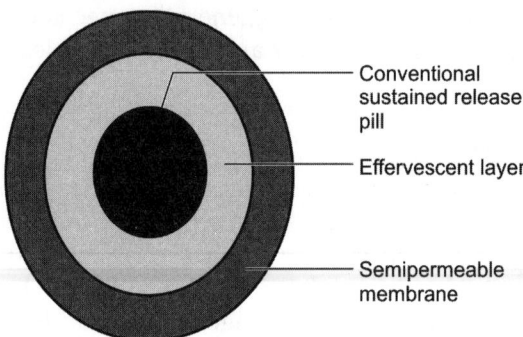

Fig. 3.5: Intragastric bilayered floating tablet

Fig. 3.6: Multiple-unit floating oral pill

in the inner sublayer, while tartaric acid is in outer layer. When the system is immersed in buffer system at 37°C, it sinks at once in the solution and forms swollen pills, like balloons (density <1 g/ml), which float as they have lower density. This lower density is due to generation and entrapment of CO_2 within this system.

2. ***Volatile liquid or vacuum-containing systems:*** *Intragastric osmotically controlled floating delivery systems:* The osmotic pressure controlled floating systems containing two compartments: A drug reservoir compartment and an osmotically active compartment. It is shown in Fig. 3.7.

The drug reservoir compartment is enclosed by a pressure responsive collapsible bag, which is impermeable to vapour and liquid. This compartment also has a drug delivery orifice. On the other hand, the osmotically active compartment consists of osmotically active salts and is enclosed within a semipermeable housing. The water in the gastric fluid is continuously absorbed through the semipermeable membrane into osmotically active compartment to dissolve the osmotically active component in the stomach. The osmotic pressure is then generated, which acts on the collapsible bag and in turn forces the drug reservoir

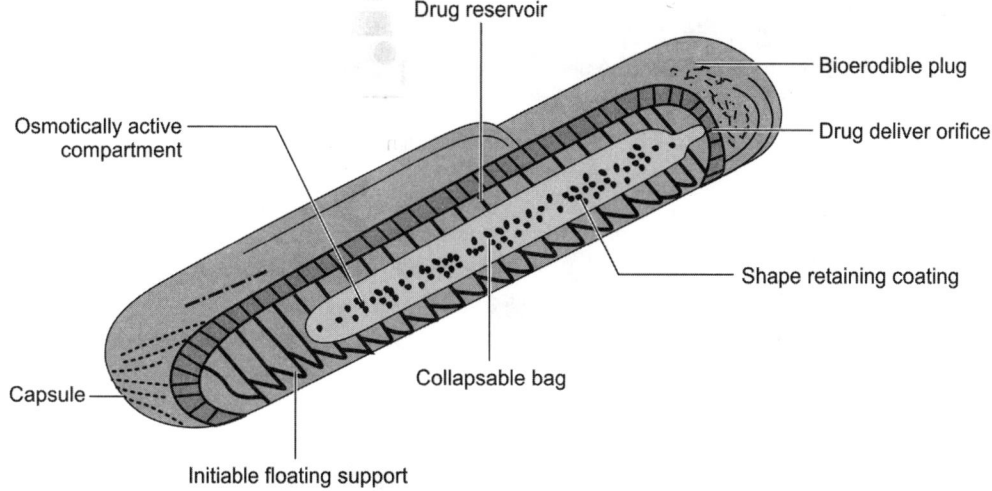

Drug reservoir

Bioerodible plug

Osmotically active compartment

Drug deliver orifice

Shape retaining coating

Capsule

Collapsable bag

Initiable floating support

Fig. 3.7: Intragastric osmotically controlled floating delivery systems

compartment to decrease its volume and activate the release of drug candidates in form of solution through the delivery orifice. The floating support consists of a bioerodible plug that erodes after a predicted time period to deflate the support. The drug delivery system is then emptied from the stomach.

b. **Non-effervescent systems:** Non-effervescent FDDSs are normally prepared from gel-forming or highly swellable cellulose type hydrocolloids, polysaccharides or matrix forming polymers like polyacrylate, polycarbonate, polystyrene, polymethacrylate, carbopol, HPMC, sodium alginate, chitosan, etc. These systems can be further divided into following subtypes:

1. *Hydrodynamically balanced systems (HBS):* HBSs have gained a lot of importance in recent days to improve absorption of drugs especially those are absorbed from stomach and small intestine or drugs such as weak bases, which dissolve better in the acid environment of the stomach. These systems contain drug with gel-forming hydrocolloids meant to remain buoyant on the stomach content. These are single-unit dosage forms, containing one or more gel-forming hydrophilic polymers. HPMC, hydroxyethyl cellulose (HEC), hydroxypropyl cellulose (HPC), sodium carboxymethyl cellulose (NaCMC), polycarbophil, polyacrylate, polystyrene, agar, carrageenans and alginic acid are commonly used excipients to develop these systems (Fig. 3.8).

2. *Microballoons (hollow microspheres):* Microballoons (hollow microspheres) loaded with drugs in their other polymer shelf were prepared by simple solvent evaporation or solvent diffusion/evaporation method to create a hollow inner core 43, which prolongs the GRT of the dosage form. Commonly used polymers to develop these systems are polycarbonate, cellulose acetate, calcium alginate, eudragit S, agar and low methoxylated pectin, etc. The polymer is dissolved or dispersed in the organic solvent and the drug is either dissolved or dispersed in the polymer solution.

3. *Alginate beads:* Researchers recently developed a multiple-unit floating system based on cross-linked beads. They are made by using Ca^{2+} and low methoxylated pectin (anionic polysaccharide), or Ca^{2+} low methoxylated pectin and sodium

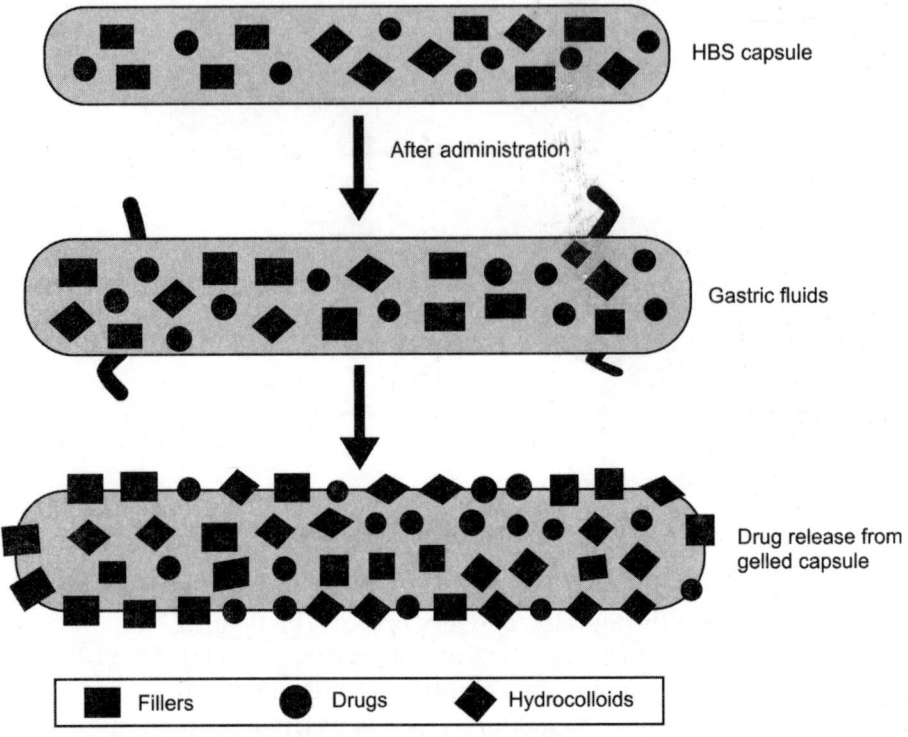

Fig. 3.8: Mechanism of hydrodynamically balanced systems as FDDS

alginate. In this approach, normally sodium alginate solution is dropped into aqueous solution of calcium chloride and causes the precipitation of calcium alginate. In another investigation, multiple-unit floating alginate beads are developed from freeze-dried calcium alginate using sodium alginate as the polymer and calcium chloride as a cross-linking agent (Fig. 3.9).

4. *Gas-filled floating delivery systems:* Gas-filled floating delivery systems include incorporation of a gas filled floatation chamber, which may be vacuum or filled with air or a harmless gas into a microporous component that houses a drug reservoir. Apertures or openings are present along the top and bottom walls through which the gastric fluid enters to dissolve the drug, while the other two walls in contact the fluid are sealed, so that the undissolved drug remains therein.

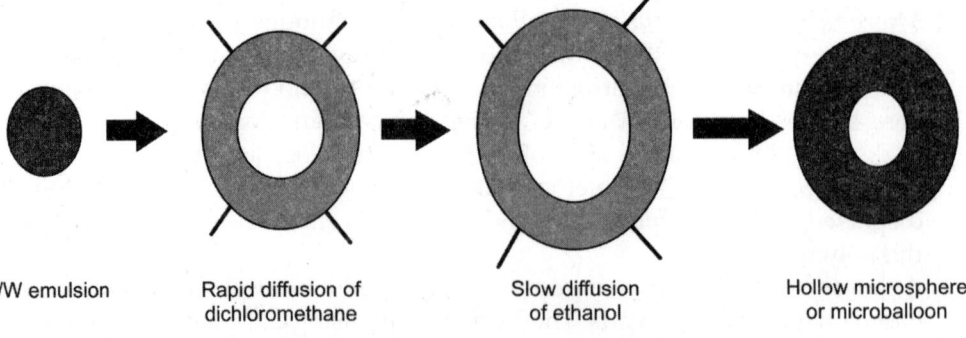

Fig. 3.9: Formulation of floating hollow microsphere or microballoon

Bioadhesive or Mucoadhesive Drug Delivery Systems (Gastroadhesive Systems)

These systems are used as a delivery device within the human to enhance drug absorption in a site-specific manner. Bioadhesive polymers are used and they may adhere to the epithelial surface in the stomach. Thus, these systems improve the prolongation of gastric retention. The basis of adhesion in that a dosage form may stick to the mucosal surface by different mechanisms. These mechanisms are:

1. The wetting theory which is based on the ability of bioadhesive polymers to spread and develop intimate contact with the mucus layers.
2. The diffusion theory, which proposes physical entanglement of mucin strands, the flexible polymer chains, or an interpenetration of mucin strands into the porous structure of the polymer substrate.
3. The absorption theory suggests that bioadhesion is due to secondary forces such as van der Waals forces and hydrogen bonding.
4. The electron theory which proposes attractive electrostatic forces between the glycoprotein mucin network and the bioadhesive material. Materials commonly used for bioadhesion are polyacrylic acid, chitosan, cholestyramine, sodium alginate, hydroxypropyl methylcellulose (HPMC), sucralfate, tragacanth, dextrin, polyethylene glycol (PEG), polylactic acids, etc. Although some of these polymers are effective at producing bioadhesive, it is very difficult to maintain it effective because of the rapid turnover of mucus in the GI tract.

High-Density Systems

These systems are intended to lodge in the rugae of the stomach withstanding the peristaltic movements. Systems with a density of 1.3 g/ml or higher are expected to be retained in the lower part of the stomach. The formulation of heavy pellets is based on the assumption that the pellets might be positioned in the lower part of the antrum because of their higher density. It is reported that the pellets with density of at least 1.5 g/ml have significantly higher gastric residence time both in fasted and fed states. However, *in vivo* data do not confirm the effectiveness of this system, as the primary determining factor of gastric emptying is the state of stomach when it is administered.

Expandable, Unfoldable and Swellable Systems

A dosage form in the stomach will withstand gastric transit, if it is bigger than pyloric sphincter. However, the dosage form must be small enough to be swallowed and must not cause gastric obstruction either singly or by accumulation. Thus, their configurations are required to develop an expandable system to prolong gastric retention time:

1. A small configuration for oral intake,
2. An expanded gastroretentive form, and
3. A final small form enabling evacuation following drug release from the device.

Thus, gastroretentivity is improved by the combination of substantial dimension with high rigidity of dosage form to withstand peristalsis and mechanical contractility of the stomach. Unfoldable and swellable systems are investigated and recently tried to develop an effective gastroretentive drug delivery. Unfoldable systems are made of biodegradable polymers. They are available in different geometric forms like tetrahedron, ring or planner membrane (4-label disc or 4-limbed cross form) of bioerodible polymer compressed within a capsule which extends in the stomach, swellable systems are also retained in the GI tract due to their mechanical properties.

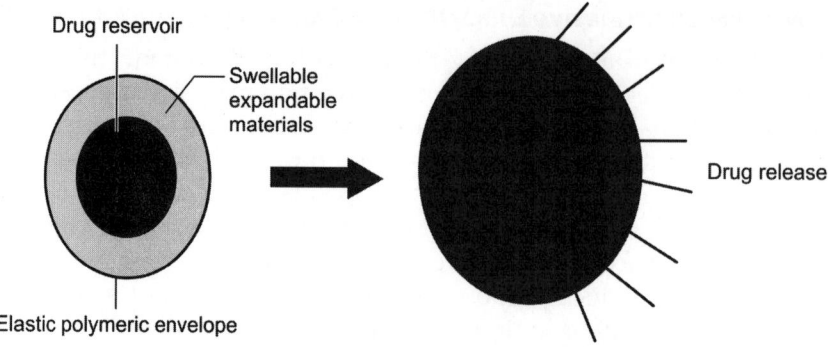

Fig. 3.10: Drug release from swellable systems

The swelling usually results from osmotic absorption of water and the dosage form is small enough to be swallowed by the gastric fluid (Fig. 3.10). Expandable systems have some drawbacks like problematical storage of much easily hydrolysable, biodegradable polymers relatively short-lived mechanical shape memory for the unfolding system most difficult to industrialize and not cost-effective. Again, permanent retention of rigid, large single-unit expandable drug delivery dosage forms may cause brief obstruction, intestinal adhesion and gastropathy.

NASOPULMONARY DRUG DELIVERY SYSTEM

Nasal Drug Delivery

In ancient times, the Indian Ayurvedic System of Medicines used nasal route for administration of drug and the process is called 'Nasya'. Intranasal drug delivery is now recognized to be a useful and reliable alternative to oral and parenteral routes. Undoubtedly, the intranasal administration of medicines for the symptomatic relief and prevention or treatment of topical nasal conditions is widely used for a long period of time. However, recently, the nasal mucosa has seriously emerged as a therapeutically viable route for the systemic drug delivery.

In general, among the primary targets for intranasal administration are pharmacologically active compounds with poor stability in gastrointestinal fluids, poor intestinal absorption and/or extensive hepatic first-pass elimination, such as peptides, proteins and polar drugs. The nasal delivery seems to be a favourable way to circumvent the obstacles for blood-brain barrier (BBB) allowing the direct drug delivery in the biophase of central nervous system (CNS)—active compounds. It is also considered to the administration of vaccines.

Nasal Enzymes

Cytochrome p-450 dependent oxygenase, lactate dehydrogenase, oxydoreductase, acid hydrolases, esterases, lactic dehydrogenases, malic enzymes, lysosomal proteinases, steroid hydroxylases, etc.

Nasal pH

- Adult nasal secretion pH: 5.5–6.5
- Infants and children: 5–6.7.

- It becomes alkaline in conditions such as acute rhinitis, acute sinusitis.
- Lysosome in the nasal secretion helps as antibacterial and its activity is diminished in alkaline pH.

Advantages

- Hepatic first pass metabolism avoided.
- Rapid drug absorption and quick onset of action.
- Bioavailability of larger drug molecules may be improved by means of absorption enhancer.
- Convenient for long-term therapy, compared to parenteral medication.
- Drugs possessing poor stability GI tract fluids given by nasal route.
- Easy and convenient.
- Easily administered to unconscious patients.

Disadvantages

- Pathologic conditions such as cold or allergies may alter significantly the nasal bioavailability.
- The histological toxicity of absorption enhancers used in nasal drug delivery system is not yet clearly established.
- Relatively inconvenient to patients when compared to oral delivery systems since there is a possibility of nasal irritation.
- Nasal cavity provides smaller absorption surface area when compared to GI tract.

Pulmonary Drug Delivery

Pulmonary delivery is used from ancient times in the delivery of drug for both local and systemic drug deliveries. The inhaled therapies started for 4000 years ago in India, from that time leaves of the *Atropa belladonna* plant smoke, aromatic plants are used to treat cough and other respiratory disorders. Pulmonary drug delivery is mainly used in the treatment of asthma, cystic fibrosis and cough. It minimizes systemic side effects, requires small dose and provides fast response. The inhalation therapies involved the use of leaves from plants, vapours from aromatic plants and balsams. Around the turn of the 19th century, the invention of liquid nebulizers as a newer treatment developed into valid pharmaceutical therapies. In 1920, adrenaline was introduced as a nebulizer solution, in 1925 nebulizer porcine insulin was used in investigational studies in diabetes, and in 1945 pulmonary delivery of the newly revealed penicillin was investigated. Steroids had been introduced in 1950 in the form of nebulizers for the treatment of asthma. In 1956, the pressurized metered-dose inhaler (pMDI) was introduced and become the major stay for the asthma treatment. It may find that certain drugs taken by pulmonary route are readily absorbed by the alveolar region direct into blood circulation because of some unique physiological characteristics of the respiratory route of drug administration.

Advantages

- Pulmonary drug delivery requires small fraction of oral dose (i.e. drug content of one 4 mg tablet of salbutamol equals to 40 doses of metered doses.)
- It delivers drug locally at low concentration that reaches systemic circulation thus reducing systemic side effects.
- Onset of action is very quick with pulmonary drug delivery.

- It avoids first pass metabolism (e.g. budesonide almost completely absorbed from the GI tract but its bioavailability is low, i.e. about 10% due to extensive first-pass metabolism in the liver).
- Large surface area around 100 m^2 and thin 0.1 to 0.2 µm thickness of pulmonary epithelium increase the permeation of the drug.
- Bioavailability of larger drug molecules may be improved by means of absorption enhancer.

Disadvantages

- Oropharyngeal deposition causes local side effects.
- Patient faces difficulty in using the pulmonary drug devices correctly.
- The total amount of drug per puff delivered to the lung is less than 1000 µg.

Devices for Pulmonary Drug Delivery

There are three main methods of delivering respiratory drugs for most of the asthma patients metered-dose inhaler (MDI), dry powder inhaler (DPI) and nebulizers. In case of dry powder inhalers, active pharmaceutical ingredient (API) powder with or without carrier (e.g. lactose) fine micronized particles are inhaled. The aggregates are converted into an aerosol by inspiratory airflow and this minimizes the problem of coordination between the delivery of the drug and the initiation of inspiration. But it is unsuitable for patients who are unable to generate high inspiratory flow rates. Active drug particles have a typical length-scale of 5 µm, while the carrier particles (usually a form of lactose) have a much wider size distribution. The most common carrier blend, lactose monohydrate, has particles ranging between order of magnitude larger and smaller than the active drug particles. This powder is stored within the device in different ways depending on the design.

Nebulizer is a device used to administer aerosolized medication in the form of a mist inhaled into the lungs. Nebulizer uses oxygen, compressed air or ultrasonic powder to break up medical solutions and suspensions into small aerosol droplet called mists that can be directly inhaled from the mouthpiece of the device. Nebulizers have also many disadvantages such as operation noise especially with jet nebulizers, bulky design, long administration period, unportable, variable performance because of gas flow for jet nebulizers, reservoir volume and drug physicochemical properties such as viscosity for ultrasonic nebulizers.

In the metered-dose inhaler (MDI), the API dispersed or solubilized in a high vapour pressure propellant and metered accurately in tens to hundreds of micrograms and administered directly to the lungs. pMDIs are most widely used device for drug delivery to the lungs. With this method, a medication is mixed in a canister with a propellant, and the preformed mixture is expelled in precise measured amounts upon actuation of the device (Fig. 3.11).

Advantages

- It delivers specified amount of dose.
- It is small in size, portable and convenient for use.
- It is usually less expensive as compared to dry powder inhalers and nebulizers.
- Quick to use.
- The contents are protected from contamination by pathogens.
- It is having multidose capability more than 100 doses available.

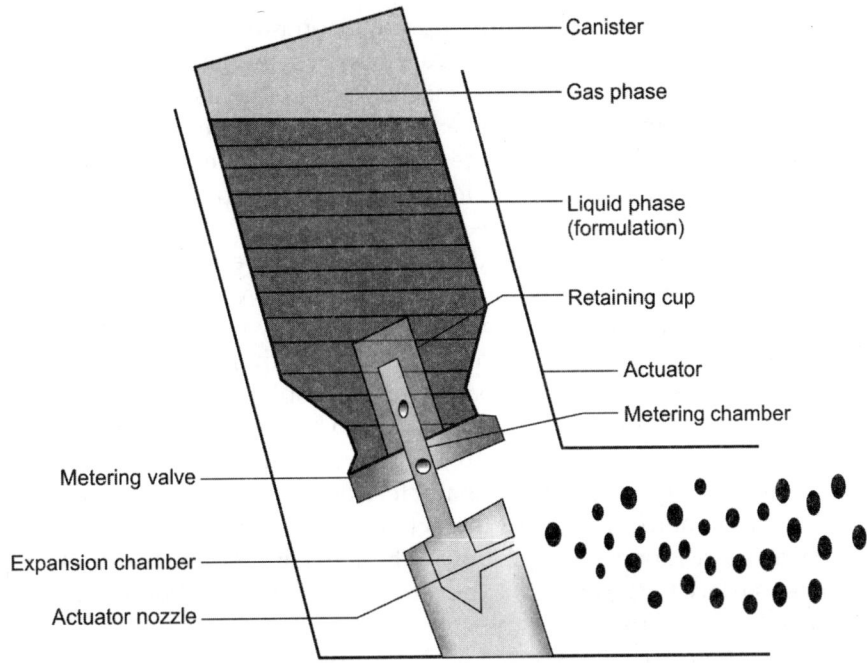

Fig. 3.11: Pressurized metered-dose inhaler

Disadvantages

- It is difficult to deliver high doses through pMDI.
- Accurate co-ordination between actuation of a dose and inhalation is required.
- Drug delivery is dependent on patient technique.

Components

The key components of pMDI are drug formulation, propellant, metering valve, actuator, and container. All play an important role in the formation of aerosol plume and in determining amount of drug to the lung.

1. **Canister:** The pMDI container should be able to withstand the high pressure generated by the propellant and it should be made of inert materials. Aluminium container is nowadays preferred because it is lighter, more compact, less fragile and light-proof. Coatings on the internal surfaces of canister can be useful to prevent drug adsorption, corrosion and drug degradation. Common coatings include epoxy resins, anodized aluminium, epoxy-phenol and perfluoroalkoxy alkane.

   Ideal properties:
   - Material used for canister should be compatible with formulation.
   - It should have ability to withstand pressure up to 1500 kPa.
   - It should have light weight.
   - It should be break resistant.
   - It should protect concentrate from sunlight.

2. **Metering valve:** The metering valve of a pMDI is critical component in the effectiveness of the delivery system. The function of the metering valve is to deliver dose accurately and reproducibly. The volume measured by it ranges from 20–100 µl and form a propellant-tight seal for high pressure in the canister. The

elastomeric seals and the gaskets are important components of the metering valve. The valves must be constructed from a variety of inert materials to ensure the compatibility of the formulation with the valve components. They form the barrier to the external environment and prevent the leakage of the product. The solvency properties of the propellant and storage temperature can affect the degree of swelling of valve elastomer. The valve regulates the flow of the content from the container and determines the spray characteristics of the aerosol.

3. **Actuator:** The actuator which is fitted to the aerosol valve stem is a device which on depression or any other required movement opens the valve and directs the spray to the desired area. The actuator of a pMDI is generally made from polyethylene or polypropylene materials. The design of actuator is important for the production of appropriate aerosols including the particle size, droplet size and the characteristics of the aerosol plume emitted from a pMDI. The design of an actuator which incorporates an orifice of varying size, shape and expansion chamber are crucial factors in influencing the physical characteristics of the spray particularly in the case of inhalation aerosols, where the active ingredient must be delivered in the proper particle size range. A proportion of the active ingredient is usually deposited on the inner surface of the actuator, the amount available is, therefore, less than the amount released by actuation of the valve.

4. **Formulation:** There are two types of MDI formulations:
   i. Solution formulations, in which the drug is dissolved in either the propellant or a combination of propellant and co-solvent.
   ii. Suspension formulations, in which micronized drugs are dispersed in a propellant or combination of propellants.

   a. *Solution formulation:* Drug is completely dissolved in HFA propellant and appropriate co-solvent (e.g. ethanol) is added to produce the solution. This is a two-phase system of gas and liquid.

   Advantages:
   - Homogeneous and uniform drug delivery.
   - Enhance efficiency of aerosolization and increase lung deposition.
   - No issue of particle growth and aggregation.
   - Very less drug particle deposition on component.

   Disadvantages:
   - Sufficient solubility is required in vehicle.
   - Possible reduction in chemical stability.
   - Few options of co-solvent for inhalation formulation.
   - Co-solvent decreases vapour pressure which is required for automation.

   b. *Suspension formulation:* Micronized drug is suspended in propellant or combination of propellant. Drug should be insoluble in propellant. This is a three-phase system consisting of gas, liquid and solid.

   Advantages:
   - Formulation resulting good chemical stability.
   - No additional excipients need to add which may be toxic.

   Disadvantages:
   - The density difference between propellant and drug affects dose uniformity.
   - Difference in hydrophilicity and hydrophobicity causes flocculation.

Formulation Components

1. **Active pharmaceutical ingredient:** Active pharmaceutical ingredient first checked for pre-formulation studies and particle size (D97) should be below 10 µm in case of suspension formulation.

2. **Propellant:** The propellant is used to provide the energy to produce a fine aerosol of drug particles and to expel the concentrate from the container and deliver to lung. The liquefied compressed gases are mainly used because discharge of aerosol undergoes evaporation of propellant to give aerosol of very small particles. A compressed liquefied gas gives consistent pressure throughout the use of content.

   The traditional pMDI propellant is chlorofluorocarbon (CFC). However, nowadays CFC is replaced by hydrofluoroalkane (HFA) due to concern about the environmental effects of CFCs on the ozone layer which filters ultraviolet (UV) radiation posing an increased risk of skin disease and global warming. HFAs do not contain chlorine and thus have no ozone-depleting potential. The Montreal Protocol was adopted in 1987 because of complete phase-out of the CFCs. From 2005, the Food and Drug Administration (FDA) ruled out the sale of CFC. pMDI would be prohibited in the United States after 2008. HFAs have greenhouse gas potential less than that of CFCs.

   Ideal properties of propellant:
   a. Boiling point should be between 100°C and 30°C.
   b. Density should be in between 1.2 and 1.5 g/cm^2.
   c. Vapour pressure 40 to 80 psig.
   d. Non-flammable.
   e. It should be non-toxic and pure.
   f. It should be inert and not reactive in formulation.
   g. It should have acceptable taste and odour.
   h. It should be compatible with primary packaging material.
   i. It should have acceptable solvency properties.
   j. Low cost.

3. **Stabilizing agent:** Surfactants are used to stabilize the suspension formulation. It also helps in solubilizing drug and prevents crystal growth during the storage period. It improves valve lubrication. Surfactants such as oleic acid, sorbitan trioleate and soya derived lecithin are highly soluble in CFC but are not soluble in HFAs, therefore, co-solvents are used to dissolve these surfactants in the HFA propellants.

4. **Co-solvent:** Surfactants are highly soluble in CFC but are not soluble in HFA, therefore, co-solvent is used to dissolve the surfactants in the HFA propellants. Ethanol is one of the most commonly used co-solvents in pMDI formulation. It lowers the vapour pressure of HFA propellants which produce smaller particle and more respirable drug fractions. It can even increase the solubility of certain APIs which lead to an increased problem of crystal growth. Also increase in ethanol causes decrease in volatility and vapour pressure of the formulation inside the container.

Manufacturing of Pressurized Metered-Dose Inhaler

Cold Filling Method

In cold filling method, the product concentrate is chilled to temperature of –30 to –40°F. The chilled product concentrate is added to the chilled aerosol container. The chilled propellant is added through an inlet valve present under side of the valve of the aerosol container. In this method, cold temperatures are used to convert the drug formulation to a liquid phase.

Initially, active pharmaceutical ingredient (API) and solvent are mixed to form either a homogenous suspension or a solution. Simultaneously, the propellant is placed into a pre-chilled vessel. The low temperature ensures that the propellant is in liquid form in the batching vessel. The concentrate is then transferred into the manufacturing vessel and the entire formulation is mixed. In the next step of the cold filling process, formulation is dispensed into appropriate-sized canisters by pumping the formulation to a filling head and feeding a predetermined portion of the chilled liquid formulation into an open canister. The valve is placed on top of each canister and then crimped into place.

Pressure Filling Method

In this method, the product concentrate is filled to the aerosol container through the metering pressure filling burette at room temperature. In contrast to cold filling, the pressure fill process uses pressure instead of low temperature to condense the propellant.

Pressure filling manufacturing can follow two methods. In one method, known as two-stage pressure filling method, the drug concentrate is placed in an open canister. A valve is then placed on top of the canister and crimped into position to form the seal. The propellant is then driven under pressure through the valve and into the canister. Using this method, the mixing of the concentrate and propellant actually happens in the canister.

The other method of pressure fill manufacturing is referred as single-stage pressure filling. In this process, the API and propellant are mixed and held under pressure in the vessel. An empty canister is then fed onto the filling table and a valve is placed on top and crimped into place. The complete formulation is then filled under pressure into the canister.

Nasal Sprays

Nasal sprays are used to deliver medications locally in the nasal cavities or systemically. They are used locally for conditions such as nasal congestion and allergic rhinitis. In some situations, the nasal delivery route is preferred for systemic therapy because it provides an agreeable alternative to injection or pills. Substances can be assimilated extremely quickly and directly through the nose. Many pharmaceutical drugs exist as nasal sprays for systemic administration (e.g. treatment for pain, migraine, osteoporosis and nausea). Other applications include hormone replacement therapy, treatment of Alzheimer's disease and Parkinson's disease. Nasal sprays are seen as a more efficient way of transporting drugs with potential use in crossing the blood–brain barrier.

Types of Nasal Sprays

There are three types to choose from:

1. **Decongestants:** We can buy these over the counter or with a prescription from doctor. They get rid of stuffiness by narrowing blood vessels in the lining of nose, which shrinks swollen tissues. It can be used these for more than 3 days, or cold symptoms could get worse. Doctors call this the 'rebound effect'.

2. **Salt-water solutions:** They are also called 'saline' nasal sprays, and we can buy them without a prescription. They loosen up your mucus and keep it from getting crusty. Since they do not contain any medications, feel free to use them as often you like.

3. **Steroid nasal sprays:** We can get these over the counter or with a prescription. They are approved to relieve allergy symptoms, but they are sometimes used to help clear a stuffed-up nose that comes from a sinus infection.

Nebulizers

In medicine, a nebulizer is a drug delivery device used to administer medication in the form of a mist inhaled into the lungs. Nebulizers are commonly used for the treatment of asthma, cystic fibrosis, cough and other respiratory diseases or disorders. Analytical nebulizers are another form of nebulizer that is used primarily in laboratory settings for elemental analysis. Nebulizers use oxygen, compressed air or ultrasonic power to break up solutions and suspensions into small aerosol droplets that can be directly inhaled from the mouthpiece of the device. An aerosol is a mixture of gas and solid or liquid particles.

Types of Nebulizers

1. **Soft mist inhaler:** The medical company Boehringer Ingelheim also invented a new device named Respimat Soft Mist Inhaler in 1997. This new technology provides a metered dose to the user, as the liquid bottom of the inhaler is rotated clockwise 180 degrees by hand, adding a build up tension into a spring around the flexible liquid container. When the user activates the bottom of the inhaler, the energy from the spring is released and imposes pressure on the flexible liquid container, causing liquid to spray out of 2 nozzles, thus forming a soft mist to be inhaled. The device features no gas propellant and no need for battery/power to operate. The average droplet size in the mist is measured to 5.8 µm, which could indicate some potential efficiency problems for the inhaled medicine to reach the lungs. Subsequent trials have proven this was not the case. Due to the very low velocity of the mist, the soft mist inhaler in fact has a higher efficiency compared to a conventional pMDI. In 2000, arguments were launched towards the European Respiratory Society (ERS) to clarify/expand their definition of a nebulizer, as the new soft mist inhaler in technical terms both could be classified as a 'hand-driven nebulizer' and a 'hand-driven pMDI'.

2. **Electrical jet nebulizer:** The most commonly used nebulizers are jet nebulizers, which are also called 'atomizers'. Jet nebulizers are connected by tubing to a compressor that causes compressed air or oxygen to flow at high velocity through a liquid medicine to turn it into an aerosol, which is then inhaled by the patient. Currently there seems to be a tendency among physicians to prefer prescription of a pressurized metered-dose inhaler (pMDI) for their patients, instead of a jet nebulizer that generates a lot more noise (often 60 dB during use) and is less portable due to a greater weight. However, jet nebulizers are commonly used for patients in hospitals who have difficulty using inhalers, such as in serious cases of respiratory disease, or severe asthma attacks. The main advantage of the jet nebulizer is related to its low operational cost. If the patient needs to inhale medicine on a daily basis, the use of a pMDI can be rather expensive. Today several manufacturers have also managed to lower the weight of the jet nebulizer down to 635 grams (22.4 oz), and

thereby started to label it as a portable device. Compared to all the competing inhalers and nebulizers, the noise and heavy weight is, however, still the biggest drawback of the jet nebulizer. Trade names for jet nebulizers include Maxin.

3. **Ultrasonic wave nebulizer:** Ultrasonic wave nebulizers were invented in 1965 as a new type of portable nebulizer. The technology inside an ultrasonic wave nebulizer is to have an electronic oscillator generate a high frequency ultrasonic wave, which causes the mechanical vibration of a piezoelectric element. This vibrating element is in contact with a liquid reservoir and its high frequency vibration is sufficient to produce a vapor mist. As they create aerosols from ultrasonic vibration instead of using a heavy air compressor, they only have a weight around 170 grams (6.0 oz). Another advantage is that the ultrasonic vibration is almost silent. Examples of these more modern types of nebulizers are: Omron NE-U17 and Beurer Nebulizer.

Aerosols

Pharmaceutical aerosols including metered-dose inhalers (MDIs) and dry powder inhalers (DPIs) are devices that deliver a specific quantity of drug to the lungs. The particle size distribution and shape of the delivered dose is more critical for inhalation aerosols than for most other conventional drug products because these factors greatly influence the deposition profile in the lungs of the patient. The optimum aerodynamic particle size distribution for most inhalation aerosols has generally been recognized as being in the range of 1–5 μm.

Advantages

Pharmaceutical aerosols are gaining popularity due to certain advantages. These are as follows:

- Pharmaceutical aerosols are easy to apply.
- Aerosol administration gives very efficient and quick relief.
- The stability of drug is enhanced by storing in MDIs and DPIs since the drug is not come in contact with atmospheric oxygen and moisture.
- The drug can be directly applied to the affected areas.
- Administration of drug by aerosol is a rapid process.
- It protects the drug from gastrointestinal tract degradation.
- Hepatic first pass metabolism can be avoided.
- Aerosols can be used for both systemic and local applications.
- A sterile dose of drug is dispensed and also the contamination of drug is prevented.

Types of Pharmaceutical Aerosols

Generally, pharmaceutical aerosols are stored in two types of inhalers, viz. metered-dose inhalers (MDIs) and dry powder inhalers (DPIs). MDIs and DPIs deliver a specific quantity of drug to the lungs through pulmonary tracks on external surface of body parts. Both types of product are used to treat lung diseases characterized by obstruction of airflow and shortness of breath, including asthma and chronic obstructive pulmonary disease (COPD), as well as respiratory infections and cystic fibrosis. The inhalation route offers further potential for systemic drug delivery

1. **Metered-dose inhalers:** The MDI device consists of a canister, and actuator, and sometimes a spacer. The canister itself consists of a metering dose valve with an

actuating stem. The formulation resides within the canister and is made up of the drug, a liquefied gas propellant, and often stabilizing excipients. Actuation of the device releases a single metered dose of liquid propellant that contains the medication. The volatile propellant breaks up into droplets which then evaporate, creating an aerosol-containing micronized drug that is inhaled into the lungs (Fig. 3.12).

The dose delivered by an MDI can be analyzed using a microscope, or preferable an automated image analyzer. A bronchodilator MDI is examined using the PSA300 image analysis system.

2. **Dry powder inhalers:** DPIs are an alternative to the aerosol-based inhalers commonly MDIs, that deliver a powder dosage form to the lungs. Most DPIs include an active ingredient and one or more excipient to aid powder dispersion and flow. The powder dose from a DPI can be analyzed on the PSA300 image analysis system. Results from a bronchodilator DPI containing salmeterol and fluticasone.

Components of Pharmaceutical Aerosol

An aerosol product consists of (Fig. 3.12):
1. Propellants
2. Containers
3. Valve and actuator

1. Propellants

It is most important components and called heart of aerosol because it generates required pressure to expel the content outside the container in required amount.

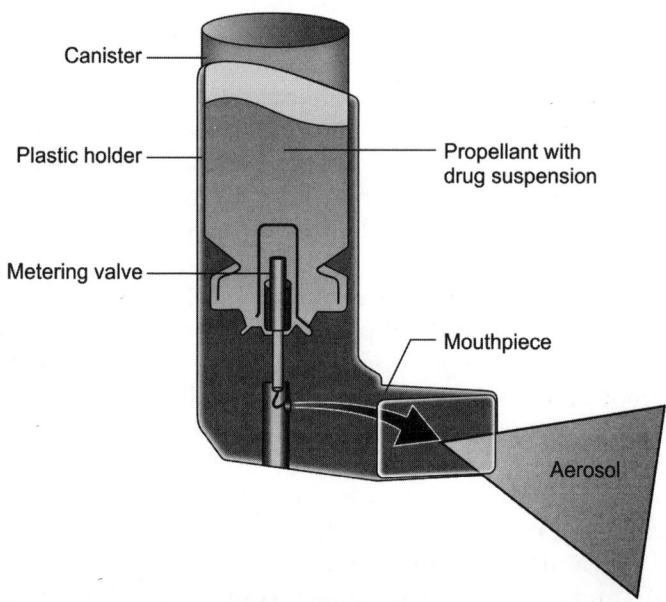

Fig. 3.12: Diagram of MDI device

Types of propellants

a. *Liquefied gas propellant:* It should have greater atmospheric pressure and low boiling point.

For example: Fluorinated hydrocarbons (halo carbons) for oral inhalants, e.g. trichloromono-fluoromethane (propellant-11), dichlorodifluoromethane (propellant-12), dichlorotetrafluoroethane (propellant-114).

Hydrocarbons (for topical): It has characteristic odour, taste and high degree of inflammability. These are not much used but in combination with fluorinated hydrocarbons, e.g. propane, butane and isobutane.

b. *Compressed gas propellants:*
   i. Insoluble in water compressed type: Argon, nitrogen - used in vitamin ointments
   ii. Soluble in water type: CO_2, NO_2, etc.—has usually acidic pH and used mainly in veterinary aerosols.

2. Containers

Various materials are used for containers, which must withstand pressure as high as 140 to 180 psi at 13°F, e.g.

   i. Tin plate containers—consist a sheet of steel plate that has been electroplated on both sides with tin thickness is described in terms of weight, e.g. #25, #50, #75, #100.
   ii. Aluminium containers—for seamless aerosol containers.
   iii. Stainless steel containers and glass containers.

3. Valves and Actuators

Valves for pharmaceutical use, material of construction must be approved by FDA. The valve assemblies consist of following parts.

a. *Ferrule and mounting cup:* Ferrule attaches valve with mounting cup. It has 1 inch opening, made up of thin-plated stainless steel or aluminium, used to place the valve assembly in the container. Since the underside of the valve cap is exposed to the contents of the container and to the effects of oxygen trapped in the head space, a single or double epoxy or vinyl coating can be added to increase resistance to corrosion. Ferrules are used with glass bottles or small aluminium tubes and are usually made from a softer metal such as aluminium or brass. Ferrule is attached to the container either by rolling the end under the lip of the bottle or by clinching the metal under the lip.

b. *Valve body or housing:* It is made from nylon or Delrin and contains an opening at the point of the attachment of the dip tubes, which range from 0.013 to 0.080 inch. This may contain or not another opening referred to as 'vapour tap' to escape of vapourized propellant along with liquid product. The vapour tap further produces a fine particle size, prevents valve clogging with product containing insoluble materials.

c. *Stem:* It is made from nylon or Delrin, but materials such as brass and stainless steel can be also utilized. It may contain aperture or hole 1–4 number, having size range 0.013 to 0.030 inch and set into the stem.

d. *Gasket:* Buna-N and neoprene rubber is used commonly in gasket material. It should be compatible with pharmaceutical formulation.

e. *Spring:* It helps to hold the gasket in place. When the actuator is depressed and released. It returns the valve to its closed position. Spring is made up of stainless steels.

f. *Dip tubes:* Dip tubes are made up of polyethylene or polypropylene. More rigid dip tube is due to polypropylene. The inside diameter of commonly used dip tube is 0.120–0.125 inch.

g. *Metering valves:* It is applicable to dispensing of potent medication. These operate on the principle of a chamber whose size determines the amount of medicaments dispensed. Approximately 50 to 150 mg ± 10% of the liquid material can be dispensed at one time using such valves.

h. *Actuators:* The actuator allows for easy opening and closing of the valve and is an integral part of almost every aerosol package.

Types of actuator:

1. Spray actuator—product dispense in small amount
2. Foam actuator—has larger aperture size, 0.07 to 0.125 inch orifices to deliver foam.
3. Solid-stream actuators—larger than foam actuator (.0125)—use to delivery of product in the form of ointment or cream.
4. Special type actuator—specially designed to deliver drugs into body cavity.

Working of Aerosols

Container is made up of metal, viz. aluminium, tin-plated alloys, glass or plastic depending on the nature of drug and its size is designed as per the number of doses and other requirements. The purpose of the container is to hold or store the aerosols. Normally, it is perfectly and safely sealed. No drug or propellant can escape (Fig. 3.13).

A *deep pipe* is inserted from the bottom most position of the container. A suitable *valve* is attached at the top through which the deep pipe is attached. The function of the valve is delivering the contents. Different types of valves are used. Continuous spray valves continuously spray the medicine, metering valves, when open it spray metered amount of medicine through the exit tube on the side of the valve normally remain safely closed.

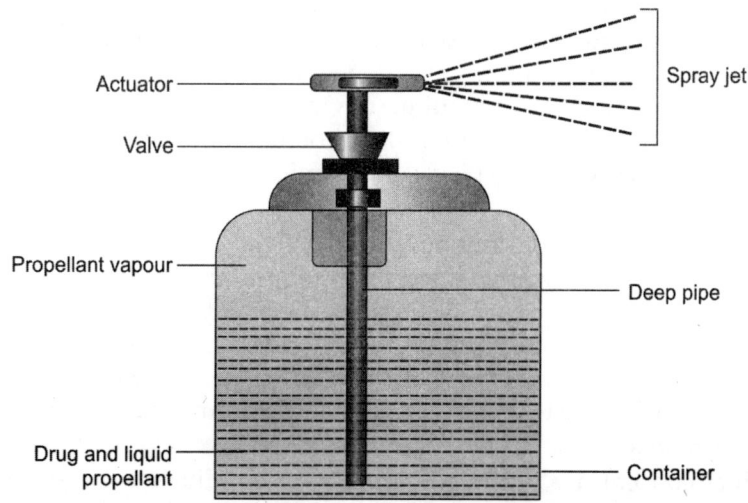

Fig. 3.13: The various components of an aerosol

A spring holds the valve tightly in place. The valve is operated through a push button type *actuator* which is normally remaining in its 'up' position. The function of the actuator is to open the valve and produce required types of discharge. The *drug* (either liquid or solid powder) is kept in suspense or in solution of a *propellant* whose vapour occupies the empty space of the container and its vapour creates pressure inside the container. The function of the propellant is to develop pressure within the container and to expel the product. Different types of propellants are used. Trichlorofluoromethane, and dichlorodifluoromethane are most commonly used.

When the actuator button is pressed towards bottom, the spring is compressed and it allows opening the valve. The pressurized drug and propellant escape through an opening at the top of the valve as aerosol or mist jet. Again, when the actuator button released, the spring expands and closes the valve.

Drug delivery to the lungs is an attractive route for local treatment of pulmonary disease such as asthma, and chronic obstructive pulmonary disorder (COPD), and also delivering drugs systemically. In particular, significant research and development efforts have been put into dry powder aerosols, which require no propellant, have superior chemical stability compared with solution, and are easy for patients to use. There are two types of dry powder inhalers, passive or breath-actuated devices, and active devices. With passive devices, the energy for dispersion is generated by the patient's inspiratory effort. In contrast, active devices minimize inspiratory effort by using an independent means (motor or compressed gas) to fluidize the powder. In the literature, the active devices have also been referred to the third generation DPI.

Clinical efficacy of inhaled therapeutics is governed by lung deposition, which depends on the aerosol properties. For DPIs, the aerosol properties are related to the dispersion of the powder, governed by the complex interaction between patient inspiratory flow rate, the device, and the formulation. The effect of these variables on deposition in the lungs can be examined by *in vivo* lung deposition studies.

Inline DPIs are pharmaceutical aerosol produced using a gas stream supplied from a positive pressure source, such as an air-filled syringe or manual ventilation bag. Advantages of these devices compared with conventional inhalation driven DPIs include high quality aerosol generation, use in subjects that cannot generate sufficient inspiratory flow, reproducible aerosol delivery, assistance with deep inspiration and breath hold. As aerosol generation is not dependent on patient inspiratory effort and following inspiration instructions, inline devices may be useful for administering aerosols to infants and young children. Based on operation with a positive pressure gas source, these devices can also be used to administer aerosols during invasive and non-invasive ventilation.

A vast majority of studies considering aerosol delivery during mechanical ventilation have implemented nebulizers and metered-dose inhalers. In contrast, a few studies have considered DPI delivery during mechanical ventilation. This limited use may be because of the perception that humidity in the ventilation system will degrade the powder quality and aerosolization performance. However, successful inline DPI devices for use with humidified systems have separated the humidified ventilation and DPI actuation gas streams.

The product concentrate in the container is in equilibrium between liquid and gaseous state. When actuator is pressed the valve opens. Since the product is under pressure, the vapour above the liquid concentrate pushes the products down. Then the product gets expelled through dip-tube from the container.

Formulation of Aerosol Preparation

An aerosol formulation consists of two essential components, i.e. product concentrate and propellants. Physiological properties and pharmacological properties of drug are considered to utilize different systems of aerosol. The product concentrate consists of active ingredients, or a mixture of active ingredients, and other required agents such as solvents, antioxidants, and surfactants. The propellants may be a single propellant or a blend of various propellants.

Depending on the type of aerosol system utilized, the pharmaceutical aerosol may be dispensed as a fine mist, wet spray, quick-breaking foam, stable foam, semi-solid, or solid. The type of system selected depends on many factors, including the following: Physical, chemical, and pharmacological properties of active ingredients, and site of application.

Types of System

Solution system: This system is also referred to as a two-phase system and consists of a vapour and liquid phase. When the active ingredients are soluble in the propellants, no other solvent is required. Depending on the type of spray required, the propellant may consist of propellant-12 or A-70 (which produces very fine particles), or a mixture of propellant-12 and other propellants such as propellant-12/11 in ratio 50:50 produces 37.4 psig at 70°F with 1.412 g/ml (density). As other propellants with vapour pressures lower than that of propellant-12 are added to propellant-12, the pressure of the system decreases, resulting in the production of larger particles.

For example: Active ingredients—10–20%w and propellant-12/11 mixture (50:50) to produce 100 ml. These sprays are also useful for topical preparation, since they tend to coat the affected area with a film of active ingredients. Depending on the boiling point of solvent used, the rate of vaporization of the propellant is decreased, thereby increasing any chilling effect that may present.

Aqueous system (or 3-phase system): Relatively large amount of water can be used to replace all or part of the non-aqueous solvents used in aerosols. These products are generally referred to as 'water-based' aerosols, and depending on the formulation, are emitted as a spray or foam. To produce a spray, the formulation must consist of a dispersion of active ingredients and other solvents in an emulsion system in which the propellant is in the external phase. In this way, when the product is dispensed, the propellant vapourizes and disperses the active ingredients into minute particles. Since propellant and water are not miscible, a three-phase aerosol forms (propellant phase, water phase, and vapour phase). Ethanol has been used as a cosolvent to solubilize some of the propellant in the water. By virtue of its surface tension lowering properties, ethanol also aids in the production of small particles.

Surfactants have been used to larger extents to produce a satisfactory homogeneous dispersion, about 0.5 to 2% of surfactants are used. The propellants content varies from about 25–60%, but can be low as 5% depending on the nature of the product. To achieve the desired fine particle size with products containing large amounts of water and a low proportion of propellant, a mechanical breakup actuator must be used along with a 'vapour tap valve'.

Suspension or dispersion system: This system is primarily developed for use with oral inhalation. Various methods have been used to overcome the difficulties encountered that are due to the use of a cosolvent. This system involves a dispersion of active ingredients in the propellant or a mixture of propellants. To decrease the rate of settling of the dispersed particles, various surfactants or suspending agents have been added to the system.

For example: Epinephrine bitartrate (within 1 to 5 μ): 0.5%w/v

Foam system: Emulsion and foam aerosols consist of active ingredients, aqueous or non-aqueous vehicle, surfactant, and propellant, and are dispensed as a stable or quick-braking foam, depending on the nature of the ingredients and the formulation. The liquefied propellant is emulsified and is generally found in the internal phase. Non-aerosol emulsions are usually in lotion or viscous liquid forms, but aerosol emulsions are dispensed as foams, and this can be advantageous for varoius applications involving irritating ingredients, or when the material is applied to a limited area.

1. *Aqueous stable foams:* These can be formulated as follows:
   - *Active ingredients:* Oil-waxes, o/w surfactant, and water: 95.0–96.5%w/w
   - *Hydrocarbon propellants:* 3.5–5.0%w/v

   While the total propellant content may be as high as 5% in certain cases, it usually is about 8–10%v/v or 3 or 5%w/w. As the amount of propellant A-70, A-46, etc. increases, stiffer and dryer foam is produced. Lower propellant concentrations yield wetter foams.

2. *Non-aqueous stable foams:* Non-aqueous stable foams may be formulated through the use of various glycols such as polyethylene glycol, which may be formulated according to the following.
   - *Glycol:* 91.0–92.5%w/w
   - *Emulsifying agent:* 4.0%w/w
   - *Hydrocarbon propellant:* 3.5–5.0%w/w

   The emulsifying agents found most effective were from the class of glycol esters, e.g. propylene glycol monostearate. Various medicinal agents can be incorporated into this base.

3. *Quick-breaking foams:* In this system, the propellant is in the external phase. When dispensed, the product is emitted as foam, which then collapses into a liquid. This type of system is especially applicable to topical medication, which can be applied to limited or to large areas without the use of a mechanical force to dispense the active ingredients. Quick-breaking aerosol foams may be formulated starting with the following.
   - *Ethyl alcohol:* 46.0–66.0%w/w
   - *Surfactant:* 0.5–5.0% w/w
   - *Water:* 28.0–42.0% w/w
   - *Hydrocarbon propellant:* 3.0–15.0%w/w

   The surfactant can be of the non-ionic, anionic, or cation type. It should be soluble in both alcohol and water. If the proportion of ingredients is varied, foams may be obtained having a wide range in stability.

4. *Thermal foams:* This is used to produce warm foam for shaving. They are not readily accepted by the consumer, however, and are soon discontinued, owing to inconvenience of use, expense, and lack of effectiveness. The same technology is

used to dispense hair colours and dyes corrosion problems, and is, therefore, unsuccessful. Suitable for dispensing medicated foam in which the application of heat would be desirable.

Intranasal Aerosols

Drug delivery systems intended for the deposition of medication into the nasal passageways have long been used as a most effective means of administering drugs intended to produce either a local or systemic effect. Recently, the modes of administering intranasal preparation have been limited to nasal drops, non-pressurized nasal sprays (mist), inhalants, and intranasal gels, creams and ointments. A new alternative is pressurized metered nasal aerosol.

Production of Aerosol

Pressure filling method: In this method, the products concentrate is placed in the container and closed with the valve. The product is maintained below critical temperature/slightly below boiling point. (Critical temperature is defined as the temperature above which the liquid can no longer exist as liquid or in easy term, temperature above which liquid shows properties which are intermediate between gas and liquid.) The propellant gets liquefied in the container.

Evaluation

1. Flammability and combustibility:
   - Flash point
   - Flame extension, including flashback
2. Physicochemical characteristics:
   - Vapour pressure
   - Density
   - Moisture content
   - Identification of propellant(s)
   - Concentrate-propellant ratio
3. Performance:
   - Aerosol valve discharge rate
   - Spray pattern
   - Dosage with metered valves
   - Net contents
   - Foam stability
   - Particle size determination
   - Leakage
4. Biologic characteristics

Flame projection: Effect of an aerosol formulation on an open flame. The product is sprayed for about 4 sec into a flame depending on the nature of the formulation, the flame is extended, the exact length is measured with a ruler.

Flash point: Determined by using the standard tag open cup apparatus. The aerosol product is allowed to chill to a temperature of about –25°F and transferred to test apparatus. The test liquid is allowed to increase slowly in a temperature and the temperature at which the vapour ignites is taken as the flash point. Calculated for flammable components, which in case of topical hydrocarbons.

Measurement of vapour pressure: To determine pressure variation from container to container. Determine by pressure gauge or can puncturing device. Variation in pressure indicates the presence of air in headspace.

Measurement of density: Determination by hydrometer or a pycnometer.

Procedure: A pressure tube is fitted with metal fingers and hoke valve, which allow for the introduction of liquids under pressure. The hydrometer is placed into the glass pressure tube. Sufficient sample is introduced through the valve to cause the hydrometer to rise half way up the length of the tube. The density can be read directly.

Identification of propellants: By GC and IR spectroscopy. These methods are used for the identification as well as measurement for proportion of each component in blend.

Moisture: By Karl Fischer method and GC.

Aerosol valve discharge rate: This is determined by taking an aerosol product of known weight and discharge the content for a given period of time using standard apparatus. By reweighing the container after the time limit has expired, the change in weight per time dispensed is the discharge rate, which can then be expressed as grams per second.

Spray pattern: Method is based on the impingement of the spray on a piece of paper that has been treated with a dye–talc mixture. Depending on the nature of the aerosol, an oil-soluble or water-soluble dye is used. The particles that strike the paper cause the dye to go into solution and to be absorbed onto the paper. These give the record of the spray, which can then be used for comparison.

Dosage with metered valve: Reproducibility of dosage each time the valve is depressed. Amount of medication actually received by the patient. It is done by assay method either by spraying the content into the solvent or on the material which absorb the API.

Net content:
- Weight of empty container = W_1 g
- Weight of the filled container = W_2 g
- Difference in the weight = W_1–W_2 g net content.

Distractive method: Weight the filled container, dispensing the content and then contents are weighed.

Foam stability: Visual evaluation time for a given mass to penetrate the foam time for a given rod that is inserted into the foam to fall rotational viscometer.

Particle size determination:
- *Cascade impactor:* It operates on the principle that in a stream of particles projected through a series of nozzles and glass slides at high velocity, larger particles become impacted first on the lower velocity stages and the smaller particles pass on and are collected at higher velocity stages. Particle size = 2–8 μ.
- *Light scatter decay:* As the aerosol settles under turbulent conditions, the change in the light intensity of a Tindal beam is measured.

Leakage: Select 12 pressurized containers at random, and record the date and time to the nearest half-hour. Weigh each container to the nearest mg, and record the weight, in mg, of each as W_1. Allow the container to stand in an upright position at room temperature for not less than 3 days, and again weigh each container, recording the weight, in mg, of each as W_2 recording the date and time to the nearest half-hour.

Determine the time, T, in hours, during which the containers are under test. Calculate the leakage rate, in mg per year, of each container from the expression.

Biological Test

- Therapeutic activity
- Toxicity

Applications

Administration of drugs from aerosols is very easy and they can be applied directly on the affected parts or abraded skin introduced into body cavity and passages. When sprayed on skin, some of propellants (e.g. ethyl chloride) cool the tissue due to sudden expansion of propellant. For these reasons, a pharmaceutical aerosol has a wide range of applications in the treatment of a patient due to its beneficial effect over the other dosage form. It is used as very effective treatment of asthma and chronic obstructive pulmonary disease (COPD). In a recent study, it has been observed that inline dry powder inhalers offer a potentially effective option to deliver high dose inhaled medications simultaneously with mechanical ventilation. Inline DPI which is actuated using a low volume of air (LV-DPI) is available for efficiently deliver pharmaceutical aerosols during low flow nasal cannula (LFNC) therapy. Pharmaceutical aerosols are also very effective in the treatment of diseases like diabetes, angina pectoris and many others.

QUESTIONS

A. Short Answer Type Questions

1. Give a short note on nasal spray.
2. What are the basic components used for transdermal drug delivery system?
3. Write about the manufacturing of pressurized metered-dose inhaler.
4. What are nebulizers?
5. Describe drug penetration through the skin.
6. Describe the property of drug candidates for transdermal delivery system.
7. Discuss gastroretentive drug delivery systems and their advantages.
8. What are the approaches used to prolong gastric residence time?
9. Discuss on devices for pulmonary drug delivery system.
10. What is nasal spray? Discuss their different types.

B. Long Answer Type Questions

1. What are the approaches used for gastroretentive drug delivery system?
2. Discuss in detail about aerosols.
3. Define nasal drug delivery system. Give their advantages and disadvantages.
4. What are the factors affecting transdermal drug permeation?
5. Describe in detail about pulmonary drug delivery system.
6. What is transdermal drug delivery system? Give their advantages and disadvantages.

Targeted Drug Delivery System

INTRODUCTION

Targeted drug delivery system, also known as smart drug delivery system, is a method of treatment that involves the increase in medicament in one or few body parts in comparison to others. Two strategies are widely used for drug targeting to the desired organ/tissue: Passive targeting and active targeting.

Targeted drug delivery system is a kind of smart drug delivery system which is miraculous in delivering the drug to a patient. This conventional drug delivery system is done by the absorption of the drug across a biological membrane, whereas the targeted release system is that in which drug is released in a dosage form. Targeted drug delivery system is based on a method that delivers a certain amount of a therapeutic agent for a prolonged period of time to a targeted diseased area within the body. This helps maintain the required plasma and tissue drug levels in the body; therefore, avoiding any damage to the healthy tissue via the drug. The drug delivery system is highly integrated and requires various disciplines, such as chemists, biologist and engineers, to join forces to optimize this system. When implementing a targeted release system, the following design criteria for the system need to take into account: The drug properties, side effects of the drugs, the route taken for the delivery of the drug, the targeted site, and the disease.

Carriers used should be biodegradable or readily eliminated from the body without any problem. The preparation of the delivery system should be easy or reasonably simple, reproductive and cost-effective. A targeted drug delivery system is preferred over conventional drug delivery systems due to three main reasons. Conventional drugs have low solubility and more drug instability in comparison to targeted drug delivery systems. Conventional drugs also have poor absorption, shorter half-life and require large volume of distribution. These constitute its pharmacokinetic properties. The third reason constitutes the pharmacodynamic properties of drugs. The conventional drugs have low specificity and low therapeutic index as compared to targeted drug delivery system. Due to these reasons, targeted drug delivery system is preferred over conventional drug delivery systems.

Drug delivery vehicles transport the drug either within or in the vicinity of target. An ideal drug delivery vehicle is supposed to cross even stubborn sites such as a blood-brain barrier. Recently, nano-medicine has emerged as the medical application of nanotechnology. Since nanoparticles are very small in size, nano-drug delivery can allow for the delivery of drugs with poor solubility in water and also aid in avoiding the first pass metabolism of liver. Nanotechnology derived drug delivery can cause the drug to remain in blood circulation for a long time, thereby leading to lesser fluctuations in plasma levels and, therefore, minimal side effects.

It differs from the conventional drug delivery system in that, it releases in a dosage form while the former functions by the absorption of drug across biological membrane. Greogoriadis, in 1981, described the use of novel drug delivery for drug targeting as "old drug in new clothes". Conventional dosage forms such as injections, oral formulations comprising solutions and suspensions, tablets, capsules, and topical creams and ointments possess certain innate disadvantages. Parenteral delivery of drugs is highly invasive with ephemeral effects. Oral administration of drug, in spite of being immensely popular and appropriate, cannot be used for certain drugs, such as protein or peptide drugs, owing to their poor absorption by the oral route. These may be degraded in the gastrointestinal tract. Topical creams and ointments have a drawback of being limited to local effects, rather than systemic ones. Currently drug delivery technology has become refined and it takes into consideration several factors such as bioavailability, drug absorption processes, pharmacokinetic processes, timing for optimal drug delivery, etc.

There are four principal requirements for a successful targeted drug delivery system: Retain, evade, target and release, i.e. there should be proper loading of the drug into an appropriate drug delivery vehicle, it must possess an ability to escape the body's secretions that may degrade it, leading to a long residence time in circulation and thereby reaching the site of interest and, should release the drug at the specific site within the time that calls for effective drug functioning. Different sites of interest within the body necessitate the use of different drug delivery systems, depending upon the route to be followed.

STRATEGIES OF DRUG TARGETING

Drug targeting to an area of interest within the body increases the therapeutic effectiveness as well as it reduces the toxicity that may arise otherwise.

Two strategies are widely used for drug targeting to the desired organ/tissue.

Passive Targeting

This is based on the accumulation of drug at areas around the site of interest, such as in case of tumour tissues. This is called enhanced permeability retention (EPR) effect. Such a type of targeting occurs with almost all types of drug delivery carriers. Passive targeting is actually a misnomer because it cannot really be described as a form of selective targeting. Although the EPR effect applies for nanoparticle administered, the majority (>95%) of these nanoparticles tend to accumulate in organs other than those of interest such as liver, lungs and spleen. Thus, it is the distribution of drug by blood circulation. Examples include the use of anti-malarial drugs being targeted for the treatment of microbial infections such as leishmaniasis, candidiasis and brucellosis.

Active Targeting

Through the use of ligand-receptor interactions, active targeting describes the drug targeting interactions. However, interactions between a ligand and a receptor are possible only when the two are in close propinquity (i.e. less than about 0.5 mm). The currently available drug delivery systems are able to reach the target by the virtue of blood circulation and extravasation. Therefore, we can conclude that active receptor targeting actually means ligand–receptor interaction but that takes place only after blood circulation and extravasation. Active targeting can further be divided into three different targeting levels.

First order targeting: This is the distribution of drug to capillary beds of target sites—organ or tissue, e.g. in case of lymphatic tissue, peritoneal cavity, pleural cavity, cerebral ventricles, eyes, joints, etc.

Second order targeting: This is the targeting of drugs to specific sites such as the tumour cells, e.g. to Kupffer cells in liver.

Third order targeting: It is the type of drug targeting wherein the drug is intracellularly localized at the target site via endocytosis or through receptor-based ligand mediated entry (Fig. 4.1).

Components of Drug Targeting

Any drug delivery system comprises a target and the drug carriers or markers required for it.

Target: Target means an organ or a tissue or a cell, which is in need of treatment.

Drug carrier or marker: Drug delivery is possible only by means of a carrier system. Carriers are molecules or any other systems responsible for the successful transportation of a drug to the site of interest. Carriers are vectors specifically engineered for the purpose of holding a drug inside them. This is possible by means of encapsulation.

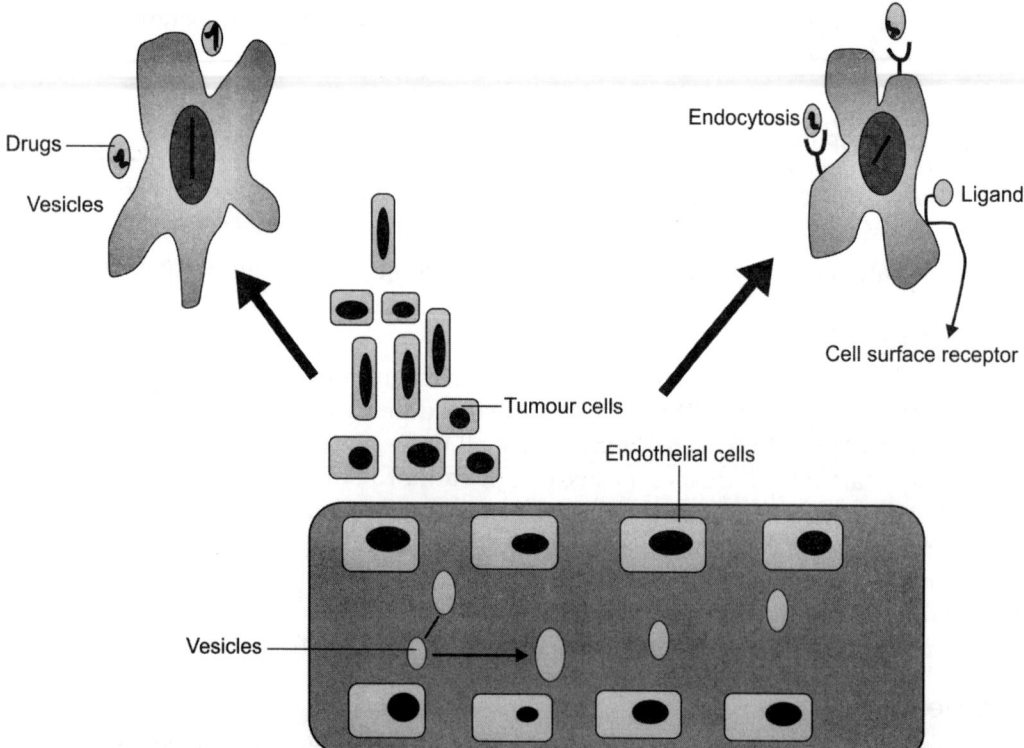

Fig. 4.1: Target site via endocytosis or through receptor-based ligand mediated entry

Drug Delivery Vehicles

These transport the drug either within or in the vicinity of target. An ideal drug delivery vehicle is supposed to cross even stubborn sites such as a blood–brain barrier. It should be easily recognized by the target cells and the drug–ligand complex hence formed should be stable. These need to be non-toxic, and biodegradable as well. The biodegradable nature of drug carrier enables them to be easily cleared away by the body and physiological mechanism, and thus avoids any chance of their accumulation within cells that may lead to cytotoxicity.

Ideal Characteristics

- It should be non-toxic, biocompatible, biodegradable and physicochemical stable *in vivo* and *in vitro*.
- Restrict drug distribution to target cells or tissue or organ should have uniform capillary distribution.
- Controllable and predicate rate of drug release.
- Drug release does not affect the drug action.
- Therapeutic amount of drug release.
- Minimal drug leakage during transit.
- Carriers used must be biodegradable or readily eliminated from the body without any problem and no carrier induced modulation of diseased state.
- The preparation of delivery system should be easy or reasonably simple, reproductive and cost-effective.

Advantages

- Drug administration protocols may be simplified.
- Toxicity is reduced by delivering a drug to its target site, thereby reducing harmful systemic effect.
- Drug can be administered in a smaller dose to produce the desire effect.
- Avoidance of hepatic first pass metabolism.
- Enhancement of the absorption of target molecules such as peptides and particulates.
- Dose is less compared to conventional drug delivery system.
- No peak and valley plasma concentration.
- Selective targeting to infections cells that compare to normal cells.

Disadvantages

- Rapid clearance of targeted systems.
- Immune reactions against intravenously administered carrier systems.
- Insufficient localization of targeted systems into tumour cells.
- Diffusion and redistribution of released drugs.
- Requires highly sophisticated technology for the formulation.
- Requires skill for manufacturing storage administration.
- Drug deposition at the target site may produce toxic symptoms.
- Difficult to maintain stability of dosage form. For example, released erythrocytes have to be stored at 4°C.
- Drug loading is usually low, e.g. as in micelles. Therefore, it is difficult to predict/ fix the dosage regimen.

LIPOSOMES

Paul Ehrlich in 1906 initiated the era of development for targeted delivery when he envisaged a drug delivery mechanism that would target drug directly to diseased cells, what he called as magic bullets. "Liposomes are colloidal, vesicular structures composed of one or more lipid bilayers surrounding an equal numbers of aqueous compartments". The sphere-like shell encapsulated a liquid interior which contains substances such as peptides and protein, hormones, enzymes, antibiotic, antifungal and anticancer agents. A free drug injected in bloodstream typically achieves therapeutic level for short duration due to metabolism and excretion. Drug encapsulated by liposomes achieves therapeutic level for long duration as drug must first be release from liposome before metabolism and excretion (Fig. 4.2).

Types of Liposomes

Liposomes are classified as:
1. Based on structural parameters
2. Based on method of liposome preparation
3. Based upon composition

Based on Structural Parameters

1. **Unilamellar vesicles:**
   • Small unilamellar vesicles (SUV): Size ranges from 20–40 nm.
   • Medium unilamellar vesicles (MUV): Size ranges from 40–80 nm.
   • Large unilamellar vesicles (LUV): Size ranges from 100–1,000 nm.

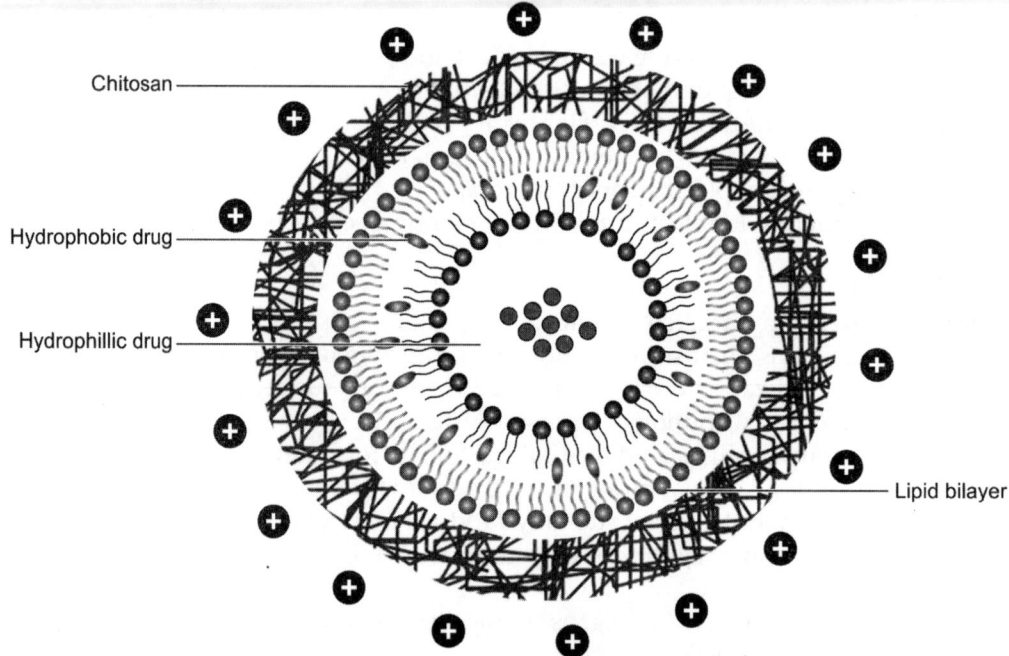

Fig. 4.2: Diagram representing liposome

2. **Oligolamellar vesicles (OLV):** These are made up of 2–10 bilayers of lipid surrounding a large internal volume.
3. **Multilamellar vesicles (MLV):** They have several bilayers. They can compartmentalize the aqueous volume in an infinite number of ways. They differ according to way by which they are prepared. The arrangements can be onion-like arrangements of concentric spherical bilayers of LUV/MLV enclosing a large number of SUV, etc.

Based on Method of Liposome Preparation

1. REV: Single or oligolamellar vesicles made by reverse-phase evaporation method.
2. MLV-REV: Multilamellar vesicles made by reverse-phase evaporation method.
3. SPLV: Stable plurilamellar vesicles
4. FATMLV: Frozen and thawed MLV
5. VET: Vesicles prepared by extrusion technique
6. DRV: Dehydration-rehydration method.

Based Upon Composition

1. **Conventional liposomes (CL):** Neutral or negatively charged phospholipids and cholesterol.
2. **Fusogenic liposomes (RSVE):** Reconstituted Sendai virus envelopes.
3. **pH sensitive liposomes:** Phospholipids such as PE or DOPE with either CHEMS or OA.
4. **Cationic liposomes:** Cationic lipids with DOPE.
5. **Long circulatory (stealth) liposomes (LCL):** They have polyethylene glycol (PEG) derivatives attached to their surface to decrease their detection by phagocyte system (reticuloendothelial system; RES). The attachment of PEG to liposomes decreases the clearance from bloodstream and extends circulation time of liposomes in the body. The attachment of PEG is also known as pegylation.
6. **Immunoliposomes:** CL or LCL with attached monoclonal antibody or recognition sequence.

Structural Components of Liposome

Liposomes are globular lipid bilayers of 50–1000 nm in diameter that serve as convenient delivery vehicles for biologically active compounds. Topical application of liposomes has large possibilities in dermatology and in the delivery of anticancer agents in order to reduce the toxic effects of the drugs when given alone, or to increase the circulation time and effectiveness of the drugs. Liposomes might be used to target precise cells by attaching amino acid fragments such as antibodies or proteins or appropriate fragments that target specific receptor sites. DNA vaccination and improved efficiency of gene therapy are just a few of the upcoming applications of liposomes. Liposomes are especially effective in treating diseases that affect the phagocytes of the immune system because they tend to accumulate in the phagocytes, which know them as strange attackers. There are a number of structural and non-structural components of liposomes. The main structural parts of liposomes are: Phospholipids and cholesterol.

Phospholipids

Phospholipids are the major structural component of biological coverings, and two sorts of phospholipids exist—phosphodiglycerides and sphingolipids. The most common phospholipid is the phosphatidylcholine (PC) molecule. Particles of phosphatidylcholine are not soluble in water and in aqueous media, they align themselves closely in planar bilayer sheets in order to minimize the unfavourable action between the bulk aqueous phase and the long hydrocarbon fatty series. The glycerols, including phospholipids, are the most commonly used component of liposome formulation and represent greater than 50% of the weight of lipid in biological membranes. These are derivatives of phosphatidic acid. Examples of phospholipids are:

- Phosphatidylcholine (lecithin)—PC
- Phosphatidylethanolamine (cephalin)—PE
- Phosphatidylserine (PS)
- Phosphatidylinositol (PI)
- Phosphatidylglycerol (PG)

Cholesterol

Cholesterol does not form a bilayer construction by itself, but is able to be included into phospholipid membranes in very high concentrations of up to 1:1 or even 2:1 molar ratio of cholesterol to phosphatidylcholine. Cholesterol positions itself in the membrane with its hydroxyl group oriented towards the aqueous surface and the aliphatic chain aligned parallel to the acyl chains in the centre of the bilayer. The high solubility of cholesterol in the phospholipid liposome has been attributed to both hydrophobic and definite head group interaction, but there is no clear indication for the arrangement of cholesterol in the bilayer.

Preparation of Liposomes

1. General method of preparation
2. Specific methods of preparation

General Method of Preparation

The lipid is dissolved in organic solvent. The solvent is evaporated leaving a small film of lipids on the wall of the container. An aqueous solution of drug is added. In first procedure, the mixture is agitated to produce multilamellar vesicle and then sonicated to get SUVs. In the second procedure, the mixture is sonicated and the solvent is evaporated to get LUVs. After extrusion, SUVs are formed. Drug can be incorporated into the aqueous solution or buffer, if it is water-soluble or included in organic solvent, if it is hydrophobic. Free drug and liposomes can be separated by gel chromatography.

Specific Methods of Preparation

These are classified into three types based on the modes of dispersion.
1. Physical dispersion methods
2. Solvent dispersion methods
3. Detergent solubilization methods

1. Physical Dispersion Methods

In these methods, the aqueous volume enclosed within lipid membranes is about 5-10%, which is very small proportion of total volume used for preparation. So large amount of water-soluble drug is wasted during preparation. But lipid-soluble drug can be encapsulated to high percentage. In these methods, MLVs are formed and further treatment is required for preparation of unilamellar vesicles.

Hand shaken method: This is the simplest and widely used method. The lipid mixture and charged components are dissolved in chloroform and methanol mixture (2:1 ratio) and then this mixture is introduced into a 250 ml round bottomed flask. The flask is attached to rotary evaporator connected with vacuum pump and rotated at 60 rpm. The organic solvents are evaporated at about 30°. A dry residue is formed at the walls of the flask and rotation is continued for 15 minutes after dry residue appeared. The evaporator is detached from vacuum pump and nitrogen is introduced into it. The flask is then removed from evaporator and fixed onto lyophilizer to remove residual solvent. Then the flask is again flushed with nitrogen and 5 ml of phosphate buffer is added. The flask is attached to evaporator again and rotated at about 60 rpm speed for 30 minutes or until all lipid has been removed from the wall of the flask. A milky white suspension is formed finally. The suspension is allowed to stand for 2 hours in order to complete swelling process to give MLVs.

Non-shaking method: This is similar to shaking method except that care is taken in swelling procedure. The solution of lipid in chloroform and methanol mixture is spread over the flat bottom of the conical flask. The solution is evaporated at room temperature by flow of nitrogen through the flask without disturbing the solution. After drying, water saturated nitrogen is passed through the flask until the opacity of the dried film disappears. After hydration, lipid is swelled by addition of bulk liquid. The flask is inclined to one side, 10 to 20 ml of 0.2M sucrose in distilled water is introduced down the side of the flask and then flask is slowly returned to upright position. The solution is allowed to run gently over the lipid layer on the bottom of the flask. The flask is flushed with nitrogen sealed and allowed to stand for 2 hours at 37°C for swelling. After that, the vesicles are mixed to yield a milky suspension. The suspension is centrifuged at 1200 rpm for 10 minutes. The layer of MLVs floating on the surface is removed. From the remaining fluid, LUVs are produced.

Freeze drying: Another method of dispersing the lipid in a finally divided form prior to addition of aqueous media is to freeze dry the lipid dissolved in a suitable organic solvent. The solvent usually used is tertiary butanol. All the above methods produce MLVs. These are too large or too heterogeneous. In order to modify the size, the prepared MLVs are further processed using the following procedures.

Processing of lipids hydrated by physical means:

- *Microemulsification of liposomes:* An equipment called microfluidizer is used to prepare small vesicles from concentrated lipid suspension. The lipids can be introduced into the fluidizer as a suspension of large MLVs. This equipment pumps the fluid at very high pressure through 5 μm screen. Then it is forced long microchannels, which direct two streams of fluids collide together at right angles at very high velocity. The fluid collected can be recycled through the pump and interaction chamber until vesicles of spherical dimensions are obtained.

- *Sonication:* This method reduces the size of the vesicles and imparts energy to lipid suspension. This can be achieved by exposing the MLV to ultrasonic irradiation. There are two methods of sonication: (a) Using bath sonicator, and (b) using probe sonicator. The probe sonicator is used for suspensions which require high energy in small volume (e.g. high concentration of lipids or viscous aqueous phase). The bath sonicator is used for large volume of dilute lipids. The disadvantage of probe sonicator is contamination of preparation with metal from tip of probe. By this method, small unilamellar vesicles are formed and they are purified by ultracentrifugation.

- *Membrane extrusion liposome:* In this method, the size is reduced by passing those through a membrane filter of defined pore size. There are two types of membrane filter: The tortuous path type and the nucleation track type. The former is used for sterile filtration. In this random path arise between the crisscross fibres. The average diameter of these fibres is controlled by the density of fibres in the matrix. Liposomes that are larger than the channel diameter get struck when one tries to pass them through such membrane. The nucleation track type is composed of thin continuous sheet of polycarbonate. They will offer less resistance to passage of liposomes as these consist of straight-sided pore holes of exact diameter bored from one side to another. This method can be used to process both LUVs and MLV.

- *Freeze and thaw sonication:* This is a method in which rupture and refusing of SUVs are done during which the solute equilibrates between the inside and outside. This process increases the entrapment volume and entrapment efficiency. This method will result in the formation of vesicles within vesicles and vesicle between lamellae. This method can increase the entrapment volume up to 30%.

2. Solvent Dispersion Methods

In these methods, lipids are first dissolved in an organic solution and then brought into contact with aqueous phase containing materials to be entrapped within liposome. At the interface between the organic and the aqueous phases, the phospholipids align themselves to form a monolayer, which is important step to form the bilayer of liposome.

Ethanol injection method: This is a simple method. In this method, an ethanol solution of the lipids is directly injected rapidly to an excess of saline or other aqueous medium through a fine needle. The ethanol is diluted in water and phospholipid molecules are dispersed evenly through the medium. This procedure yields a high proportion of SUVs (about 25 nm diameter).

Ether injection: This method is similar to above one. It involves injecting the immiscible organic solution very slowly into an aqueous phase through a narrow needle at temperature of vapourizing of organic solvent. In this method, the lipids are carefully treated and there is very less risk of oxidative degradation. The disadvantage is that long time is required for the process and careful control is needed for introduction of lipid solution.

3. Detergent Solubilization Technique

In this method, the phospholipids are brought into close contact with the aqueous phase via detergents, which associate with phospholipids molecules. The structures formed as a result of this association are known as micelles. They are composed of several hundreds of component molecules. The concentration of detergent in water at which micelles start to form is called CMC. Below CMC, the detergent molecules exist in free solution. As the detergent molecule is dissolved in water at concentrations higher than the CMC, micelles form in large amounts. As the concentration of detergent added is increased, more amount of detergent is incorporated into the bilayer, until a point is reached where conversion from lamellar form to spherical micellar form takes place. As detergent concentration is further increased, the micelles are reduced in size.

Mechanism of Formation of Liposomes

Lipids capable of forming liposomes exhibit a dual chemical nature. Their head groups are hydrophilic and their fatty acyl chains are hydrophobic. It has been estimated that each Zwitter ionic head group of phosphatidylcholine has on the order of 15 molecules of water weakly bound to it, which explain its overwhelming preference for the water phase. The hydrocarbon fatty acid chains on the other hand vastly prefer each others company to that of H_2O. This can be understood by taking the CMC of PC into account. The CMC of dipalmitoyl PC found to be 4.6–10 M in water, which is a small number indicating the overwhelming preference of this molecule for a hydrophobic environment such as that found in the core of micelle or bilayer. The free energy of transfer from water to micelle is 15.3 kcal/mol for dipalmitoyl PC and 13.0 kcal/mol for dimyristoyl PC. These results clearly point out the thermodynamic basis for bilayer assembly that has been termed the hydrophobic effect. The large free energy change between a water and a hydrophobic environment explains the overwhelming preference of typical lipids to assemble in bilayer structures, including water as much is possible from the hydrophobic core in order to achieve the lowest energy level, hence the highest stability for the aggregate structure.

Purification of Liposomes

Liposomes are generally purified by gel filtration chromatography, dialysis and centrifugation. In chromatographic separation, Sephadex-50 is most widely used. In dialysis method, hollow fibre dialysis cartridge may be used. In centrifugation method, SUVs in normal saline may be separated by centrifuging at 200000 g, for 10–20 hours. MLVs are separated by centrifuging at 100000 g for less than 1 hour.

Evaluation of Liposomes

Liposomal formulation and processing for specified purpose are characterized to ensure their predictable *in vitro* and *in vivo* performance. The characterization parameters for purpose of evaluation could be classified into three broad categories which include physical, chemical and biological parameters.

- Physical characterization evaluates various parameters including size, shape, surface features, lamellarity, phase behaviour and drug release profile.
- Chemical characterization includes those studies which establish the purity and potency of various lipophilic constituents.
- Biological characterization parameters are helpful in establishing the safety and suitability of formulation for therapeutic application. Some of parameters are:
    1. **Vesicle shape and lamellarity:** Vesicle shape can be assessed using electron microscopic techniques. Lamellarity of vesicles, i.e. number of bilayers presents in liposomes is determined using freeze-fracture electron microscopy and p-31 nuclear magnetic resonance analysis.
    2. **Vesicle size and size distribution:** Various techniques are available for determination of size and size distribution. These include light microscopy, fluorescent microscopy, electron microscopy (specially transmission electron

microscopy), laser light scattering photon correlation spectroscopy, field flow fractionation, gel permeation and gel exclusion. The most precise method to determine size of liposome is electron microscopy since it permits one to view each individual liposome and to obtain exact information about profile of liposome population over the whole range of sizes.

3. **Encapsulation efficiency and trapped volume:** These determine amount and rate of entrapment of water-soluble agents in aqueous compartment of liposomes.

   a. *Encapsulation efficiency:* It describes the percent of the aqueous phase and hence percent of water-soluble drug that become ultimately entrapped during preparation of liposomes and is usually expressed as % entrapment/mg lipid.

   b. *Trapped volume:* It is an important parameter that governs morphology of vesicles. The trapped or internal volume is aqueous entrapped volume per unit quantity of lipids. This can vary from 0.5 to 30 microlitre/micro mol. Various materials including spectroscopically inert fluid, radioactive markers and fluorescent markers are used to determine trapped/internal volume.

4. **Phase response and transitional behaviour:** Liposome and lipid bilayers exhibit various phase transitions that are studied for their role in triggered drug release or stimulus-mediated fusion of liposomal constituents with target cell.

5. **Drug release:** The mechanism of drug release from liposomes can be assessed by use of well calibrated *in vitro* diffusion cell. The liposome-based formulation can be assisted by employing *in vitro* assays to predict pharmacokinetics and bioavailability of drug before employing costly and time-consuming *in vivo* studies.

Applications

- Cancer chemotherapy
- Gene therapy
- Liposomes as carrier for vaccines
- Liposomes as carrier of drug in oral treatment
- Liposomes for topical applications
- Liposomes for pulmonary delivery
- Against leishmaniasis
- Lysosomal storage disease
- Cell biological application
- Metal storage disease
- Ophthalmic delivery of drugs

Applications of Liposomes in Food Science

Liposomes and nano-liposomes are used for improving and/or developing new taste, controlling the release of flavour, improving the food colour and altering the texture of food components. They are also able to increase the absorption and bioavailability of nutraceutical and health supplements and develop food antimicrobials.

In the following sections, some applications of the liposomes in the food industry are explained:

- One of the first reported liposome applications in food products was in cheese manufacture, in order to decrease the time and cost of the cheese ripening by adding the proteinases encapsulated in liposome to cheese mixes. Researchers have shown that encapsulated enzymes in liposome improve the stability and activity of enzymes and control their release time and improve the flavour of cheese and reduce the cost of production.

- The enzyme bromelain (used as a meat tenderizer) in liposomes and they also found that the stability and bioavailability of enzyme significantly increase.
- Liposome-entrapped galactosidase in order to aid the digestion of dairy foods by the lactose intolerance. They found out that liposomes can stabilize the enzyme during the storage.
- Vitamins are also encapsulated in liposomes to enhance their retention.
- Liposomes have also been used to increase the nutritional quality of dairy products by entrapping the vitamin D in cream and cheese.

Applications of Liposomes in Cosmetics

Liposome applications in skin treatment are based on the similarity of the bilayer structure of liposome to that of the natural membranes, so depending on the lipid composition of liposome; they can alter cell membrane fluidity and deliver active drugs to the target site.

1. Anti-inflammatory agents, immunostimulants, and enhancers of molecular and cellular detoxification within liposomes could avoid age spots, dark circles, wrinkles, and other clinical aspects of skin aging.
2. Nutricosmetics are an emerging class of health and beauty aid products that combine the herbs and liposomes to maintain and enhance human beauty because of their beneficial properties, such as sunscreen, antiaging, moisturizing, antioxidant, anticellulite, and antimicrobial effects.

NANOPARTICLES

Nanoparticles are defined as particulate dispersions or solid particles with a size in the range of 10–1000 nm. The drug is dissolved, entrapped, encapsulated or attached to a nanoparticle matrix. Depending upon the method of preparation, nanoparticles, nanospheres or nanocapsules can be obtained. Nanocapsules are systems in which the drug is confined to a cavity surrounded by a unique polymer membrane, while nanospheres are matrix systems in which the drug is physically and uniformly dispersed. In recent years, biodegradable polymeric nanoparticles, particularly those coated with hydrophilic polymer such as poly (ethylene glycol) (PEG) known as long-circulating particles, have been used as potential drug delivery devices because of their ability to circulate for a prolonged period time target a particular organ, as carriers of DNA in gene therapy, and their ability to deliver proteins, peptides and genes.

Nanoparticles are being used for diverse purposes, from medical treatments, using in various branches of industry production such as solar and oxide fuel batteries for energy storage, to wide incorporation into diverse materials of everyday use such as cosmetics or clothes.

Types of Nanoparticles

Silver: Silver nanoparticles have proved to be most effective because of its good antimicrobial efficacy against bacteria, viruses and other eukaryotic micro-organisms. They are undoubtedly the most widely used nanomaterials among all, thereby being used as antimicrobial agents, in textile industries, for water treatment, sunscreen lotions, etc. Studies have already reported the successful biosynthesis of silver nanoparticles by plants such as *Azadirachta indica, Capsicum annuum* and *Carica papaya*.

Gold: Gold nanoparticles (AuNPs) are used in immunochemical studies for identification of protein interactions. They are used as lab tracer in DNA fingerprinting to detect presence of DNA in a sample. They are also used for detection of aminoglycoside antibiotics like streptomycin, gentamicin and neomycin. Gold nanorods are being used to detect cancer stem cells, beneficial for cancer diagnosis and for identification of different classes of bacteria.

Alloy: Alloy nanoparticles exhibit structural properties that are different from their bulk samples. Since Ag has the highest electrical conductivity among metal fillers and, unlike many other metals, their oxides have relatively better conductivity, Ag flakes are most widely used. Bimetallic alloy nanoparticle properties are influenced by both metals and show more advantages over ordinary metallic NPs.

Magnetic: Magnetic nanoparticles like Fe_3O_4 (magnetite) and Fe_2O_3 (maghemite) are known to be biocompatible. They have been actively investigated for targeted cancer treatment (magnetic hyperthermia), stem cell sorting and manipulation, guided drug delivery, gene therapy, DNA analysis, and magnetic resonance imaging (MRI).

Preparation of Nanoparticles

Nanoparticles can be prepared from a variety of materials such as proteins, polysaccharides and synthetic polymers. The selection of matrix materials is dependent on many factors including:

- Size of nanoparticles required
- Inherent properties of the drug, e.g. aqueous solubility and stability
- Surface characteristics such as charge and permeability
- Degree of biodegradability, biocompatibility and toxicity
- Drug release profile desired
- Antigenicity of the final product.
- Nanoparticles have been prepared most frequently by three methods:
  a. Dispersion of preformed polymers
  b. Polymerization of monomers
  c. Ionic gelation or coacervation of hydrophilic polymers.

Dispersion of Preformed Polymers

Dispersion of preformed polymers is a common technique used to prepare biodegradable nanoparticles from poly (lactic acid) (PLA); poly (D, L-glycolide) (PLG); poly (D, L-lactide-co-glycolide) (PLGA); and poly (cyanoacrylate) (PCA). This technique can be used in various ways as described below.

a. **Solvent evaporation method:** In this method, the polymer is dissolved in an organic solvent such as dichloromethane, chloroform or ethyl acetate which is also used as the solvent for dissolving the hydrophobic drug. The mixture of polymer and drug solution is then emulsified in an aqueous solution containing a surfactant or emulsifying agent to form oil in water (o/w) emulsion. After the formation of stable emulsion, the organic solvent is evaporated either by reducing the pressure or by continuous stirring. Particle size was found to be influenced by the type and concentrations of stabilizer, homogenizer speed and polymer concentration. In order to produce small particle size, often a high-speed homogenization or ultrasonication may be employed.

b. **Spontaneous emulsification or solvent diffusion method:** This is a modified version of solvent evaporation method. In this method, the water miscible solvent along with a small amount of the water immiscible organic solvent is used as an oil phase. Due to the spontaneous diffusion of solvents, an interfacial turbulence is created between the two phases leading to the formation of small particles. As the concentration of water miscible solvent increases, a decrease in the size of particle can be achieved.

Both solvent evaporation and solvent diffusion methods can be used for hydrophobic or hydrophilic drugs. In the case of hydrophilic drug, a multiple w/o/w emulsion needs to be formed with the drug dissolved in the internal aqueous phase.

Polymerization Method

In this method, monomers are polymerized to form nanoparticles in an aqueous solution. Drug is incorporated either by being dissolved in the polymerization medium or by adsorption onto the nanoparticles after polymerization completed. The nanoparticle suspension is then purified to remove various stabilizers and surfactants employed for polymerization by ultracentrifugation and re-suspending the particles in an isotonic surfactant-free medium. This technique has been reported for making poly (butyl cyanoacrylate) or poly (alkyl cyanoacrylate) nanoparticles. Nanocapsules formation and their particle size depend on the concentration of the surfactants and stabilizers used.

Coacervation or Ionic Gelation Method

Much research has been focused on the preparation of nanoparticles using biodegradable hydrophilic polymers such as chitosan, gelatin and sodium alginate. Calvo and coworkers developed a method for preparing hydrophilic chitosan nanoparticles by ionic gelation. The method involves a mixture of two aqueous phases, of which one is the polymer chitosan, a di-block copolymer ethylene oxide or propylene oxide (PEO-PPO) and the other is a polyanion sodium tripolyphosphate. In this method, positively charged amino group of chitosan interacts with negative charged tripolyphosphate to form coacervates with a size in the range of nanometer. Coacervates are formed as a result of electrostatic interaction between two aqueous phases, whereas, ionic gelation involves the material undergoing transition from liquid to gel due to ionic interaction conditions at room temperature.

Applications

Nanomedicine has tremendous prospects for the improvement of the diagnosis and treatment of human diseases. Use of microbes in biosynthesis of nanoparticles is an environmentally acceptable procedure. Nanotechnology has potential to revolutionize a wide array of tools in biotechnology so that they are more personalized, portable, cheaper, safer, and easier to administer. Nanoparticles will be able to deliver a concentrate dose of drug in the vicinity of the tumour targets via the enhanced permeability and retention effect or active targeting by ligands on the surface of nanoparticles. Nanoparticles will reduce the drug exposure of health tissues by limiting drug distribution to target organ.

- *In drugs and medications:* Nano-sized inorganic particles of either simple or complex nature, display unique, physical and chemical properties and represent an increasingly important material in the development of novel nanodevices which can be used in numerous physical, biological, biomedical and pharmaceutical applications.

- *In manufacturing and materials:* Nanocrystalline materials provide very interesting substances for material science since their properties deviate from respective bulk material in a size dependent manner. Manufacture NPs display physicochemical characteristics that induce unique electrical, mechanical, optical and imaging properties that are extremely looked-for in certain applications within the medical, commercial, and ecological sectors.

- *In the environment:* The increasing area of engineered NPs in industrial and household applications leads to the release of such materials into the environment. Assessing the risk of these NPs in the environment requires on understanding of their mobility, reactivity, ecotoxicity and persistency.

- *In electronics:* There has been growing interest in the development of printed electronics in last few years because printed electronics offer attractive to traditional silicon techniques and the potential for low cost, large area electronics for flexible displays, sensors. Printed electronics with various functional inks containing NPs such as metallic NPs, organic electronic molecules, CNTs and ceramics NPs have been expected to flow rapidly as a mass production process for new types of electronic equipment.

- *In energy harvesting:* Recent studies warned us about the limitations and scarcity of fossil fuels in coming years due to their non-renewable nature. Therefore, scientists shifting their research strategies to generate renewable energies from easily available resources at cheap cost. They found that NPs are the best candidate for this purpose due to their, large surface area, optical behaviour and catalytic nature. Especially in photocatalytic applications, NPs are widely used to generate energy from photoelectrochemical (PEC) and electrochemical water splitting.

AQUASOMES

Aquasomes are one of the most recently developed delivery systems that are finding a niche as peptide and protein carriers. These are nanoparticulate carrier systems with three-layered self-assembled structures. They comprise a central solid nanocrystalline core coated with polyhydroxy oligomers onto which biochemically active molecules are adsorbed. The solid core provides the structural stability, while the carbohydrate coating protects against dehydration and stabilizes the biochemically active molecules. This property of maintaining the conformational integrity of bioactive molecules has led to the proposal that aquasomes have potential as a carrier system for delivery of peptide-based pharmaceuticals. The delivery system has been successfully utilized for the delivery of insulin, haemoglobin, and various antigens. Oral delivery of enzymes like serratiopeptidase has also been achieved. This article discusses the problems faced in the delivery of clinically important peptides and presents aquasomes as a reliable approach to troubleshoot them.

A new class of solid drug carriers, aquasomes, has emerged during the last decade. Aquasomes are three-layered structures (i.e. core, coating, and drug) that are self-assembled through non-covalent bonds, ionic bonds, and van der Waals forces. They consist of a ceramic core whose surface is non-covalently modified with carbohydrates to obtain a sugar ball, which is then exposed to adsorption of a therapeutic agent. The core provides structural stability to a largely immutable solid. Aquasomes offer an attractive mode of delivery for therapeutic agents belonging to the class of proteins and peptides, since they are able to overcome some inherent problems associated with these molecules. These problems include suitable route of delivery, physical as well as chemical instability, poor bioavailability, and potent side effects. The surface modification with carbohydrates creates a glassy molecular stabilization film that adsorbs therapeutic proteins with minimal structural denaturation. Thus, these particles provide complete protection of an aqueous nature to the adsorbed drugs against the denaturing effects of external pH and temperature, because there are no swelling and porosity changes with change in pH or temperature.

Rationale

Aquasomes are like 'bodies of water' and their water-like properties protect and preserve fragile biological molecules, and this property of maintaining conformational integrity as well as high degree of surface exposure is exploited in targeting of bioactive molecules like peptide and protein hormones, enzymes, antigens and genes to specific sites.

Properties

1. Aquasomes possess large size and active surface hence can be efficiently loaded with substantial amount of agents through ionic, non-covalent bonds, van der Waals forces and entropic forces. As solid particles dispersed in aqueous environment, exhibit physical properties of colloids.
2. Aquasomes' mechanism of action is controlled by their surface chemistry. Aquasomes deliver contents through combination of specific targeting, molecular shielding, and slow and sustained release process.
3. Aquasomes' water-like properties provide a platform for preserving the conformational integrity and biochemical stability of bioactives.
4. Aquasomes, due to their size and structure stability, avoid clearance by reticuloendothelial system or degradation by other environmental challenges.

Method of Preparation

The method of preparation of aquasomes involves three steps. The general procedure consists of:
1. Formation of an inorganic core
2. Coating of the core with polyhydroxy oligomer
3. Loading of the drug of choice to this assembly.

The first step involves the fabrication of a ceramic core, and the procedure depends upon the materials selected. The two most commonly used ceramic cores are calcium phosphate and diamond. These can be fabricated by colloidal precipitation and sonication, inverted magnetron sputtering, or plasma condensation, among other methods. Ceramic materials, being structurally highly regular, are most widely used for core fabrication. The high degree of order in crystalline ceramics ensures only a limited effect on the nature of atoms below the surface layer when any surface modification is being done, thus preserving the bulk properties of ceramics. This high degree of order also offers a high level of surface energy that favours the binding of polyhydroxy oligomeric surface film. The precipitated cores are centrifuged and then washed with enough distilled water to remove sodium chloride formed during the reaction. The precipitates are resuspended in distilled water and passed through a fine membrane filter to collect the particles of desired size. The equation for the reaction is as follows:

$$2Na_2HPO_4 + 3CaCl_2 + H_2O \rightarrow Ca_3(PO_4)_2 + 4NaCl + 2H_2 + Cl_2 + (O)$$

In the second step, ceramic cores are coated with carbohydrate (polyhydroxy oligomer). The coating is carried out by addition of carbohydrate into an aqueous dispersion of the cores under sonication. These are then subjected to lyophilization to promote an irreversible adsorption of carbohydrate onto the ceramic surface. The unadsorbed carbohydrate is removed by centrifugation. Finally, the drug is loaded to the coated particles by adsorption. For that, a solution of known concentration of drug is prepared in suitable pH buffer, and coated particles are dispersed into it. The dispersion is then either kept overnight at low temperature for drug loading or lyophilized after some time so as to obtain the drug-loaded formulation (i.e. aquasomes). The preparation thus obtained is then characterized using various techniques. The procedure for preparation of aquasomes is depicted in Fig. 4.3.

Characterization

Aquasomes are characterized chiefly for their structural and morphological properties, particle size distribution, and drug loading capacity.

Characterization of Ceramic Core

Size distribution: For morphological characterization and size distribution analysis, scanning electron microscopy (SEM) and transmission electron microscopy (TEM) are generally used. Core, coated core, as well as drug-loaded aquasomes are analyzed by these techniques. Mean particle size and zeta potential of the particles can also be determined by using photo correlation spectroscopy.

Structural analysis: FT-IR spectroscopy can be used for structural analysis. Using the potassium bromide sample disk method, the core as well as the coated core can be

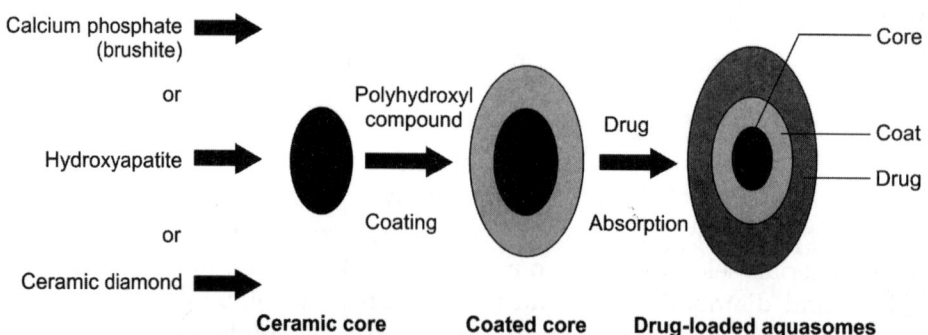

Fig. 4.3: The procedure for preparation of aquasomes

analyzed by recording their IR spectra in the wave-number range 4000–400 cm^{-1}; the characteristic peaks observed are then matched with reference peaks. Identification of sugar and drug loaded over the ceramic core can also be confirmed by FT-IR analysis of the sample.

Crystallinity: The prepared ceramic core can be analyzed for its crystalline or amorphous behaviour using X-ray diffraction. In this technique, the X-ray diffraction pattern of the sample is compared with the standard diffractogram, based on which the interpretations are made.

Characterization of Coated Core

Carbohydrate coating: Coating of sugar over the ceramic core can be confirmed by concanavalin A-induced aggregation method (determines the amount of sugar coated over core) or by anthrone method (determines the residual sugar unbound or residual sugar remaining after coating). Furthermore, the adsorption of sugar over the core can also be confirmed by measurement of zeta potential.

Glass transition temperature: DSC can be used to analyze the effect of carbohydrate on the drug loaded to aquasomes. DSC studies have been extensively used to study glass transition temperature of carbohydrates and proteins. The transition from glass to rubber state can be measured using a DSC analyzer as a change in temperature upon melting of glass.

Characterization of Drug-Loaded Aquasomes

Drug payload: The drug loading can be determined by incubating the basic aquasome formulation (i.e. without drug) in a known concentration of the drug solution for 24 hours at 4°C. The supernatant is then separated by high-speed centrifugation for 1 hour at low temperature in a refrigerated centrifuge. The drug remaining in the supernatant liquid after loading can be estimated by any suitable method of analysis.

In vitro **drug release studies:** The *in vitro* release kinetics of the loaded drug is determined to study the release pattern of drug from the aquasomes by incubating a known quantity of drug-loaded aquasomes in a buffer of suitable pH at 37°C with continuous stirring. Samples are withdrawn periodically and centrifuged at high speed for certain lengths of time. Equal volumes of medium must be replaced after each withdrawal. The supernatants are then analyzed for the amount of drug released by any suitable method.

In-process stability studies: SDS-PAGE can be performed to determine the stability and integrity of protein during the formulation of the aquasomes.

Applications

1. Aquasomes are used as vaccines for delivery of viral antigen, i.e. Epstein-Barr and immune deficiency viruses to evoke correct antibody, objective of vaccine therapy must be triggered by conformationally specific target molecules.
2. Aquasomes as red blood cell substitutes, haemoglobin immobilized on oligomer surface because release of oxygen by haemoglobin is conformationally sensitive. By this, toxicity is reduced, haemoglobin concentration of 80% achieved and reported to deliver blood in non-linear manner like natural blood cells.
3. Aquasomes have been used for successful targeted intracellular gene therapy, a five-layered composition comprised ceramic core, polyoxyoligomeric film,

therapeutic gene segment, additional carbohydrate film and a targeting layer of conformationally conserved viral membrane protein.

4. Aquasomes for pharmaceuticals delivery, i.e. insulin, developed because drug activity is conformationally specific. Bio-activity preserved and activity increased to 60% as compared to IV administration and toxicity not reported.

5. Aquasomes are also used for delivery of enzymes like DNase and pigments/dyes because enzymes activity fluctuates with molecular conformation and cosmetic properties of pigments are sensitive to molecular conformation.

PHYTOSOME

The phytosomes, a patented technology developed by Indena (Milan, Italy), are for the significant improvement of bioavailability, substantial better clinical advantages, and guaranteed deliverance to the tissues with improved nutrient capacity. The term "phyto" means plant while "some" means cell-like. Phytosomes are little cell-like structure. This is advanced forms of herbal formulations which contains the bioactive phytoconsituents of herb extract surrounds and bound by a lipid. Most of the bioactive constituents of phytomedicines are water-soluble compounds like flavonoids, glycosides. Because of water-soluble herbal extract and lipophilic outer layer, phytosomes show better absorption and as a result produce better bioavailability and actions than the conventional herbal extracts containing dosage form. In other word, phytosomes; complex of natural bioactive materials and phospholipids, mostly phosphatidylcholine, increase absorption of herbal extracts or isolated active ingredients when applied topically or orally. Phospholipids are selected from the group consisting of soy lecithin, from bovine or swine brain or dermis, phosphatidylcholine (PC), phosphatidylethanolamine (PE), phosphatidylserine (PS) in which acyl group may be same or different, and is mostly derived from palmitic, stearic, oleic and linoleic acid. Selection of flavonoids is done from the group consisting of quercetin, kaempferol, quercretin-3, rhamnoglucoside, quercetin-3-rhamnoside, hyperoside, vitexin, diosmine, 3-rhamnoside, (+) catechin, (–) epicatechin, apigenin-7-glucoside, luteolin, luteolin glucoside, ginkgonetine, isoginkgetin and bilobetin. Phytosomes are amphiphilic substances, having specific melting point, and generally soluble in lipids. Encapsulation is a process that entraps one substance within another substance, and, therefore, produces particles with diameters of a few nm to a few mm. The encapsulated components may be called the base material, the active agent, fill, internal phase, or payload phase. Phytosomes are examples of these encapsulating systems that are suitable in food and pharmacokinetic applications. Phytosome is a technology developed by incorporating standardized plant extracts or water-soluble phytoconstituents into phospholipids to form complexes that have the ability to increase the extract's bioactivity and antioxidant effects. Phytosome technology has been applied to herbal extracts (ginkgo, milk thistle, and green tea) successfully as well as phytochemicals (curcumin and silybin) with remarkable results both in animals and in human pharmacokinetic studies.

Mechanism of Action

The free radical scavenging capacity of the extract accounts for most of the biological activities. Phytosome is also reported to trigger other mechanisms of action:

- Increasing the antioxidant defense systems
- Stimulation of alpha1 adrenergic stimulated glucose transport
- Interference with the formation of proinflammatory response function cytokines

Phytosome Preparation Method

There are some methods for production of phytosomes including:
- Anti-solvent precipitation
- Solvent evaporation
- Precipitation
- Anhydrous cosolvent lyophilization

Phytosomes are prepared by reacting 3–2 moles or preferably 1 mole of phosphatidylcholine with 1 mole of active phytoconstituents mostly the flavonoids and the terpenoids in an aprotic solvent such as dioxane or acetone from which complex can be isolated by precipitation with non-solvent such as aliphatic hydrocarbons or by lyophilization or by spray drying. In the phyto-phospholipid complex formation, the ratio between these two components is in the range of 0.5–2 moles. The most preferable ratio of phospholipid to phytoconstituents is 1:1. Spectroscopic techniques reveal that the molecules of the phytoconstituents are bonded to phospholipid moiety by means of a chemical bond (Fig. 4.4).

Phytosome production consists of blending biomaterial, inorganic solvent and phospholipid until clear solution creation, solvent evaporation and creating thin layer, hydration and sonication, respectively.

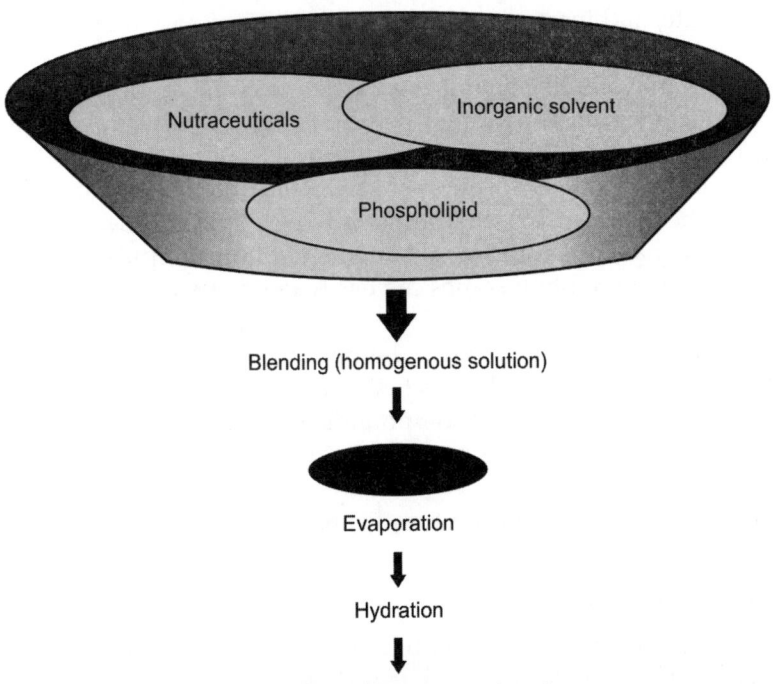

Fig. 4.4: The procedure for preparation of phytosome

Properties of Phytosomes

Chemical Properties

- Phytosome is a complex between a natural product and natural phospholipids.
- The phytosome complex is obtained by reaction of suitable amounts of phospholipid and the substrate in an appropriate solvent such as glycerol.
- The main phospholipid–substrate interaction is due to the formation of hydrogen bonds between the polar head of phospholipids (i.e. phosphate and ammonium groups) and the polar functionalities of the substrate.
- When treated with water, phytosomes assume a micellar shape forming liposome-like structures.

Biological Properties

- Phytosomes are advanced forms of herbal products that are better absorbed, utilized and as a result produce better results than conventional herbal extracts.
- Phytosomes are lipophilic substances with definite melting point, freely soluble in non-polar solvents, and moderately soluble in fats.
- Phytosomes can accommodate the active principle that is anchored to the polar head of the phospholipids, which finally becomes an integral part of the membrane.
- The increased bioavailability of the phytosome over the non-complexed botanical derivatives has been demonstrated by pharmacokinetic studies or by pharmacodynamic tests in experimental animals and in human subjects.

Advantages of Phytosomes

- Phytosomes enhance the absorption of hydrophilic polar phytoconstituents through oral topical route, and increasing the bioavailability.
- They improve active constituent absorption and reduce the dose requirement.
- Besides phosphatidylcholine acting as a carrier, they act as a hepatoprotective.
- Because chemical bonds are formed between phosphatidylcholine molecule and phytoconstituents, phytosomes show good stability profile.
- Phytosomes improve skin absorption of phytoconstituents, and are widely used in cosmetics for their more skin penetration and high lipid profile.
- Phytosomes also have the nutritional benefits of phospholipids.
- The phytoconstituent in phytosomes can easily permeate the intestinal walls and is better absorbed.
- Drug entrapment is not a problem with herbosome as the complex is biodegradable.
- They improve the solubility of bile to herbal constituent.
- They intensify the effect of herbal compounds by improving absorption, enhancing biological activity, and delivering to the target tissue; therefore, phytosomes are suitable for a delivery system.
- They transit from the cell membrane and enter the cell easily.
- Duration of action is increased.

Applications of Phytosomes

- Most of the phytosomes are focused to *Silybum marianum* which contains premier liver-protectant flavonoids.
- The fruit of the milk thistle plant (*S. marianum*; family: Steraceae) contains flavonoids known for hepatoprotective effects.

- Silymarin has been shown to have positive effects in treating liver diseases of various kinds, including hepatitis, cirrhosis, fatty infiltration of the liver (chemical and alcohol-induced fatty liver) and inflammation of the bile duct, e.g. Silymarin phytosome.
- Grape seed phytosome is composed of oligomeric polyphenols of varying molecular size complexed with phospholipids.
- The main properties of procyanidin flavonoids of grape seed are an increase in total antioxidant capacity and stimulation of physiological defenses of plasma.
- Green tea leaves (*Thea sinensis*) are characterized by presence of a polyphenolic compound epigallocatechin 3-O-gallate as the key component.
- These compounds are potent modulators of several biochemical processes linked to the breakdown of homeostasis in major chronic-degenerative diseases such as cancer and atherosclerosis.
- Green tea also furnishes us with a number of beneficial activities such as antioxidant, anticarcinogenic, antimutagenic, hypocholesterolaemic, cardioprotective effects.
- Researchers have been developed the phytosomes of curcumin (flavonoid from turmeric, *Curcuma longa linn*) and naringenin (flavonoid from grape, *Vitis vinifera*).
- Phytosome of naringenin produces better antioxidant activity than the free compound with a prolonged duration of action.

Differences between liposome and phytosome are described in Table 4.1 and depicted in Fig. 4.5.

Table 4.1: Difference between phytosome and liposome

Phytosome	*Liposome*
In phytosome, the phosphatidylcholine and the plant components actually form a 1:1 or a 2:1 molecular complex depending on the substance(s) complexes. Phytosome involves chemical bonds	A liposome is formed by mixing a water-soluble substance with phosphatidylcholine in definite ratio under specific conditions
	Here, no chemical bond is formed; the phosphatidylcholine molecules surround the water-soluble substance.
Phytosomes are much better absorbed than liposomes showing better bioavailability	Bioavailability of liposomes is less than phytosomes

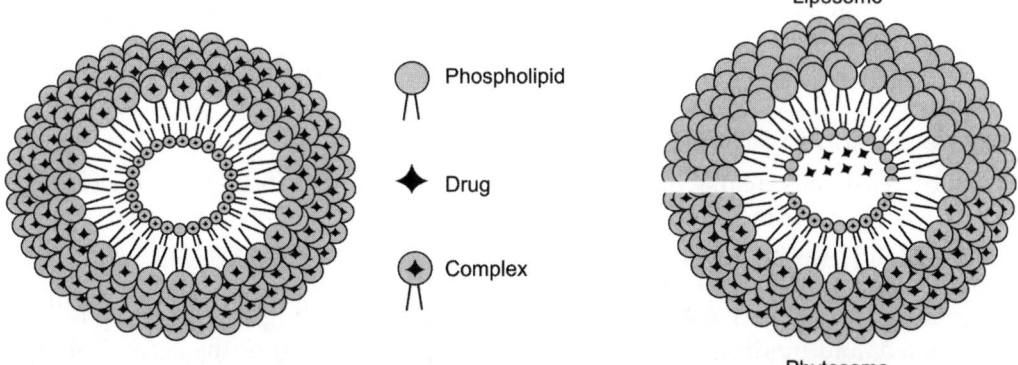

Fig 4.5: Structural differences between liposome and phytosome

ELECTROSOMES

The electrosomes, a novel surface-display system based on the specific interaction between the cellulosomal scaffoldin protein and a cascade of redox enzymes that allows multiple electron-releases by fuel oxidation. The electrosome is composed of two compartments: (i) A hybrid anode, which consists of dockerin-containing enzymes attached specifically to cohesin sites in the scaffoldin to assemble an ethanol oxidation cascade, and (ii) a hybrid cathode, which consists of a dockerin-containing oxygen-reducing enzyme attached in multiple copies to the cohesin-bearing scaffoldin. The electrosome was designed for use both in an anode and a cathode compartment; in each compartment, the unique attributes of the cellulosome scaffoldin give a different advantage.

In the anode, the ethanol oxidation cascade consists of two enzymes, ADH and formaldehyde dehydrogenase (FormDH), both containing a different dockerin modules of *Acetivibrio cellulolyticus* and of *Clostridium thermocellum, C. thermocellum* (zADH-Ac and pFormDH-Ct), respectively, assembled on a 'designer'-scaffoldin chimera displayed on the surface of *S. cerevisiae*. At the cathode, copper oxidase (CueO) is selected for surface-display. CueO is a multi-copper oxidase enzyme expressed by *E. coli* that catalyzes the oxidation of Cu(I) ions coupled to oxygen reduction to water. The different constructs used for assembly are depicted. We report the characterization of the dockerin-containing enzymes and their electrochemical activity using a diffusing redox mediator.

Method of Preparation

- Strains and constructs method
- Enzyme binding to scaffoldin
- Biofuel-cell assembly and characterization

Strains and Constructs Method

The genes encoding dockerins of *Acetivibrio cellulolyticus* and *Clostridium thermocellum* are cloned and ligated to the C-terminus of *Zymomonas mobilis* alcohol dehydrogenase and to *Pseudomonas putida* formaldehyde dehydrogenase by standard methods. The dockerin module of *C. thermocellum* is also ligated to the C-terminus of CueO (CueO-Ct) of *E.coli*. All the dockerin-containing enzymes encoding genes have been cloned into the pET15b vector for expression in *E. coli*, yielding the pET15b-zADH-Ac, pET15b- pFormDH-Ct, and pET15b-CueO-Ct vectors. For controls, the genes encoding the native enzymes without an appended dockerin module are also cloned in the same vector, yielding plasmids pET15b- zADH, pET15b-pFormDH, and pET15b-CueO.

Enzyme Binding to Scaffoldin

2.0 ml of yeast cells displaying scaffoldin, for which absorbance at a wavelength of 600 nm was 1.0, were incubated with bacterial lysates containing the expressed enzymes at room temperature for 1 h. 1.0 ml of the bacterial lysates were used for the binding, which was performed in a final volume of 15 ml. As a binding buffer, 50 mM Tris buffer at pH 8.0 with 1 mM CaCl$_2$ was used. Upon binding, the yeast cells were precipitated, and binding was repeated using fresh lysate. After the second binding cycle, the yeast cells were washed four times in the buffer to remove non-specifically bound enzymes. For the CueO-Ct binding, the yeast cells were suspended in 0.1m acetate buffer pH 5.0 containing 1 mM $CaCl_2$ after the last washes. Following binding, the yeast cells were resuspended in 2.0 ml of buffer.

Biofuel-Cell Assembly and Characterization

Air was continuously purged to the fuel-cells. A potentiostatically controlled anode set to –0.2 V versus Ag/AgCl was used. In all experiments, the cells were left to stabilize overnight, following fuel cell assembly, before characterization was performed. The characterization of fuel cell performance was done by measuring the voltage of the cells under variable external loads. A background current cell was used as a negative control for all fuel cell experiments and did not contain any yeast. Graphite rods of 5 mm diameter served as both anodes and cathodes. The counterelectrode that served for the potentiostatically controlled electrode was of a larger surface area, as described for the CV and CA measurements.

Advantages

- It perpetuates the endurance of active drug molecule in the systemic circulation.
- Deferments the elimination reactions of promptly metabolize drugs and contributes to controlled release.
- Incorporates both hydrophilic and lipophilic drugs.
- Intensifies the stability of medicament.
- Cost of therapy is minimized by reducing the dose per unit formulation.
- Elevate bioavailability especially in water disfavouring drugs.
- Selective uptake by tissues due to direct drug delivery.

Disadvantages

- The production costs of electrosomes are generally high since these come under the class of nanotherapeutics.
- The constituent phospholipids present in lipid vesicular structures may undergo oxidation or hydrolysis.

Applications

- They use enzymatic reactions to catalyze the conversion of chemical energy to electricity in a fuel cell.
- The use of enzymatic cascades in enzymatic fuel cell anodes resulted in very high power outputs, as the electron density achieved was much higher when the fuel was fully oxidized.
- It is used as a carrier in drug targeting.
- Used in the treatment of cancer.
- Used in studying immune response.
- Ear targeting
- Muscle targeting

NIOSOMES

Niosomes are synthetic microscopic vesicles consisting of an aqueous core enclosed in a bilayer consisting of cholesterol and one or more nonionic surfactants. Vesicles are prepared from self-assembly of hydrated non-ionic surfactant molecules.

General Characteristics of Niosome

- Biocompatible, biodegradable, non-toxic, non-immunogenic and non-carcinogenic.
- The ability of non-ionic surfactant to form bilayer vesicles is dependent on the HLB value of the surfactant, the chemical structure of the components and the critical packing parameter.
- Niosomes can be characterized by their size distribution studies.
- High resistance to hydrolytic degradation
- The properties of niosome depend both on composition of the bilayer and on method of their production.

Advantages of Niosomes

- Targeted drug delivery can be achieved using niosomes, the drug is delivered directly to the body part where the therapeutic effect is required.
- Reduced dose is required to achieve the desired effect.
- Subsequent decrease in the side effects.
- The therapeutic efficacy of the drugs is improved by reducing the clearance rate, targeting to the specific site and by protecting the encapsulated drug.
- Niosomes are amphiphilic, i.e. both hydrophilic and lipophilic in nature and can accommodate a large number of drugs with a wide range of solubilities.
- Improve the oral bioavailability of poorly soluble drugs.
- Enhance the skin permeability of drugs when applied topically.
- Provide advantage of usage through various routes, viz. oral, parenteral, topical, ocular, etc.
- The bilayers of the niosomes protect the enclosed active pharmaceutical ingredient from the various factors present both inside and outside the body.
- The surfactants used and also the prepared niosomes are biodegradable, biocompatible and non-immunogenic.
- They are osmotically active and stable.

Disadvantages of Niosome

- Aqueous suspension of niosome may exhibit fusion, aggregation leaching or hydrolysis of entrapped drug, thus limiting the shelf life of niosome dispersion.
- Time consuming
- Requires specialized equipment
- Inefficient drug loading

Composition of Niosomes

Cholesterol and non-ionic surfactants are the two major components used for the preparation of niosomes. Cholesterol provides rigidity and proper shape. The surfactants play a major role in the formation of niosomes. Non-ionic surfactants like spans (span 20, 40, 60, 85, 80), tweens (tween 20, 40, 60, 80) and brij (brij 30, 35, 52, 58, 72, 76) are generally used for the preparation of niosomes (Fig. 4.6). A few other surfactants that are reported to form niosomes are as follows.

- Ether-linked surfactant
- Dialkyl chain surfactant
- Ester linked
- Sorbitan esters
- Polysorbates

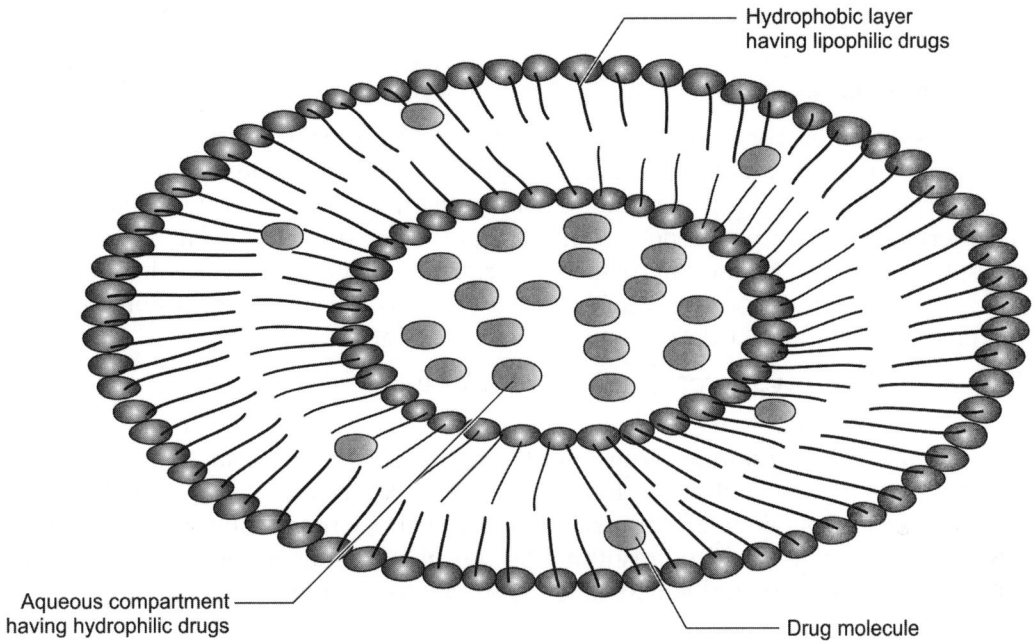

Hydrophobic layer
having lipophilic drugs

Aqueous compartment
having hydrophilic drugs

Drug molecule

Fig 4.6: Diagrammatic represention of niosome

Method of Preparation

1. Ether injection (LUV) based on the vesicle size; niosomes can be divided into three groups.
2. Hand-shaking method (MLV). These are small unilamellar vesicles (SUV, size = 0.025–0.05 μm).
3. The "bubble" method. Multilamellar vesicles (MLV, size → 0.05 μm), and large
4. Reverse phase evaporation (LUV). Unilamellar vesicles (LUV, size → 0.10 μm).
5. Sonication (SUV)
6. Multiple membrane extrusion method
7. Transmembrane pH gradient drug uptake process (remote loading) (MLV)
8. Microfluidization method (SUV)
9. Formation of niosomes from proniosomes

1. Ether-injection method

This method is based on slow injection of surfactant: Cholesterol solution in ether through gauge needle into a preheated aqueous phase maintained at 60°C. Vaporization of ether resulting into a formation of ether gradient at ether–water interface which leads to formation of single-layered vesicles. Depending upon the conditions used the diameter of the vesicle range from 50 to 1000 nm.

2. Hand-shaking method (Thin Film Hydration Technique)

Surfactant and cholesterol are dissolved in a volatile organic solvent (diethyl ether, chloroform or methanol) in a round bottom flask. The organic solvent is removed under vacuum at room temperature using rotary evaporator leaving a thin layer of solid mixture deposited on the wall of the flask. The dried surfactant film can be rehydrated with aqueous phase at temperature slightly above the phase transition temperature of the surfactant used, with gentle agitation. This process forms large multilamellar niosomes.

3. The "Bubble" Method

It is novel technique for the one step preparation of liposomes and niosomes without the use of organic solvents. The bubbling unit consists of round-bottom flask with three necks positioned in water bath to control the temperature. Water-cooled reflux and thermometer are positioned in the first and second neck and nitrogen supply through the third neck. Cholesterol and surfactant are dispersed together in this buffer (pH 7.4) at 70°C, the dispersion mixed for 15 seconds with high shear homogenizer and immediately afterwards bubbled at 70°C using nitrogen gas.

4. Reverse Phase Evaporation (REV) Technique

Cholesterol and surfactant (1:1) are dissolved in a mixture of ether and chloroform. An aqueous phase containing drug is added to this and the resulting two phases are sonicated at 4–5°C. The clear gel formed is further sonicated after the addition of a small amount of phosphate buffered saline (PBS). The organic phase is removed at 40°C under low pressure. The resulting viscous niosome suspension is diluted with PBS and heated on a water bath at 60°C for 10 min to yield niosomes.

5. Sonication

In this method, an aliquot of drug solution in buffer is added to the surfactant/ cholesterol mixture in a 10 ml glass vial. The mixture is probe sonicated at 60°C for 3 minutes using a sonicator. The resultant vesicles are of small unilamellar type niosomes (Fig. 4.7).

6. Multiple Membrane Extrusion Method

In this method, a mixture of surfactant, cholesterol and diacetyl phosphate is prepared and then solvent is evaporated using rotary vacuum evaporator to leave a thin film. The film is then hydrated with aqueous drug solution and the suspension thus obtained

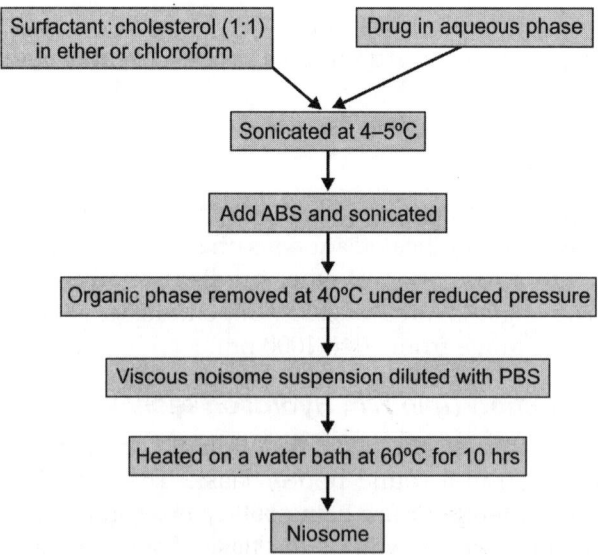

Fig. 4.7: Method of preparation of niosomes by sonication

is extruded through the polycarbonate membrane (mean pore size 0.1 mm) and then placed in series up to eight passages to obtain uniform size niosomes. Good method of controlling niosome size.

7. Transmembrane pH Gradient (Inside Acidic) Drug Uptake Process (Remote Loading)

Surfactant and cholesterol are dissolved in chloroform. The solvent is then evaporated under reduced pressure to get a thin film on the wall of the round bottom flask. The film is hydrated with 300 mM citric acid (pH 4.0) by vortex mixing. The multilamellar vesicles are frozen and thawed 3 times and later sonicated. To this niosomal suspension, aqueous solution containing 10 mg/ml of drug is added and vortexed. The pH of the sample is then raised to 7.0–7.2 with 1M disodium phosphate. This mixture is later heated at 60°C for 10 minutes to give niosomes.

8. Microfluidization Method

In this method, two fluidized streams (one containing drug and the other surfactant) interact at ultra-high velocity, in precisely defined microchannels within the interaction chamber in such a way that the energy supplied to the system remains in the area of niosomes formation. This is called submerged jet principle. It results in better uniformity, smaller size and reproducibility in the formulation of niosomes.

9. Formation of Niosomes from Proniosomes

Another method of producing niosomes is to coat a water-soluble carrier such as sorbitol with surfactant. The result of the coating process is a dry formulation. In which each water-soluble particle is covered with a thin film of dry surfactant. This preparation is termed "proniosomes". The niosomes are formed by the addition of aqueous phase at $T > T_m$ and brief agitation: T = Temperature, T_m = mean phase transition temperature

General Steps of Niosome Preparation

- Hydration of mixture of surfactant/lipid at elevated temperature
- Sizing of niosomes
- Removal of unentrapped material from vesicles

Common Stages of all Methods of Preparation of Niosomes

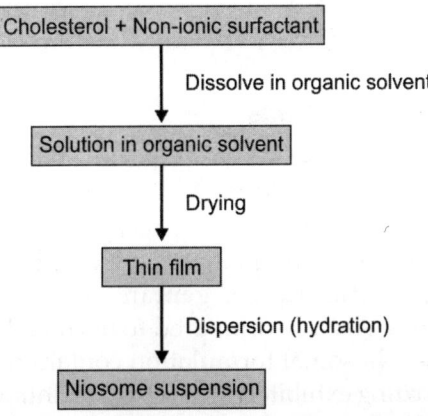

Evaluation

Entrapment efficiency: After preparing niosomal dispersion, unentrapped drug is separated by dialysis, centrifugation and gel filtration. The drug remains entrapped in niosomes determined by complete vesicle disruption using 50% *n*-propanol or 0.1% Triton X-100 and analyzed resultant solution by appropriate assay method using following equation.

$$\text{Entrapment efficiency} = (\text{Amount entrapped}/\text{total amount}) \times 100$$

Bilayer formation: Assembly of non-ionic surfactants to form a bilayer vesicle is characterized by an X-cross formation under light polarization microscopy.

Size: Shape of niosomal vesicles is assumed to be spherical, and their mean diameter can be determined by using laser light scattering method. Also, diameter of these vesicles can be determined by using electron microscopy, molecular sieve chromatography, ultracentrifugation, photon correlation microscopy, optical microscopy and freeze fracture electron microscopy.

Numbers of lamellae: This is determined by using nuclear magnetic resonance (NMR) spectroscopy, small angle X-ray scattering and electron microscopy.

Membrane rigidity: Membrane rigidity can be measured by means of mobility of fluorescence probe as a function of temperature.

***In vitro* release:** A method of *in vitro* release rate study includes the use of dialysis tubing. A dialysis sac is washed and soaked in distilled water. The vesicle suspension is pipetted into a bag made up of the tubing and sealed. The bag containing the vesicles is placed in 200 ml of buffer solution in a 250 ml beaker with constant shaking at 25°C or 37°C. At various time intervals, the buffer is analyzed for the drug content by an appropriate assay method.

Microscopic evaluation: Transmission electron microscopy (TEM) is used for microscopic evaluation of niosomes dispersion. TEM used for determination of size and used to identify whether it is spherical or not.

Therapeutic Applications of Niosomes

The applications of niosomes can be mainly classified into three categories:
1. For controlled release of drugs
2. To improve the stability and physical properties of the drugs
3. For targeting and retention of drug in blood circulation

To Prolong the Release Rate of Drugs

- *For controlled release:* The release rate of drugs, like withaferin and gliclazide from the niosomes, is found slower as compared to other dosage forms.
- *In ophthalmic drug delivery:* Experimental results of the water-soluble antibiotic gentamicin sulphate showed a substantial change in the release rate. Beside this, the percent entrapment efficiency of gentamicin sulphate was altered when administered as niosomes. Also, as compared to normal drug solution, niosomes of drug show slow release. Niosomal formulation containing timolol maleate (0.25%) prepared by chitosan coating exhibited more effect on intraocular tension with fewer side effects as compared to the marketed formulation.

To Improve the Stability and Physical Properties of the Drugs

- *To increase oral bioavailability:* With the formulation of niosomes, the oral bioavailability of the acyclovir as well as griseofulvin was increased as compared to the drug alone. Similarly, the absorptivity of poorly absorbed peptide and ergot alkaloid can be increased by the administration in the bile duct of rats when administered as micellar solution together with the POE-24-cholesteryl ester.
- *For improvement of stability of peptide drugs:* 8-arginin vasopressin, 9-glycinamide. The *in vitro* release of insulin from niosomes formulated by span 40 and span 60 in simulated intestinal fluid was lower than the niosomes formulated by span 20 and span 80. Niosomes prepared by the span 60 has high resistance against proteolytic enzyme and exhibit good stability in storage temperature and in presence of sodium deoxycholate.
- *To promote transdermal delivery of drugs:* Many drugs such as lidocaine, estradiol, cyclosporine, etc. are used for topical and transdermal drug delivery system by formulating them as niosomes. The niosomes of natural compound, ammonium glycyrrhizinate were formulated for effective anti-inflammatory activity using new non-ionic surfactant, bola surfactant-span 80-cholesterol (2:3:1 ratio). Experimental study showed that the bola niosomes were able to promote the intracellular uptake of ammonium glycyrrhetinic acid.
- *As a tool for improvement of stability of immunological products:* Important tool for immunological selectivity, low toxicity and more stability of the incorporated active moiety.
- *To improve anti-inflammatory activity:* Niosomal formulation of diclofenac sodium prepared with 70% cholesterol showed greater anti-inflammatory effect as compared to the free drug. Similarly, nimesulide and flurbiprofen showed greater activity than the free drug.

For Targeting and Retention of Drug in Blood Circulation

- *For increased uptake by A431 cells [a model cell line (epidermoid carcinoma) used in biomedical research]:* Chitosan-based vesicles incorporating transferrin and glucose as ligand has been reported. These vesicles bind CoA to their surface. Chitosan containing vesicles are then taken up by A431 cells and the uptake was found to be enhanced by transferrin.
- *For liver targeting:* Methotrexate was reported to be selectively taken up by liver cells after administration as a niosomal drug delivery system.
- *To improve the efficacy of drugs in cancer therapy:* Niosomes can also be used as a suitable delivery system for the administration of drugs like 5-FU. Niosomes of doxorubicin prepared from C16 monoalkyl glycerol ether with or without cholesterol, exhibited an increased level of doxorubicin in tumour cells, serum and lungs, but not in liver and spleen. Niosomal preparation of methotrexate exhibited greater antitumour activity as compared to plain drug solution.
- *In treatment of localized psoriasis:* In the treatment of localized psoriasis, niosomes of methotrexate taking chitosan as polymer have shown promising results.
- *In leishmaniasis:* The Leishmania parasite mainly infects liver and spleen cells. The commonly used drugs, antimonials, may damage the body organ like heart, liver, kidney, etc. The efficiency of sodium stibogluconate has been found to be enhanced by incorporation in niosomes. The additive effect was observed for two doses given on successive days. Moreover, the distribution of antimony in mice showed the

higher level of antimony in liver after its intravenous (IV) administration via niosomes drug formulation.

- *In diagnostic imaging:* It has been studied that niosomes can also act as a carrier radiopharmaceutical and showed site specificity for spleen and liver for their imaging studies using ^{99m}Tc-labelled DTPA (diethylenetriaminepenta-acetic acid) containing niosomes. Conjugated niosomal formulations of gadobenate with (N-palmitoyl-glucosamine, NPG), PEG 4400 and both PEG and NPG can be used to increase tumour targeting of a paramagnetic agent.
- *Carrier for haemoglobin:* Niosomes play an important role as a carrier for haemoglobin. The niosomal haemoglobin suspension was found to give superimposable curve on free haemoglobin curve usefulness of niosomes in cosmetics. Niosomes of N-acetyl glucosamine are prepared due to its potential in the delivery of hydrophilic and hydrophobic drugs in topical form and improved penetration into the skin. Prepared formulations improved the extent of drug localized in the skin, as needed in hyperpigmentation disorders. Elastic niosomes showed increased permeation through the skin which will be beneficial for topical antiaging application. Suitable for skin moisturizing and tanning products. Niosomes were prepared as possible approach to improve the low skin penetration and bioavailability shown by conventional topical vehicle for minoxidil. Niosomes with added solubilizers enhanced the permeation of ellagic acid (a potent antioxidant phytochemical substance which has limited use due to poor biopharmaceutical properties, low solubility and low permeability) into the skin with 55 increased efficacies of ellagic acid.

Similarity of Niosomes and Liposomes

- However, niosomes are similar to liposomes in functionality.
- Niosomes also increase the bioavailability of the drug and reduce the clearance like liposomes.
- Niosomes can also be used for targeted drug delivery, similar to liposomes.
- As with liposomes, the properties of the niosomes depend both—on the composition of the bilayer, and the method of production used.

Contrast of Niosomes vs Liposomes (Table 4.2)

Table 4.2: Contrast of niosomes vs liposomes	
Niosomes	*Liposomes*
Less expensive	More expensive
Chemically stable	Chemically unstable
Niosomes are prepared from uncharged single-chain surfactant	Liposomes are prepared from double-chain phospholipids
They do not require special storage and handling	They require special storage, handling and purity of natural phospholipid is variable
Non-ionic drugs carriers are safer	The ionic drug carriers are relatively toxic and unsuitable

PHARMACOSOMES

Pharmacosomes are the colloidal dispersions of drugs covalently bound to lipids, and may exist as ultrafine vesicular, micellar, or hexagonal aggregates, depending on the chemical structure of drug–lipid complex. Pharmacosomes are amphiphilic phospholipid complexes of drugs bearing active hydrogen that bind to phospholipids. Pharmacosomes impart better biopharmaceutical properties to the drug, resulting in improved bioavailability. Pharmacosomes have been prepared for various non-steroidal anti-inflammatory drugs, proteins, cardiovascular and antineoplastic drugs. Developing the pharmacosomes of the drugs has been found to improve the absorption and minimize the gastrointestinal toxicity.

In pharmacosomes, membrane fluidity depends upon the phase transition temperature of the drug–lipid complex, but it does not affect release rate since the drug is covalently bound. The drug is released from pharmacosome by hydrolysis (including enzymatic). The physicochemical stability of the pharmacosome depends upon the physicochemical properties of the drug–lipid complex. Following absorption, their degradation velocity into active drug molecule depends to a great extent on the size and functional groups of drug molecule, the chain length of the lipids, and the spacer. They can be given orally, topically, extra- or intravascularly.

Importance

Pharamcosomes have some importance in escaping the tedious steps of removing the free unentrapped drug from the formulation. Pharmacosomes provide an efficient method for delivery of drug directly to the site of infection, leading to reduction of drug toxicity with no adverse effects and also reduces the cost of therapy by improved bioavailability of medication, especially in case of poorly soluble drugs. Pharmacosomes are suitable for incorporating both hydrophilic and lipophilic drugs. Entrapment efficiency is not only high but predetermined, because drug itself in conjugation with lipids forms vesicles. There is no need of following the tedious, time-consuming step for removing the free, unentrapped drug from the formulation. Since the drug is covalently linked, loss due to leakage of drug, does not take place. No problem of drug incorporation. Encaptured volume and drug-bilayer interactions do not influence entrapment efficiency, in case of pharmacosomes.

Preparation

Two methods have been used to prepare vesicles:
1. The hand-shaking method
2. The ether-injection method

In the hand-shaking method, the dried film of the drug–lipid complex (with or without egg lecithin) is deposited in a round-bottom flask and upon hydration with aqueous medium, readily gives a vesicular suspension. In the ether-injection method, an organic solution of the drug–lipid complex is injected slowly into the hot aqueous medium, wherein the vesicles are readily formed.

Evaluation of Pharmacosomes

- Solubility
- Drug content
- Entrapment efficiency
- Dissolution study
- Scanning electron microscopy (SEM)
- Differential scanning calorimetry (DSC)
- X-ray powder diffraction (XRPD)

Applications

- The approach has successfully improved the therapeutic performance of various drugs, i.e. pindolol maleate, bupranolol hydrochloride, taxol, acyclovir, etc.
- The phase transition temperature of pharmacosomes in the vesicular and micellar state could have significant influence on their interaction with membranes.
- Pharmacosomes can interact with bimembranes enabling a better transfer of active ingredient. This interaction leads to change in phase transition temperature of bimembranes thereby improving the membrane fluidity leading to enhance permeations.
- Amphiphilic prodrug
- Pharmacosomes of aceclophenac
- Pharmacosomes of diclophenac
- Pharmacosomes of didnosine
- Pharmacosomes of acyclovir

RESEALED ERYTHROCYTES

Erythrocytes have been the most extensively investigated and found to possess great potential in novel drug delivery. Erythrocytes are loaded with drug/enzymes and provide target drug delivery system. Such drug-loaded carrier erythrocytes are prepared simply by collecting blood samples from the organism of interest, separating erythrocytes from plasma, entrapping drug in the erythrocytes, and resealing the resultant cellular carriers. Hence, these carriers are called resealed erythrocyte. Erythrocytes are potential biocompatible vectors for different bioactive substances, biological carriers of drugs, and enzymes. Erythrocytes loaded with drugs and other substances allow for different release rates to be obtained. Encapsulation in erythrocytes significantly changes the pharmacokinetic properties of drugs in both animals and humans, enhancing liver and spleen uptake and targeting the reticuloendothelial system (RES). Encapsulation of new prodrugs increases with increased duration of action, etc. Erythrocytes are biocompatible, biodegradable, possess long circulation half-lives, and can be loaded with a variety of biologically active compounds using various chemical and physical methods. Erythrocytes, the most abundant cells in the human body, have potential carrier capabilities for the delivery of drugs. They have capability for prevention of premature degradation or inactivation.

Resealed Erythrocytes Properties as Carrier

- Appropriate size, shape to permit passage through the capillaries.
- Biocompatible and minimum toxic side effects.
- Minimum leakage before target site is achieved, should be able to carry broad-spectrum of drugs.
- Appreciable stability during storage period.
- Should have sufficient space and should carry adequate amounts of drugs.

Advantages of Erythrocyte as Carrier

- Biodegradable
- Isolation is easy
- Non-immunogenic
- Large volume of drug can be encapsulated in small volume of erythrocytes

- Prolong systemic activity of drug
- Protection from premature degradation
- Prodrug concept (bioreactor)
- Reduced adverse effect
- Peptide and enzyme delivery
- Biocompatibility
- Circulate throughout the circulatory system
- Inert environment
- Prevention of undesired immune response
- Can be utilized for organ targeting within RES
- A longer lifespan as compared to synthetic carriers
- Decrease in side effect of drugs
- Increase in drug dosing interval
- Easy control during lifespan ranging from minutes to months
- Large quantity of material can be encapsulated within small volume of cells.

Disadvantages
- Possibility of leakage of cells and dose dumping.
- Molecule alter physiology of cell.
- They are removed *in vivo* by RES so may cause toxicological problems.
- Lesser standardization in their preparation, compared to other carrier systems.
- The storage of the loaded erythrocytes is a further problem involving carrier erythrocytes.
- Liable to biological contamination due to the origin of the blood, the equipment and the environment.

Methods of Drug Loading
Methods of drug loading in erythrocytes are:
1. Hypo-osmotic lyses method
   a. Dilution haemolysis
   b. Pre-swell dilutional haemolysis
   c. Isotonic osmotic lysis
   d. Dialysis
2. Chemical perturbation of membrane
3. Electroencapsulation
4. Entrapment by endocytosis

1. Hypo-Osmotic Lyses Method
- Erythrocytes have an exceptional capability for reversible shape change.
- They do not have internal membrane and no capacity to synthesize additional plasma membranes, the surface area is inevitably fixed.
- So, increase in volume initially leads to conversion of normal biconcave, discocyte (normal erythrocyte) to spherocytes.
- Thus, the cells become spheres as they accommodate additional volume with a fixed surface area.

- The swollen erythrocytes when placed in solution –150 mOsm/kg, the membrane ruptures, permitting escape of the cellular component.
- These ruptured membranes can be resealed by raising the salt concentration to its isotonic levels and upon incubation, the resealed erythrocytes assemble their normal biconcave shape and recover impermeability.

a. **Dilution haemolysis:**
  - Erythrocytes exposed to hypotonic medium (0.4% NaCl)
  - Membrane ruptures and becomes permeable to macromolecules and ions.
  - One volume of washed erythrocytes can be treated with 2–20 volumes of material to be loaded.
  - Further incubation at 25°C in an isotonic medium (0.9% NaCl) and reseal them

b. **Pre-swell dilutional haemolysis:**
  - Initial controlled swelling in a hypotonic buffered solution
  - Supernatant is discarded.
  - Mixture is centrifuged.
  - Lysis occurs.
  - Mixture is centrifuged at low g values.
  - Addition of 100–150 ml aqueous solution of drug and cell brought to lysis point.
  - Addition of isotonic medium suspension is incubated at 37°C to form the resealed erythrocytes.

c. **Isotonic osmotic lysis:**
  - If erythrocytes are incubated in solutions of a substance with high membrane permeability, the solute will diffuse into the cells because of the concentration gradient.
  - This process is followed by an influx of water to maintain osmotic equilibrium.
  - Chemicals such as urea solution, polyethylene glycol, and ammonium chloride have been used for isotonic haemolysis.

d. **Dialysis:**
  - Washed erythrocytes are mixed with phosphate buffer saline, pH 7.4.
  - This mixture is placed in dialysis bag.
  - The bag is inflated with air bubble.
  - Sealed dialysis bag is placed in a bottle containing at least 200 ml of lysis buffer (0.1% NaCl, 0°C).
  - Placed in a mechanical rotator for 2 hours at 4°C.
  - Resealing at RT for 30 minutes
  - Mixer stirrer

2. Chemical Perturbation of Membrane

This method is based on the observation that the permeability of the erythrocytic membrane is increased when exposed to certain chemicals, e.g. daunomycin by amphotericin B.

3. Electroencapsulation

Also known as electroporation, the method is based on the observation that electrical shock brings about desirable membrane permeability for drug loading into erythrocytes, e.g. methotrexate, isoniazid.

4. Entrapment by Endocytosis

- Addition of one volume of washed packed erythrocytes to nine volumes of buffer.
- The pores created by this method are resealed by using 154 mM of NaCl.
- The bag is inflated with air bubble incubate for 2 min at RT.
- Incubate for 2 min at 37°C.

Applications of Resealed Erythrocytes

- Erythrocytes as carrier for enzymes
- Erythrocytes as carrier for drugs
- Erythrocytes for drug targeting
- Drug targeting to reticuloendothelial system
- Drug targeting to liver
    - Treatment of liver tumours
    - Treatment of parasitic diseases
    - Removal of RES iron overload
    - Removal of toxic agents
- Delivery of antiviral agents
- Oxygen deficiency therapy
- Microinjection of macromolecules
- Novel systems
    - Nanoerythrosomes
    - Erythrosome

SPECIALIZED PHARMACEUTICAL EMULSIONS

An emulsion may be defined as thermodynamically unstable biphasic system consisting of two immiscible liquids, one of which (the dispersed phase) is finely and uniformly dispersed as globules throughout the second phase (the continuous phase) stabilized with emulsifying agent. The particle size of the dispersed phase commonly ranges from 0.1 to 100 μm.

Methods of Preparation of Emulsions

Emulsification Process

Milk is a natural emulsion, which consists of fatty globules surrounded by a layer of casein, suspended in water. The theory of emulsification is based on the study of milk. When a pharmaceutical emulsion is to be prepared the principal consideration is the same as that of milk.

General Method

Generally, an O/W emulsion is prepared by dividing the oily phase completely into minute globules surrounding each globule with an envelope of emulsifying agent and finally suspends the globules in the aqueous phase. Conversely, the W/O emulsion is prepared by dividing aqueous phase completely into minute globules surrounding each globule with an envelope of emulsifying agent and finally suspending the globules in the oily phase.

1. **Continental and dry gum method:** Extemporaneously emulsions are usually made by continental or dry gum method. In this method, the emulsion is prepared by

mixing the emulsifying agent (usually acacia) with the oil which is then mixed with the aqueous phase. Continental and dry gum methods differ in the proportion of constituents—4:2:1 (oil:water:gum). Primary emulsifier is triturated with the oil in perfectly dry porcelain mortar. Two parts of water is added at once triturate immediately, rapidly and continuously (until get a cracking sound).

2. **Wet gum method:** In this method, the proportion of the constituents is same as those used in the dry gum method; the only difference is the method of preparation. Here, the mucilage of the emulsifying agent (usually acacia) is formed. The oil is then added to the mucilage drop by drop with continuous trituration.

3. **Bottle or Forbes bottle method:** Extemporaneous preparations for volatile oils or oil with low viscosity gum + 2 parts of oil (dry bottle) shake water (volume equal to oil) are added in portions and shake.

4. **Beaker method oil phase:** Heated about 5–10°C above the highest melting point of ingredient (water bath). Water phase: Heated to the same temperature of oil phase (water bath). Add internal phase into external phase, mix, constant agitation being provided throughout the time of addition.

   Caution: Not to heat the phase above 85°C—rate of cooling determining the final texture and consistency.

5. **Phase inversion method:** In this method, the aqueous phase is first added to the oil phase so as to form a W/O emulsion. At the inversion point, the addition of more water results in the inversion of emulsion which gives rise to an O/W emulsion.

Membrane emulsification method: It is a method, which is based on a novel concept of generating droplets "drop by drop" to produce emulsion. Here, a pressure is applied direct to the dispersed phase which seeps through a porous membrane into the continuous phase and in this way, the droplets formed are then detached from the membrane surface due to the relative shear motion between the continuous phase and membrane surface.

Types of Emulsion

1. Macroemulsions
   - Parenteral emulsions
   - Water-in-oil emulsions
   - Oil-in-water/oral emulsions
   - Radio-opaque
   - Fluorocarbon emulsion
2. Microemulsion
3. Nanoemulsion
4. Multiple emulsions
5. Gel emulsion

Applications of Parenteral Emulsions

Parenteral Nutrition

- A major application of lipid emulsions is the delivery of fat in parenteral nutrition. Fat is a concentrated source of energy and can supply essential fatty acids.
- Carriers for drugs and as targeted delivery systems.
- The close resemblance of fat emulsion particles to chylomicrons, the natural emulsion particles that transport ingested lipophiles such as triglycerides into the lymphatic

and circulatory systems, suggests that fat emulsions can be used as carriers for drugs and as targeted delivery systems.

- Prolonged releases of drug emulsions can affect the metabolism of the drug, which can in turn affect clearance of the particles from the blood. Positive prolonged release effects have, however, been noted for progesterone and corticosteroids.

Increased bioavailability: Intralipid has been used to incorporate valinomycin, an antitumour agent and it was found that a 20-fold lower dose was sufficient to produce the same effects as an aqueous suspension.

Decreased toxicity: Amphotericin B administered as a lipid emulsion, in comparison with a 5% aqueous dextrose solution, gave a lower incidence of fever and nephrotoxicity and was as effective.

Stability: Instability of fat emulsions can arise from changes in particle size of the oil droplets leading to creaming and coalescence, or from changes in pH, hydrolysis of emulsifier, or oxidation of the oil. Emulsions cause enhanced stability furnished by a non-aqueous environment. Many drugs including barbituric acid, diazepam, and anaesthetics have been dissolved in the oil phase and administered by all parenteral routes.

Applications of Fluorocarbon Emulsions

- They are clinically evaluated as "artificial oxygen carriers".
- In future, they will be used in the concept of ANH, i.e. acute normovolaemic haemodilution, means it is used to augment oxygen delivery during surgery.
- These are also used in treatment of diseases with compromised tissue oxygenation such as cerebral ischaemia, MI, emergency, trauma, etc.

Applications of Microemulsions

- *Oral drug delivery:* Examples include send immune neural which is commercial name for cyclosporin A. Other examples include paclitaxel and simvastatin.
- *Transdermal drug delivery:* A diverse range of drug molecules such as ketoprofen, apomorphine, oestradiol, lidocaine, indomethacin, diclofenac, and prostaglandin E1 are incorporated as ME.
- *Parenteral drug delivery:* Flurbiprofen O/W ME systems were prepared and evaluated as vehicles for parenteral drug delivery. These systems were formulated using POE 20 sorbitan monolaurate (Tween 20) as the surfactant.
- *Ocular drug delivery:* Nanoemulsion is a type of emulsion sized between 20 and 200 nm with narrow distributions. They are transparent or translucent with a bluish colouration. So, the definition is different from that of sub-micron emulsions.

Applications of Nanoemulsions

- Drug and gene delivery
- Enhancement of skin permeation
- Extended drug release
- Antimicrobial activity
- Medical applications
  - Parenteral route (propofol and diazepam)
  - Ocular route (pilocarpine hydrochloride)
  - Nasal route (peptide and vaccine)
  - Topical route

Applications of Multiemulsions

- Multiple emulsions in cancer therapy
- Vaccine/vaccine adjuvant
- Oxygen substitute
- Multiple emulsions in diabetes: Surfactant-coated insulin was dispersed in the oil by ultrasonification, this dispersion was mixed with the outer water phase with a homogenizer.
- As antidiabetic: Multiple emulsions of chloroquine, an antimalarial agent has been successfully prepared and had been found to mask the bitter taste efficiently. Taste masking of chlorpromazine, an antipsychotic drug has also been reported by multiple emulsions.
- Drug over dosage treatment: This system could be utilized for the over dosage treatment by utilizing the difference in the pH, e.g. barbiturates, salicylates, etc.
- These are used as antifungals to treat topical fungal infections, e.g. itraconazol, miconazol nitrate emulsified gel.
- Terbinafin emulsion gel is an under-eye emulsion gel and is used for:
  - Moisturizing effect
  - Provide comfort to delicate eye
  - For skin repair
  - To get rid of skin circles
  - Provide protection against excessive dehydration.

QUESTIONS

A. Short Answer Type Questions

1. Describe the strategies used in drug targeting.
2. Discuss about the components of drug targeting.
3. What are ideal characteristics of drug candidate for targeted drug delivery?
4. Define liposomes and aquasome.
5. Mention in brief evaluation of liposomes.
6. Discuss about the application of liposomes.
7. Write a short note on resealed erythrocytes specialized.
8. What are niosomes? Give their method of preparation.
9. Give a short note on electrosomes.
10. Write the uses of aquasomes.
11. Differentiate between niosomes and liposomes.

B. Long Answer Type Questions

1. What is targeted drug delivery? Give its advantages and disadvantages in detail.
2. Write different types of liposomes. Give their methods of preparation.
3. Define phytosome. Give its method of preparation.
4. Discuss the pharmaceutical application of phytosomes in detail.
5. Explain the term nanoparticles and discuss their different types and method of preparation.

Ocular and Intrauterine Drug Delivery Systems

OCULAR DRUG DELIVERY SYSTEMS

Introduction

In the past two decades, the arena of ocular drug delivery technologies has dynamically advanced and results in newer therapeutic interventions for chronic ocular disorders. The main objectives of any ocular drug delivery system are to:

- Maintain therapeutic drug concentrations at the target site
- Reduce dosage frequency
- To overcome various dynamic and static ocular barriers.

Most importantly, the drug delivery system should cause no adverse ocular reactions and aim to achieve enhance drug bioavailability. Ocular pathological disorders are generally describing as anterior segment and posterior segment disorders. Clinicians treat anterior segment disorders like dry eye disease, cataract and allergic conjunctivitis by topical eyedrops. The major disadvantage of topically applied ophthalmic formulations is relatively low ocular bioavailability. This can be accounted to high tear-fluid turnover rates and high nasolacrimal drainage. Novel ocular drug delivery approaches including nanomicelles, nanoparticles, drug eluting contact lenses, ocular inserts and ocular devices that allow enhance peroneal residence and enhance bioavailability of the therapeutic agents. Ocular pathological conditions involving the posterior segment generally result in vision loss due to damage to the retina. Hyperglycaemia for a prolonged period of time can cause damage to the retinal endothelial cells causing back of the eye disorders like diabetic retinopathy (DR), diabetic macular oedema (DME) and retinal vein occlusion (RVO). High oxidative stress, endoplasmic reticulum (ER) stress and ageing can damage the retinal pigmented epithelial cells (RPE) and Bruch's membrane in the macular region leading to the death of the photoreceptors. Such pathological conditions can cause retinal degenerative disorders like age-related macular degeneration (AMD). Retinal and choroidal neovascularization (CNV) evident in back of the eye disorders is primarily due to overexpression of vascular endothelial growth (VEGF) receptor. Before the invention of anti-VEGF agents, the gold standard treatment of these disorders was the application of laser photocoagulation to lower overall oxygen demand of the retina. This therapy allowed suppression of CNV and retinal neovascularization. Since then, clinicians have introduced a plethora of anti-VEGF agents in the market including pegaptanib, bevacizumab (off-label), ranibizumab and aflibercept for treatment of back of the eye disorders with neovascularization. Clinicians administer these agents as intravitreal injections, which has drawbacks like retinal haemorrhage and retinal detachment. Moreover, intravitreal injections lack patient compliance. Novel ocular drug delivery technologies like nanoformulations, implants and other ocular devices allow enhanced drug residence time at the target tissue along with improvements of pharmacological response. Developments in novel drug delivery technologies can ultimately improve pharmacological action of drugs at the target tissue by elevating the concentrations and ocular bioavailability of the required therapeutic agent.

Modes of Administration, Barriers, and their Significance in Ocular Drug Delivery

Compared with drug delivery to other parts of the body, ocular drug delivery has met with significant challenges posed by various ocular barriers. Many of these barriers are inherent and unique to ocular anatomy and physiology making it a challenging task for drug delivery scientists. These barriers are specific depending upon the route of administration, viz. topical, systemic, and injectable. Most of these are anatomical and physiological barriers that normally protect the eye from toxicants. Moreover, various preformulation and formulation factors need to be considered while designing an ophthalmic formulation. Table 5.1 summarizes various routes of administration, their benefits, and challenges in ocular drug delivery. Figure 5.1 represents important parts of the eye along with different routes of drug administration represented in italics.

Topical Administration

Topical administration, mostly in the form of eyedrops, is employed to treat anterior segment diseases. For most of the topically applied drugs, the site of action is usually different layers of the cornea, conjunctiva, sclera, and the other tissues of the anterior segment such as the iris and ciliary body (anterior uvea). Upon administration, precorneal factors and anatomical barriers negatively affect the bioavailability of topical formulations. Precorneal factors include solution drainage, blinking, tear film, tear

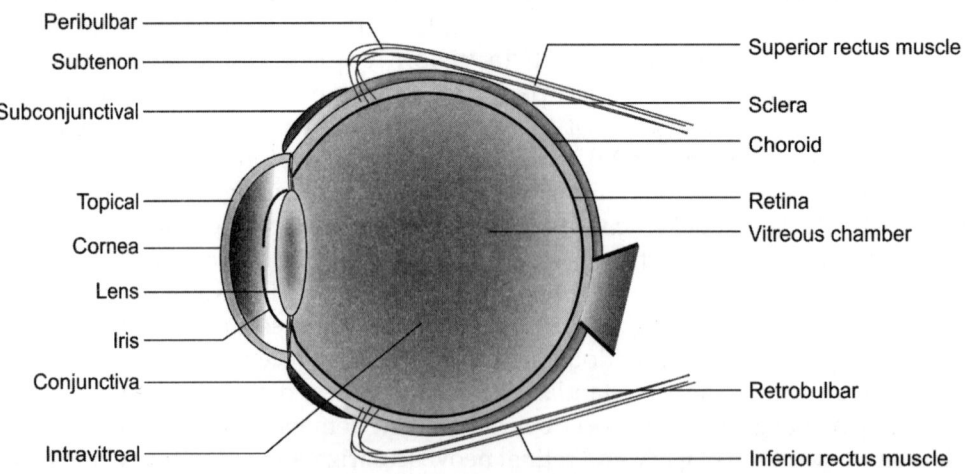

Fig 5.1: Routes of drug administration to eye

Table 5.1: Summary of routes of administration, benefits, and challenges in ocular delivery

Routes	Benefits	Challenges	Application in the treatment of disease
Topical	High patient compliance, self-administrable and non-invasive	Higher tear dilution and turnover rate, cornea act as barrier, efflux pump	Keratitis, uveitis, conjunctivitis, scleritis
Oral/systemic	Patient compliance, and non-invasive route of administration	BAB, BRB, high dosing cause toxicity	Scleritis, episcleritis, CMV retinitis, PU
Intravitreal	Direct delivery to vitreous and retina, sustains drug levels, evades, BRB	Retinal detachment, haemorrhage, contract	AMD, PU, BRVO, CRVO, DME, CME
Intracameral	Provides higher drug level in the anterior chamber, eliminates usage of topical drops, reduces corneal and systemic side effects seen with topical steroid therapy	TASS, TECDS	Anaesthesia, prevention of endophthalmitis
Subconjunctival	Delivery to anterior and posterior segments, site for depot formulation	Conjunctivital and choroidal circulation	Glaucoma, CMV retinitis, AMD, PU
Subtenon	High vitreal drug levels, relatively non-invasive, fewer complications, unlike intravitreal therapy	RPE, chemosis	Anaesthesia
Retrobulbar	Administer high local doses of anaesthetics, more effective than peribular, minimal influence on IOP	Retrobulbar haemorrhage, respiratory arrest	AMD
Posterior juxtascleral	Safe for delivery of depot formulation, sustain drug levels up to 6 months to the macula, avoids risk of endophthalmitis and intraocular damage	Requires surgery and RPE acts as barrier	

turnover, and induced lacrimation. Tear film, whose composition and amount are determinants of a healthy ocular surface, offers the first resistance due to its high turnover rate. Mucin present in the tear film plays a protective role by forming a hydrophilic layer that moves over the glycocalyx of the ocular surface and clears debris and pathogens. Human tear volume is estimated to be 7 µl, and the cul-de-sac can transiently contain around 30 µl of the administered eyedrop. However, tear film displays a rapid restoration time of 2–3 min, and most of the topically administered solutions are washed away within just 15–30 sec after instillation. Considering all the precorneal factors, contact time with the absorptive membranes is lower, which is considered to be the primary reason for less than 5% of the applied dose reaching the intraocular tissues.

In addition, various layers of the cornea, conjunctiva, and sclera play an important role in drug permeation. The cornea, the anterior most layer of the eye, is a mechanical barrier which limits the entry of exogenous substances into the eye and protects the ocular tissues. It can be mainly divided into the epithelium, stroma, and endothelium. Each layer offers a different polarity and a potential rate-limiting structure for drug permeation. The corneal epithelium is lipoidal in nature which contains 90% of the total cells in the cornea and poses a significant resistance for permeation of topically administered hydrophilic drugs. Furthermore, superficial corneal epithelial cells are joined to one another by desmosomes and are surrounded by ribbon-like tight junctional complexes (zonula occludens). Presence of these tight junctional complexes retards paracellular drug permeation from the tear film into intercellular spaces of the epithelium as well as inner layers of the cornea.

The stroma, which comprises 90% of the corneal thickness, is made up of an extracellular matrix and consists of a lamellar arrangement of collagen fibrils. The highly hydrated structure of the stroma poses a significant barrier to permeation of lipophilic drug molecules. Endothelium is the innermost monolayer of hexagonal-shaped cells. Even though endothelium is a separating barrier between the stroma and aqueous humour, it helps maintain the aqueous humour and corneal transparency due to its selective carrier-mediated transport and secretory function. Furthermore, the corneal endothelial junctions are leaky and facilitate the passage of macromolecules between the aqueous humour and stroma. Thus, corneal layers, particularly the epithelium and stroma, are considered as major barriers for ocular drug delivery. It is vital to understand that the permeant should have an amphipathic nature in order to permeate through these layers. Compared to cornea, conjunctival drug absorption is considered to be non-productive due to the presence of conjunctival blood capillaries and lymphatics, which can cause significant drug loss into the systemic circulation thereby lowering ocular bioavailability. Conjunctival epithelial tight junctions can further retard passive movement of hydrophilic molecules. The sclera, which is continuous with the cornea, originates from the limbus and extends posteriorly throughout the remainder of the globe. The sclera mainly consists of collagen fibres and proteoglycans embedded in an extracellular matrix. Permeability through the sclera is considered to be comparable to that of the corneal stroma. Recent reports indicate that the permeability of drug molecules across the sclera is inversely proportional to the molecular radius. Dextrans with linear structures were less permeable as compared to globular proteins. Furthermore, the charge of the drug molecule also affects its permeability across the sclera. Positively charged molecules exhibit poor permeability presumably due to their binding to the negatively charged proteoglycan matrix.

Systemic (Parenteral) Administration

Following systemic administration, the blood–aqueous barrier and blood–retinal barrier are the major barriers for anterior segment and posterior segment ocular drug delivery, respectively. Blood–aqueous barrier consists of two discrete cell layers located in the anterior segment of the eye, viz. the endothelium of the iris/ciliary blood vessels and the non-pigmented ciliary epithelium. Both cell layers express tight junctional complexes and prevent the entry of solutes into the intraocular environment such as the aqueous humour. Blood–retinal barrier restricts the entry of the therapeutic agents from blood into the posterior segment. It is composed of two types of cells, i.e. retinal capillary endothelial cells and retinal pigment epithelium cells (RPE) known as the inner and outer blood–retinal barrier, respectively. RPE, located between the neural retina and the choroid, is a monolayer of highly specialized cells. RPE aids in biochemical functions by selective transport of molecules between photoreceptors and choriocapillaris. Furthermore, it maintains the visual system by uptake and conversion of retinoids. However, tight junctions of the RPE efficiently restrict intercellular permeation. Following oral or intravenous dosing, drugs can easily enter into the choroid due to its high vasculature compared to retinal capillaries. The choriocapillaris is fenestrated resulting in rapid equilibration of drug molecules present in the bloodstream with the extravascular space of the choroid. However, outer blood–retinal barrier (RPE) restricts further entry of drugs from the choroid into the retina. Even though it is ideal to deliver the drug to the retina via systemic administration, it is still a challenge due to the blood-retinal barrier, which strictly regulates drug permeation from blood to the retina. Hence, specific oral or intravenous targeting systems are needed to transport molecules through the choroid into deeper layers of the retina.

Recent advancements in nanotechnology encouraged researchers to find ways to overcome blood–retinal barrier. In one such study using C57BL/6 mice, the researchers demonstrated that intravenously administered 20 nm gold nanoparticles could pass through the blood–retinal barrier and distribute in all the retinal layers without cytotoxicity. The viability of retinal endothelial cells, astrocytes, and retinoblastomal cells was also not affected. In contrast, larger 100 nm nanoparticles were not detected in the retina. A few attempts have also been made for gene delivery to the eye by intravenous route of administration. A diffuse expression of SV40/β-galactosidase gene in mouse inner retina, RPE, iris, as well as conjunctival epithelium, was observed upon intravenous administration of polyethylene glycol (PEG) conjugated immunoliposomes. A more recent report demonstrates the utility of intravenous administration of transferrin, arginine–glycine–aspartic acid peptide, or dual-functionalized poly (lactide-co-glycolide) (PLGA) nanoparticles. These functionalized PLGA nanoparticles are successful in targeted delivery of antivascular endothelial growth factor intraceptor plasmid to choroidal neovascularization (CNV) lesions. The delivery of nanoparticles to the neovascular eye is attributed to the leaky blood–retinal barrier as a result of CNV in the laser-treated rat eye. Pharmacokinetic studies involving various drugs such as micafungin, marbofloxacin, and amphotericin B demonstrated that these drugs are distributed in ocular tissues upon intravenous administration. One marketed intravenously administered formulation is Visudyne, which is used in photodynamic therapy for the treatment of wet age-related macular degeneration (AMD). However, owing to the toxicity and delivery concerns, intravenous administration is not very common in treating ocular disorders.

Oral Administration

Oral delivery or in combination with topical delivery is investigated for different reasons. Topical delivery alone failed to produce therapeutic concentrations in the posterior segment. Also, oral delivery was studied as a possible non-invasive and patient preferred route to treat chronic retinal diseases as compared to injectable route. However, limited accessibility to many of the targeted ocular tissues limits the utility of oral administration which necessitates high dosage to observe significant therapeutic efficacy. This can result in systemic side effects. Hence, parameters such as safety and toxicity need to be considered when trying to obtain a therapeutic response in the eye upon oral administration. For example, in glaucoma therapy, oral carbonic anhydrase inhibitors, such as acetazolamide and ethoxzolamide, have been discontinued in most of the cases due to their systemic toxicity. The oral route is not predominant, and only a limited number of compounds were investigated for ocular drug delivery. These include various classes of drugs such as analgesics, antibiotics, antivirals, antineoplastic agents, and omega-6 fatty acids. A major prerequisite of the oral route for ocular applications is high oral bioavailability of the drug. Following oral absorption, molecules in systemic circulation must also cross the blood–aqueous and blood–retinal barriers.

Periocular and Intravitreal Administration

Although not very patient compliant, these routes are employed partly to overcome the inefficiency of topical and systemic dosing to deliver therapeutic drug concentrations to the posterior segment. Moreover, systemic administration may lead to side effects making it a less desirable delivery route for geriatric patients. The periocular route includes subconjunctival, subtenon, retrobulbar, and peribulbar administration and is comparatively less invasive than intravitreal route (see Table 5.1). The drug administered by periocular injections can reach the posterior segment by three different pathways: Transscleral pathway; systemic circulation through the choroid; and the anterior pathway through the tear film, cornea, aqueous humour, and the vitreous humour. Subconjunctival injection obviates the conjunctival epithelial barrier, which is rate-limiting for permeation of water-soluble drugs. Thus, the transscleral route bypasses cornea–conjunctiva barrier. Nevertheless, various dynamic, static, and metabolic barriers limit drug access to the posterior segment. Dynamic barriers include conjunctival blood and lymphatic circulation. Various authors reported rapid drug elimination via these pathways following subconjunctival administration. As a result, the formulation is drained into systemic circulation thereby lowering ocular bioavailability. Thus, drug elimination from the subconjunctival space becomes a major determinant of the vitreous drug levels following subconjunctival administration. The molecules that escape conjunctival vasculature permeate through sclera and choroid to reach the neural retina and photoreceptor cells. The sclera is not a major barrier as it is more permeable than the cornea. Moreover, permeability across the sclera is independent of lipophilicity unlike corneal and conjunctival layers but depends primarily on the molecular radius. However, choroid is a significant barrier as high choroidal blood flow can also eliminate a considerable fraction of drug before it can reach the neural retina. Furthermore, blood–retinal barriers limit drug availability to the photoreceptor cells. Unlike periocular injections, the intravitreal injection offers distinct advantages as the molecules are directly inserted into the vitreous. However, drug distribution in the vitreous is non-uniform. Small molecules can rapidly distribute through the vitreous, whereas the diffusion of larger molecules is restricted. This distribution also depends on the pathophysiological condition and molecular weight of the administered drug. The vitreous also acts as a barrier for retinal gene delivery following an intravitreal injection. Hyaluronan, a negatively charged glycosaminoglycan present in the vitreous, can interact with cationic lipid, polymeric, and liposomal DNA complexes. This interaction can lead to severe aggregation and complete immobilization of DNA/cationic liposome complexes. Similarly, mobility of nanoparticles in the vitreous depends on their structure and surface charge. Polystyrene nanospheres do not diffuse freely into the vitreous due to their adherence to collagen fibrillar structures. Hence, surface modification of nanospheres with hydrophilic PEG chains has been performed. A recent study using human serum albumin nanoparticles also demonstrated that anionic nanoparticles with a zeta potential of –33.3 mV diffused more freely in the vitreous than cationic particles with a zeta potential of 11.7 mV. The inner limiting membrane (ILM), the cell layer separating the retina and the vitreous, is a barrier for retinal delivery following intravitreal administration of gene-based therapeutics. For example, the ILM poses a barrier for penetration of the adeno-associated virus into the retina from the vitreous. Mild digestion of ILM enhanced transduction of multiple retinal cell types from the vitreous indicating its high barrier property. Moreover, drug transport from vitreous to the outer segments of retina and choroid is more complex due to the presence of RPE.

The half-life in the vitreous is another factor that can determine the therapeutic efficacy. Following intravitreal injection, the drug is eliminated either by the anterior route or posterior route. The anterior elimination route involves drug diffusion across the vitreous into the aqueous humour through zonular spaces followed by elimination through aqueous turnover and uveal blood flow. The posterior elimination pathway involves drug permeation across the blood–retinal barrier and requires optimum passive permeability or active transport mechanisms. As a result, hydrophilicity and large molecular weight tend to increase the half-life of the compounds in the vitreous humour.

Posterior Juxtascleral

Safe for delivery of depot formulation, sustain drug levels up to 6 months to the macula, avoids risk of endophthalmitis and intraocular damage, requires surgery and RPE acts as barrier.

Mechanism of Drug Release

The mechanism of controlled drug release into the eye is as follows:
a. Diffusion
b. Osmosis
c. Bio-erosion

a. **Diffusion:** In the diffusion mechanism, the drug is released continuously at a controlled rate through the membrane into the tear fluid. If the insert is formed of a solid non-erodible body with pores and dispersed drug. The release of drug can take place via diffusion through the pores. Controlled release can be further regulated by gradual dissolution of solid dispersed drug within this matrix as a result of inward diffusion of aqueous solutions.

b. **Osmosis:** In the osmosis mechanism, the insert comprises a transverse impermeable elastic membrane dividing the interior of the insert into a first compartment and a second compartment; the first compartment is bounded by a semipermeable membrane and the impermeable elastic membrane, and the second compartment is bounded by an impermeable membrane and the second compartment provides a reservoir for the drug which again is in liquid or gel form. When the insert is placed in the aqueous environment of the eye, water diffuses into the first compartment and stretches the elastic membrane to expand the first compartment and contract the second compartment so that the drug is forced through the drug release aperture.

c. **Bio-erosion:** In the bio-erosion mechanism, the configuration of the body of the insert is constituted from a matrix of bio-erodible material in which the drug is dispersed. Contact of the insert with tear fluid results in controlled sustained release of the drug by bio-erosion of the matrix. The drug may be dispersed uniformly throughout the matrix but it is believed that a more controlled release is obtained, if the drug is superficially concentrated in the matrix.

Overcome in Barriers to Ocular Drug Delivery through Different Doses Forms

1. **Liquids:** Solutions, suspensions, sol to gel systems, sprays
2. **Solids:** Ocular inserts, contact lenses, corneal shield, artificial tear inserts, filter paper strips.
3. **Semisolids:** Ointments, gels
4. **Miscellaneous:** Ocular iontophoresis, vesicular systems, mucoadhesive dosage forms, particulates, ocular penetration.

Conventional Ocular Drug Delivery Systems

Topical drop instillation into the lower precorneal pocket is a patient compliant and widely recommended route of drug administration. However, most of the topically administered dose is lost due to reflux blinking and only 20% (–7 µl) of instilled dose is retained in the precorneal pocket concentration of drug available in the precorneal area acts as a driving force for its passive diffusion across cornea. However, for efficient ocular drug delivery with eyedrops, high corneal permeation with longer drug cornea contact time is required. Several efforts have been made toward improving precorneal residence time and corneal penetration. To improve corneal permeation iontophoresis, prodrugs, ion-pair forming agents and cyclodextrins are employed. There are a wide range of ophthalmic products available in the market out of which around 70% of prescriptions include conventional eyedrops. The reasons may be due to ease of bulk scale manufacturing, high patient acceptability, drug product efficacy, stability and cost-effectiveness.

Topical Liquid/Solution Eyedrops

Topical drops are the most convenient, safe, immediately active, patient compliant and non-invasive mode of ocular drug administration. An eyedrop solution provides a pulse drug permeation post-topical drop instillation, after which its concentration rapidly declines. The kinetics of drug concentration decline may follow an approximate first order. Therefore, to improve drug contact time, permeation and ocular bioavailability; various additives may be added to topical eyedrops such as viscosity enhancers, permeation enhancers and cyclodextrins. Viscosity enhancers improve precorneal residence time and bioavailability upon topical drop administration by enhancing formulation viscosity. Examples of viscosity enhancers include hydroxy methyl cellulose, hydroxy ethyl cellulose, sodium carboxy methyl cellulose, hydroxypropyl methyl cellulose and polyalcohol. Permeation enhancers improve corneal uptake by modifying the corneal integrity. Other additives such as chelating agents, preservatives, surface active agents and bile salts were studied as possible permeation enhancers. Benzalkonium chloride, polyoxyethylene glycol ethers (lauryl, stearyl and oleyl), ethylenediaminetetra-acetic acid sodium salt, sodium taurocholate, saponins and cremophor EL are the examples of permeation enhancers investigated for improving ocular delivery.

Emulsions

An emulsion-based formulation approach offers an advantage to improve both solubility and bioavailability of drugs. There are two types of emulsions which are commercially exploited as vehicles for active pharmaceuticals: Oil in water (O/W) and water in oil (W/O) emulsion systems. For ophthalmic drug delivery, O/W emulsion is common and widely preferred over W/O system. The reasons include less irritation and better ocular tolerance of O/W emulsion. Restasise™, Refresh Endura® (a non-medicated emulsion for eye lubrication) and AzaSite® are the examples of currently marketed ocular emulsions in the United States. Several studies have demonstrated applicability of emulsions in improving precorneal residence time, drug corneal permeation, providing sustain drug release and thereby enhancing ocular bioavailability.

Suspensions

Suspensions are another class of non-invasive ocular topical drop drug carrier system. Suspension may be defined as dispersion of finely divided insoluble API in an aqueous solvent consisting of a suitable suspending and dispersing agent. In other words, the carrier solvent system is a saturated solution of API. Suspension particles retain in precorneal pocket and thereby improve drug contact time and duration of action relative to drug solution. Duration of drug action for suspension is particle size dependent. Smaller size particle replenishes the drug absorbed into ocular tissues from precorneal pocket. While on the other hand, larger particle size helps retain particles for longer time and slow drug dissolution. Thus, an optimal particle size is expected to result in optimum drug activity. Several suspension formulations are marketed worldwide to treat ocular bacterial infections. TobraDex® suspension is one of the widely recommended commercial products for subjects responding to steroid therapy. TobraDex® is a combination product of antibiotic, tobramycin (0.3%), and steroid, dexamethasone (0.1%). The major drawback of this commercial product is high viscosity. Recently, Scoper et al made attempts to reduce the viscosity of TobraDex® and to improve its *in vivo* pharmacokinetics along with bactericidal activity.

Ointments

Ophthalmic ointments are another class of carrier system developed for topical application. Ocular ointment comprises mixture of semisolid and a solid hydrocarbon (paraffin) that has a melting point at physiological ocular temperature (34°C). The choice of hydrocarbon is dependent on biocompatibility. Ointments help to improve ocular bioavailability and sustain the drug release. Vancomycin hydrochloride (VCM) is a glycopeptides antibiotic with an excellent activity against aerobic and anaerobic gram-positive bacteria and methicillin and cephem resistant *Staphylococcus aureus* (MRSA). In spite of better activity of VCM, no appropriate topical formulation was available in the market. Better ocular tissue permeability of VCM was not expected in a normal eye, but a few clinical effects of VCM solution were reported in ocular disease treatment. The reason for the observed effects was hypothesized due to broken ocular barrier system, which might have improved drug permeation.

Novel Ocular Drug Delivery Systems

Nanotechnology-based ocular drug delivery in last a few decades; many approaches have been utilized for the treatment of ocular diseases. Nanotechnology-based ophthalmic formulations are one of the approaches which is currently being pursued for both anterior, as well as posterior segment drug delivery. Nanotechnology-based systems with an appropriate particle size can be designed to ensure low irritation, adequate bioavailability, and ocular tissue compatibility. Several nanocarriers, such as nanoparticles, nanosuspensions, liposomes, nanomicelles and dendrimers have been developed for ocular drug delivery. Some of them have shown promising results for improving ocular bioavailability.

Nanomicelles

Nanomicelles are the most commonly used carrier systems to formulate therapeutic agents into clear aqueous solutions. In general, these nanomicelles are made with amphiphilic molecules. These molecules may be surfactant or polymeric in nature. Currently, tremendous interest is being shown towards development of nanomicellar formulation-based technology for ocular drug delivery. The reasons may be attributed due to their high drug encapsulation capability, ease of preparation, small size, and hydrophilic nanomicellar corona generating aqueous solution. In addition, micellar formulation can enhance the bioavailability of the therapeutic drugs in ocular tissues, suggesting better therapeutic outcomes. So far, several proofs of concept studies have been conducted to investigate the applicability of nanomicelles in ocular drug delivery.

Nanoparticles

Nanoparticles are colloidal carriers with a size range of 10 to 1000 nm. For ophthalmic delivery, nanoparticles are generally composed of lipids, proteins, natural or synthetic polymers such as albumin, sodium alginate, chitosan, poly (lactide-co-glycolide) (PLGA), poly (lactic acid) (PLA) and polycaprolactone. Drug-loaded nanoparticles can be nanocapsules or nanospheres. In nanocapsules, drug is enclosed inside the polymeric shell while in nanospheres; drug is uniformly distributed throughout polymeric matrix. From past few decades, nanoparticles have gained attention for ocular drug delivery and several researchers have made attempts to develop drug-loaded nanoparticles for delivery to both anterior and posterior ocular tissues.

Nanoparticles represent a promising candidate for ocular drug delivery because of small size leading to low irritation and sustained release property avoiding frequent administration. However, like aqueous solutions, nanoparticles may be eliminated rapidly from precorneal pocket. Hence, for topical administration, nanoparticles with mucoadhesive properties have been developed to improve precorneal residence time. Polyethylene glycol (PEG), chitosan and hyaluronic acid are commonly employed to improve precorneal residence time of nanoparticles. Chitosan coating is most widely explored for improving precorneal residence of nanoparticles. The chitosan is positively charged and hence it binds to negatively charged corneal surface and thereby improves precorneal residence and decreases clearance. For instance, natamycin-loaded chitosan/ lecithin nanoparticles exhibited high ocular bioavailability at reduced dose and dosing frequency in rabbit eye compared to marketed suspension.

Nanosuspensions

Nanosuspensions are colloidal dispersion of submicron drug particles stabilized by polymer(s) or surfactant(s). It is emerged as promising strategy for delivery of hydrophobic drugs. For ocular delivery, it provides several advantages such as sterilization, ease of eyedrop formulation, less irritation, increase precorneal residence time and enhancement in ocular bioavailability of drugs which are insoluble in tear fluid. The efficacy of nanosuspensions in improving ocular bioavailability of glucocorticoids has been demonstrated in several research studies. Glucocorticoids such as prednisolone, dexamethasone and hydrocortisone are widely recommended for the treatment of inflammatory conditions affecting anterior segment ocular tissues. The current therapy with these drugs requires frequent administration at higher doses which induce cataract formation, glaucoma, and damage optic nerve. Efforts have been made toward improving ocular bioavailability of glucocorticoids by formulating as nanosuspensions. For instance, compared ocular bioavailability of various glucocorticoids (prednisolone, dexamethasone and hydrocortisone) from nanosuspensions, solutions and microcrystalline suspensions.

Liposomes

Liposomes are lipid vesicles with one or more phospholipid bilayers enclosing an aqueous core. The size of liposomes usually ranges from 0.08 to 10.00 μm and based on the size and phospholipid bilayers, liposomes can be classified as small unilamellar vesicles (10–100 nm), large unilamellar vesicles (100–300 nm) and multilamellar vesicles (contains more than one bilayer). For ophthalmic applications, liposomes represent ideal delivery systems due to excellent biocompatibility, cell membrane-like structure and ability to encapsulate both hydrophilic and hydrophobic drugs. Liposomes have demonstrated good effectiveness for both anterior and posterior segment ocular delivery in several research studies. In a recent study, for delivery of latanoprost to anterior segment ocular tissues. The single subconjunctival injection of latanoprost/liposomal formulation in rabbit eye produced sustained IOP lowering effect over a period of 50 days with IOP reduction comparable to daily eyedrop administration. For drug delivery to anterior segment of the eye, efforts are mainly put toward improving precorneal residence time by incorporating positively charged lipids or mucoadhesive polymer in liposomes.

Dendrimers

Dendrimers are characterized as nanosized, highly branched, star-shaped polymeric systems. These branched polymeric systems are available in different molecular weights with terminal end amine, hydroxyl or carboxyl functional group. The terminal functional group may be utilized to conjugate targeting moieties. Dendrimers are being employed as carrier systems in drug delivery. Selection of molecular weight, size, surface charge, molecular geometry and functional group are critical to deliver drugs. The highly branched structure of dendrimers allows incorporation of wide range of drugs, hydrophobic as well as hydrophilic. In ocular drug delivery, a few promising results were reported with these branched polymeric systems.

In Situ Gelling Systems

In situ hydrogels refer to the polymeric solutions which undergo sol-gel phase transition to form viscoelastic gel in response to environmental stimuli. Gelation can be elicited by changes in temperature, pH and ions or can also be induced by UV irradiation. For ocular delivery, research studies have been more focused toward development of thermosensitive gels which respond to changes in temperature. Several thermogelling polymers have been reported for ocular delivery which include poloxamers, multiblock copolymers made of polycaprolactone, polyethylene glycol, polylactide, polyglycolide, poly (n-isopropylacrylamide) and chitosan.

Contact Lens

Contact lenses are thin, and curved shape plastic discs which are designed to cover the cornea. After application, contact lens adheres to the film of tears over the cornea due to the surface tension. Drug-loaded contact lenses have been developed for ocular delivery of numerous drugs such as β-blockers, antihistamines and antimicrobials. It is postulated that in presence of contact lens, drug molecules have longer residence time in the post-lens tear film which ultimately led to higher drug flux through cornea with less drug inflow into the nasolacrimal duct. Usually, drug is loaded into contact lens by soaking them in drug solutions. These soaked contact lenses demonstrated higher efficiency in delivering drug compared to conventional eyedrops. Observed much higher bioavailability of dexamethasone (DX) from poly (hydroxyethyl-methacrylate) (PHEMA) contact lenses in comparison to eyedrops.

Implants

Intraocular implants are specifically designed to provide localized controlled drug release over an extended period. These devices help in circumventing multiple intraocular injections and associated complications. Usually, for drug delivery to posterior ocular tissues, implants are placed intravitreally by making incision through minor surgery at pars plana which is located posterior to the lens and anterior to the retina. Though implantation is invasive procedure, these devices are gaining interest due to their associated advantages such as sustained drug release, local drug release to diseased ocular tissues in therapeutic levels, reduced side effects and ability to circumvent blood–retinal barrier. Several implantable devices have been developed for ocular drug delivery especially for the treatment of chronic vitreoretinal diseases.

Microneedles

Microneedle-based technique is an emerging and minimally invasive mode of drug delivery to posterior ocular tissues. This technique may provide efficient treatment strategy for vision threatening posterior ocular diseases such as age-related macular degeneration, diabetic retinopathy and posterior uveitis. This new microneedle-based administration strategy may reduce the risk and complications associated with intravitreal injections such as retinal detachment, haemorrhage, cataract, endophthalmitis and pseudo-endophthalmitis. Moreover, this strategy may help to circumvent blood–retinal barrier and deliver therapeutic drug levels to retina/choroid. Microneedles are custom designed to penetrate only hundreds of microns into sclera, so that damage to deeper ocular tissues may be avoided.

Ocular Inserts

Ophthalmic insert defined as sterile preparation with solid or semisolid consisting and whose size and sharp are especially designed for ophthalmic application. They offer several advantages as increase ocular residence, possibility of releasing drug at a slow constant rate, accurate dosing and increased shelf life with respect to aqueous solutions. Ocusert®, pilocarpine ocular therapeutic system is the first product marketed by Alza incorporation USA from this category.

Advantages of Ocular Inserts

Ocular inserts offer several advantages, which can be summarized as follows:
- Diminution of complete absorption (which occurs freely with eyedrops via the nasolacrimal canal and nasal mucosa)
- Possibility of releasing drugs at a slow, steady rate
- Improved ocular habitation, hence an extended drug activity and an elevated bioavailability with respect to usual vehicles.
- Correct dosing (converse to eyedrops that can be shockingly instilled by the patient and are partially vanished after administration, each insert can be made to contain an accurate dose which is fully retained at the administration site)
- Improved shelf life with reference to aqueous solutions
- Better patient compliance, resulting from an abridged frequency of administration and a lesser incidence of visual and systemic side effects
- Exclusion of preservatives, thus plummeting the risk of sensitivity reactions
- Possibility of incorporating various novel chemical/technological approaches.

Disadvantages of Ocular Inserts

The disadvantages of ocular inserts are as follows:
- A principal disadvantage of ocular inserts resides in their 'solidity', i.e. in the fact that they are felt by the (often too sensitive) patients as a superfluous body in the eye. This may constitute a redoubtable physical and psychological obstruction to user recognition and compliance.
- Their movement in the region of the eye, in rare instances, the simple elimination is made more complicated by unnecessary movement of the insert to the upper fornix.

Formulation Methods of Ocusert

1. **Solvent casting method:** In this method using different ratios of drug and polymer, a number of batches are prepared. The polymer is dissolved in distilled water. A plasticizer is added to this solution under stirring conditions. The weighed amount of drug is added to above solution and stirred to get a uniform dispersion. After proper mixing, the casting solution is poured in clean glass petri dish and covered with an inverted funnel to allow slow and uniform evaporation at room temperature for 48 h. The dried film thus obtained is cut by cork borer into circular pieces of definite size containing drug. The ocular inserts are then stored in an airtight container (desiccator) under ambient condition.

2. **Glass substrate technique:** Drug reservoir film: 1% w/w polymer for example chitosan is soaked in 1% v/v acetic acid solution for 24 hours, to get a clear solution of chitosan in acetic acid solution. The solution is filtered through a muslin cloth to remove undissolved portion of the polymer (chitin). Required quantity of drug-β CD complex is added and vortexed for 15 minutes to dissolve the complex in chitosan solution. 1% w/v propylene glycol (plasticizer) is added to it and mixed well with stirrer. The viscous solution is kept aside for 30 minutes for complete expulsion of air bubbles. The rate controlling film is prepared. The film is casted by pouring solution into the centre of levelled glass mould and allowing it to dry at room temperature for 24 hours. After drying, films are cut into ocuserts of desired size so that each contains equal quantity of the drug. Then, the matrix is sandwiched between the rate controlling membranes using non-toxic, non-irritating, water

insoluble gum. They are wrapped in aluminium foil separately and stored in a desiccator.

3. **Melt extrusion technique:** Drugs for extraction acyclovir and the polymer are sieved through 60#, weighed and blended geometrically. The plasticizer is added and blended. The blend is then charged to the barrel of melt flow rate apparatus and extruded. The extrudate is cut into appropriate size and packed in polyethylene lined Al foil, heat sealed and sterilized by gamma radiation.

INTRAUTERINE DRUG DELIVERY SYSTEMS

Introduction

Intrauterine device (IUD) is a small object that is inserted through the cervix and placed in the uterus to prevent pregnancy. A small string hangs down from the IUD into the upper part of the vagina. The IUD is not noticeable during intercourse. IUDs can last 1–10 years. They affect the movements of eggs and sperm to prevent fertilization. They also change the lining of the uterus and prevent implantation. IUDs are 99.2–99.9% effective as birth control. They do not protect against sexually transmitted infections, including HIV/AIDS. Insertion of an IUD takes only about 5 to 10 minutes. Women health care provider will first do a pelvic exam to measure the size, shape, and position of uterus and other reproductive organs. The health care provider will then put antiseptic solution onto your cervix. The IUD will be inserted up through the opening of cervix into uterus. It is put inside using a special applicator that keeps the IUD flat and closed until it is at the top of uterus. Women may feel cramping, but it usually is not much. After the IUD has been inserted, health care provider will cut the string at the end of the IUD so that it is short enough where it would not bother partner. It will be long enough so it can check to make sure that the IUD is in place. Health care provider will then talk about what need to do about checking the string. An IUD prevents pregnancy by stopping sperm from reaching an egg that ovaries have released. It does this by not letting sperm go into the egg. An IUD also changes the lining of the uterus so an egg does not implant in the lining, if it has been fertilized. Therefore, the egg has no place to grow. IUDs are the most effective form of non-permanent birth control. They are more than 99% effective. This means that if 100 women use the copper IUD or the levonorgestrel IUS, less than one woman will become pregnant in a year.

Advantages

- Highly effective in preventing pregnancy
- Inexpensive
- Does not interrupt physical intercourse
- Does not require partner's involvement
- Can be used for a long period of time
- Can be used as an emergency method of birth control
- An IUD provides long-term contraception for 3 to 5 years and is cost-effective
- When you are ready to become pregnant, the IUD can be removed by a health care provider.
- It is convenient. You do not need to remember daily pills.

Disadvantages

- Does not protect against sexually transmitted infections (STIs). If you get a sexually transmitted infection, the IUD could increase the likelihood of developing.

- Pelvic inflammatory disease (infection of the reproductive organs), which may lead to infertility.
- May increase the likelihood of ectopic pregnancy (pregnancy outside the uterus).
- Can cause heavier and more painful periods.
- Cramping and discomfort during and 24–48 hours after insertion.
- There are risks during insertion and removal that your clinician should discuss with you before inserting an IUD.

Development of Intrauterine Devices (IUDs)

The philosophy behind the conception and development of the small T-shaped IUD is to use a device which is adapted to the size and shape of the uterine cavity rather than forcing the uterine cavity to adapt itself to the shape and size of the IUD. Although the plain T does not provide effective contraception, it provides a good platform for a potent antifertility agent. Incorporation of this drug with the plain T provided the first of the medicated IUDs. Subsequently, the Copper 7, the Nova T (Leiras Pharmaceutical, Turku, Finland), and the Multiload (Organon Pharmaceutical Company, Amsterdam, The Netherlands), in that order, are added to the copper-bearing family of IUD.

More recently, progestogens have been incorporated with the plain T, creating the second generic type of small medicated IUDs. The first of these, the Progestasert (Alza Corporation, Palo Alto, CA) contained progesterone, while the second was the Levonorgestrel T (Alza Corporation). Both of these IUDs affect a reduction in menstrual blood loss because of their suppressant action on the endometrium. There is also a possibility that their effects upon the endometrium and cervical mucus may provide a deterrent to ascending uterine and pelvic infections.

In this issue of fertility and sterility, a research paper presents clinical data from a 2-year comparison of levonorgestrel- and copper-releasing IUDs. This study illustrates a number of the generic modifications in IUDs which have been made over the past 20 years, and the authors discuss some of the advantages and disadvantages associated with them. It is apparent that while major advances have already been made in the field of intrauterine contraception, we can expect to see additional innovations and improvements in the future. It is quite possible that one of the next major modifications to be realized will be the development of a practical model of the tailless IUD.

QUESTIONS

A. Short Answer Type Questions

1. Write different barriers in ocular drug delivery system.
2. Give differences between conventional and novel ocular drug delivery system.
3. Describe the different routes uses for drug administration in ocular drug delivery system.
4. What is intrauterine drug delivery system? Discuss their advantages.

B. Long Answer Type Questions

1. What is ocusert? Describe different methods for preparation of ocusert.
2. Write in detail about the development of intrauterine devices.
3. Discuss the mechanism of drug release for ocular delivery system.
4. What do you mean by ocular drug delivery system? Give their merits and demerits in detail.

Submicron Cosmeceuticals and New Trends for Personalized Medicine

SUBMICRON COSMECEUTICALS

Introduction

Cosmetics are defined by the FDA as "articles intended to be applied to the human body or any part there of for cleansing, beautifying, promoting attractiveness, or altering the appearance". FDA does not have the legal authority to approve cosmetics before they go on the market. However, cosmetics must be safe for consumers and properly labelled. Companies and individuals who market cosmetics have a legal responsibility for the safety and labelling of their products. The word 'cosmeceutical' is used to define a product that fits the niche between a drug and cosmetics. It is used in the professional skin care arena to describe a product that has measurable biological action in the skin, like a drug, but is regulated as a cosmetic since it claims to affect appearance. Cosmeceuticals are not categorized by the FDA, but this term is used by skin scientists, physicians, and skin care professionals, to encourage the consumers to continue buying cosmetic products especially antiageing and sunscreen products, marketed by many manufacturers with scientific claims and natural positioning as a way to emphasize that using these products is not only necessary but also natural. Cosmeceuticals are the fastest growing segment of the personal care industry. Cosmeceutical formulations now have expanded from skin to body to hair and a number of topical cosmeceutical treatments for conditions such as photoaging, hyperpigmentation, wrinkles, and hair damage have come into widespread use. Recent researches focusing on cosmeceutical products highlighted strong growth perspectives in the coming years. According to them, expanding at a rapid compound annual growth rate of 7.7%, the global cosmetics market is expected to garner $429.8 billion by 2022. The global cosmeceutical market offers huge potential among the Asian countries, such as Japan, China, and India which are set to attract major players in the future. Japan has already made a remarkable position in the global cosmetics market and its position in the cosmeceutical segment is effectively improving.

Among the technologies used to develop elegant and effective cosmeceuticals, nanotechnology finds special place. In the cosmetic arena, it is believed that the smaller particles are readily absorbed into the skin and repair damage easily and more efficiently. Incorporation of nanotechnology in cosmeceuticals is aimed at making incense of perfumes last longer, sunscreens to protect the skin, antiaging creams to fight back the years, and moisturizers to maintain the hydration of skin. Some of the nanotechnology-based innovations are nanoemulsions (which are transparent and have unique tactile and texture properties), nanocapsules (which are used in skin care products), nanopigments (that are transparent and increase the efficiency of sunscreen products), liposome formulations (which contain small vesicles consisting of conventional cosmetic materials that protect oxygen or light sensitive cosmetic ingredients), niosomes, nanocrystals, solid lipid nanoparticles, carbon nanotubes, fullerenes, and dendrimers. The primary advantages of using nanoparticles in cosmeceuticals include improvement in the stability of cosmetic ingredients (e.g. vitamins, unsaturated fatty acids, and antioxidants) by encapsulating within the nanoparticles; efficient protection of the skin from harmful ultraviolet (UV) rays; aesthetically pleasing products (e.g. in mineral sunscreens, using smaller particles of active mineral allows them to be applied without leaving a noticeable white cast); targeting of active ingredient to the desired site and controlled release of active ingredients for prolonged effect.

Nanoparticles in Cosmeceuticals

Liposomes

Bangham, a researcher, published the first paper on liposomes in 1963, and it was in the early 1980s that Mezei and Gulasekharam reported the efficacy of liposomes in topical drug delivery. Liposomes are spherical, self-closed vesicles of colloidal dimensions, in which phospholipid bilayers sequester part of the solvent, in which they freely float into their interior. Liposomes typically vary in size between 20 nm and a few hundred micrometers. Liposomes are used in a variety of cosmeceuticals because they are biocompatible, biodegradable, non-toxic, and flexible vesicles and can encapsulate active ingredients easily. Liposomes have an ability to protect the encapsulated drug from external environment and are suitable for delivery of hydrophobic and hydrophilic compounds. These characteristics make them ideal candidate for the delivery of vitamins and other essential molecules to regenerate the epidermis. One of the main ingredients of liposome is phosphatidylcholine which has been used in skin care products (moisturizer, lotions, creams, etc.) and hair care products (shampoo, conditioner) due to its softening and conditioning properties. Several active ingredients (e.g. vitamins A, E, and K) and antioxidants (e.g. carotenoids, lycopene, and CoQ10) have been incorporated into liposomes which increases their physical and chemical stability when dispersed in water. Lipophilic compounds such as cholesterol and ceramides have been used in topical skin creams for many years, because they are the lipids found in normal skin tissue, and are easily incorporated into liposomes to improve skin hydration and to make the skin texture softer and smoother. "Capture" was the first liposomal antiaging cream launched by Dior in 1986.

Nanocapsule

The potential dermatological use of nanocapsules was investigated when the first nanocapsule-based cosmetic product was launched by the French company L'Oreal in 1995 in order to improve the impact of their cosmetics. The term nanocapsule is used for vesicular systems that are made up of a polymeric membrane in which an inner liquid core is encapsulated at the nanoscale level (10 to 100 nm).

Solid Lipid Nanoparticles

Solid lipid nanoparticles (SLNs) are submicron colloidal carriers whose size range from 50 to 1000 nm and are composed of physiological lipid, dispersed in water or in aqueous solution of surfactant. SLNs are popular in cosmeceuticals because of various advantages: These are composed of physiological and biodegradable lipids that exhibit low toxicity; the small size of SLNs ensures close contact with the stratum corneum and increases the penetration of active ingredients through the skin; SLNs provide occlusive properties that result in increased skin hydration. The products Nano Repair Q10 cream and Nano Repair Q10 Serum (Dr. Kurt Richter Laboratorien GmbH, Berlin, Germany) introduced to the cosmetic market in October 2005 revealed the success of lipid nanoparticles in the antiaging field. It has been found that SLNs possess characteristics of physical UV blockers on their own, thus offering the choice for developing a more effective sunscreen system with reduced side effects. In an *in vivo* study, it has been shown that skin hydration increases by 31% after 4 weeks by the addition of 4% SLNs to a conventional cream. SLNs are also advantageous as topical vehicle for perfumes. By incorporating perfumes/fragrances in SLNs, the release can be slowed down to provide prolonged effect.

Nanocrystals

Nanocrystals are aggregates composed of several hundreds to thousands of atoms that combine into a cluster and are in the size range of 10–400 nm used for the delivery of poorly soluble active. Nanocrystals appeared first in the cosmeceutical market in 2000 by Juvena with the product Juvedical having rutin. In a study, it was observed that compared to the water-soluble rutin glycoside (rutin with attached glucose), the nanocrystal formulation of original rutin molecule possesses 500 times higher bioactivity. A rutin nanosuspension with 5% rutin as non-dissolved nanocrystals was applied to the skin of human volunteers and compared to a 5% solution of a water-soluble rutin glycoside regarding photoprotection of the skin. In the aqueous nanosuspension, the solubility of rutin was 500 times lower as compared to the water-soluble derivative. It was observed that despite the 500 times lower concentration of dissolved rutin in the water phase of the nanocrystal suspension, the nanosuspension was about 25% more effective in photoprotection and the concentration of actives formulated as nanocrystals in the skin were much higher compared to water-soluble derivative or using the active in normal powder form.

Dendrimers

Dendrimers are organic chemical entities with a semipolymeric tree-like structure. The terminals of the branches provide a rich source of nanoparticles surface functionality. Their dimensions are extremely small, having diameters in the range of 2 to 10 nm. Dendrimers are an exciting new class of macromolecular architecture and an important component in the area of nanotechnology-based cosmeceuticals to treat varieties of skin conditions. L'Oreal, Unilever, and The Dow chemical company have several patents for the application of dendrimers in hair care, skin care, and nail care products. A patent on cosmetic formulation containing carbosiloxane dendrimer claimed that it can provide good water resistance, sebum resistance, glossiness, tactile sensation, and/or adhesive properties to the hair and/or skin.

Nanogold and Nanosilver

Gold and silver nanoparticles have been studied as a valuable material in cosmeceutical industry for their strong antibacterial and antifungal properties. These particles are widely used in cosmeceutical products like deodorant, face pack, antiaging cream, and so forth. An ointment containing silver nanoparticle was claimed to have antibacterial activity and can be used for skin inflammation and skin wound disinfection. A study conducted by French scientist Dr. Philippe Walter and his team, published in ACS Nanoletters, describes the synthesis of fluorescent gold nanoparticles inside human hair. It involved soaking white hairs in a solution of a gold compound. The hairs turned pale yellow and then darkened to a deep brown. Using an electron microscope, the scientists confirmed that the particles were forming inside the hair's central core cortex. The colour remained even after repeated washings.

Cubosomes

Cubosomes are discrete, submicron, nanostructured particles of bicontinuous cubic liquid crystalline phase. Recent research activities on the use of cubosome in personal care product areas varied from skin care to hair care and antiperspirants. The number of researches in association with cosmetic companies like L'Oreal and Nivea is trying to use cubosome particles as oil-in-water emulsion stabilizers and pollutant absorbents in cosmeceuticals.

Niosomes

Niosomes are non-ionic surfactant vesicles devised by using non-ionic surfactants. These vesicles possess high entrapment efficiency, improved chemical stability, and enhanced penetration, as well as lower production cost as compared to liposomes. In morphology, a niosome is a nanostructure with 100 nm to 200 μm in diameter, whose centre is an aqueous cavity enveloped by layers of non-ionic surfactant in lamellar phase. These have been evaluated as vesicular carriers for variety of drugs and cosmetics topically. Niosomes are found to be efficient in topical delivery of active ingredients as they can enhance residence time of the active ingredients in the stratum corneum as well as epidermis and also reduce the system absorption. By using niosomes, targeted delivery can also be achieved as the active ingredient is directly delivered to the specific site where therapeutic effect is desired.

Fullerene

Other nanoscale materials, such as carbon fullerene, have been used in some cosmetic products because of their antioxidative properties. They display potent scavenging capacities against radical oxygen species and they have been considered for their use in the preparation of skin rejuvenation cosmeceutical formulations. These structures are comprised of carbon rings and contain odd-numbered (like pentagon and heptagon) carbon rings, conferring a three-dimensional spherical shape. These structures have thus been called fullerenes or "Bucky balls". Fullerenes are highly hydrophobic and thus are not soluble in aqueous solutions, which initially limited their applications, but the use of surfactants or surface modifications has increased the ability of fullerenes to solubilize in water and brought more attention to their potential pharmaceutical uses.

Major Classes of Nanocosmeceuticals

Moisturizers

Stratum corneum is the primary barrier of the skin whose main purpose is to keep inside in and outside out. Water from the stratum corneum gets evaporated quickly leading to dehydration. This dehydration of skin can be averted by using moisturizers which provide flexibility to the skin. When moisturizers are applied to the skin, a thin film of humectant is formed which retains moisture and gives better appearance to the skin. Liposomes, nanoemulsions, SLNs are widely used moisturizing formulations because of their prolonged effects. These are considered to be the most useful product for the management of various skin conditions (e.g. atopic dermatitis, psoriasis, and pruritus).

Sunscreens

Sunscreens are widely used to protect the skin from harmful effects of sunrays on exposure. Zinc oxide (ZnO) and titanium dioxide (TiO$_2$) is the most effective approved mineral-based ingredient which protects the skin from sun damage. This mineral forms a materialistic barrier on the skin, reflects UVA and UVB rays from penetrating down to the deeper layers of skin, and is less irritating. The main drawback of traditional or conventional sunscreen is that, when applied, it leaves a white chalky layer on the skin. This is where nanoparticles come in. Improved sunscreens are just one of the many innovative uses of nanotechnology. Sunscreen products using nanoparticles of ZnO or TiO$_2$ are transparent, less greasy, and less smelly and have increased aesthetic appeal.

Antiaging Products

Chemical products, pollution, stress, irradiation from infrared (IR) and ultraviolet (UV) sources, and abrasion are involved in skin aging. Collagen plays an important role in skin rejuvenation and wrinkle reversal effect. The quantity of collagen in the skin decreases along with age. The aging of the skin manifests itself in many ways: Drying out, loss of elasticity and texture, thinning, damaged barrier function, appearance of spots, modification of surface line isotropy, and, finally, wrinkles. Most of the cosmeceuticals have been developed with claims of antiwrinkle and firming, moisturizing and lifting, and skin toning and whitening activity. Antiaging products are the main cosmeceuticals in the market currently being made using nanotechnology. L'Oreal has employed nanotechnology in products such as Revitalift antiwrinkle cream which contains nanosomes of pro-retinol A, and claims that it instantly retightens the skin and reduces the appearance of wrinkles. Application of retinol can increase epidermal water content, epidermal hyperplasia, and cell renewal while enhancing collagen synthesis. Retinol also interferes with melanogenesis and inhibits matrix metalloproteinases, which are involved in collagen breakdown. The clinical benefits include a reduction in the appearance of fine lines and wrinkles and lightening of lentigines. Lancôme introduces Hydra Zen Cream to renew the skin's healthy look which contains nanoencapsulated triceramide.

Hair Care

Hair care is another promising field for nanotechnology. Companies are using nanotechnology in hair care products and research is ongoing to discover the ways of how nanoparticles can be used to prevent hair loss and to maintain shine, silkiness, and health of hairs. Unlike ordinary hair straightening products, nanoemulsion in hair cosmetics does not destroy the outer structure of the hair fibres, called cuticles, to penetrate into the hair strands. Sericin (composed of cationic sericin nanoparticles) is an active area of hair cosmeceuticals. Studies have shown that sericin nanoparticles in hair cosmeceuticals easily adhere to the surface of hair seal and treat the damaged cuticles.

Skin Cleanser

The skin is covered with a hydrolipid film that, depending on the area of the body, comprises secretions from sebaceous glands and from apocrine and eccrine sweat glands. Decomposition products from corneocytes and cornification (cellular debris and stratum corneum lipids) in the process of being shed are also present. This film provides a natural defense against pathogenic organisms but also attracts dirt and pollutants from the environment. Sometimes the microorganisms present on the skin surface act on components of the surface film and create undesirable byproducts, such as those resulting from the metabolism of compounds found in apocrine sweat that create body odour. Thus, periodic cleansing to remove debris, dirt, and odour is essential to maintain skin health. Cleansing is also necessary to remove soil (which may include bacteria) from the skin surface that is acquired by incidental contact or by intentional application (medications or makeup and other cosmetic products). Silver nanoparticles are used as skin disinfectant and decontamination. Nano Cyclic Inc. produces Nano Cyclic cleanser pink soap which is a scientifically balanced blend of nanosilver and natural ingredients and claims that it kills harmful bacteria and fungi, fights acne, and diminishes age spots and sun-damaged skin.

Lip Care

Lip care is another promising class of cosmeceuticals. Different nanoparticles can be incorporated into lipstick and lip gloss which will soften or soothe the lips by preventing transepidermal water loss. Korea Research Institute of Bioscience and Biotechnology holds a patent that described that it is possible to prepare pigments exhibiting wide range of colours using gold or silver nanoparticles by mixing in various compositional ratios and whose colour can be maintained for a long period of time. Silica nanoparticles used in lipsticks improve the homogenous distribution of pigments. Once applied, they prevent the pigments from migrating or bleeding into the fine line of lips.

Nail Care

Nanotechnology-based nail cosmeceuticals have various advantages over conventional products. A study revealed that nail paints having nanosized particles improve toughness, mar resistance, and impact resistance of the mammalian nails. Nano Labs Corp (a nanotechnology research and development company) was awarded a provisional patent for its original nano-nail polish and lacquer having advantages that it dries to a very hard state, resists shock, cracking, scratching, and chipping and its elasticity offers superior ease of application without cracking. One of the new strategies which may have great potential in the cosmeceuticals is the incorporation of nanoparticles having antifungal activity (like silver and metal oxide nanoparticles) in nail polish to treat fungal toenail infections.

Regulatory Aspects

The claims made about drugs are subject to high scrutiny by the FDA review and approval process, but cosmetics are not subject to mandatory FDA review. Much confusion exists regarding the status of 'cosmeceuticals'. Although there is no legal class called cosmeceuticals, this term has found application and recognition to designate the products at the borderline between cosmetics and pharmaceuticals. Cosmeceuticals are not subject to FDA review and the Federal Food, Drug and Cosmetic Act do not recognize the term itself. It is also often difficult for consumers to determine whether 'claims' about the actions or efficacies of cosmeceuticals are in fact valid unless the product has been approved by the FDA or equivalent agency. Some experts are calling for increased regulation of cosmeceuticals that would require only proof of safety, which is not mandatory for cosmetics. Some countries have the classes of products that fall between the two categories of cosmetics and drugs. For example. Japan has 'Quasi-drugs'; Thailand has 'controlled cosmetics' and Hong Kong has 'cosmetic-type drugs'. The regulations of cosmeceuticals have not been harmonized between the USA, European, Asian and other countries.

NEW TRENDS FOR PERSONALIZED MEDICINE

Introduction

Pharmacogenetics and pharmacogenomics are two main emerging trends in medical sciences, which influence the success of drug development and therapeutics. In present times, though pharmacogenetic studies are being done extensively for research, its application for drug development needs to get started on a large scale. Pharmacogenetic studies may be used at different stages of drug development. The effect of drug target polymorphisms on drug response may be evaluated and identified. In clinical studies, pharmacogenetic tests may be used for stratification of patients based on their genotype, which corresponds to their metabolizing capacity. These prevent the occurrence of severe adverse drug reactions and help in better outcome of clinical trials. These may also reduce attrition of drug compounds. Recognition of interindividual differences in drug response is an essential step towards optimizing therapy. Over the past decades, a lot of evidence have emerged indicating that a substantial portion of variability in drug response is genetically determined, with age, nutrition, health status, environmental exposure, and concurrent therapy playing important contributory roles. To achieve individual drug therapy with a reasonably predictive outcome, one must further account for different patterns of drug response among geographically and ethnically distinct populations.

Pharmacogenomics is the study of how genes affect a person's response to drugs. This relatively new field combines pharmacology (the science of drugs) and genomics (the study of genes and their functions) to develop effective, safe medications and doses that will be tailored to a person's genetic make-up. Several drugs that are recently available are "one size fits all", but they do not work the same way for everyone. It may be difficult to predict who will benefit from a medication, who will not respond at all, and who will experience negative side effects (called adverse drug reactions).

Pharmacogenomics Affecting Drug Design, Development

The Food and Drug Administration, which monitors the safety of all drugs in the United States, has included pharmacogenomic information on the labels of more than 150 medications. This information which can cover dosage guidance, possible side effects or differences in effectiveness for people with certain genomic variations can help doctors tailor their drug prescriptions for individual patients. Many pharmaceutical companies are beginning to use pharmacogenomic knowledge to develop and market drugs for people with specific genetic profiles. Studying a drug only in those likely to benefit from it could speed up and streamline its development and greatly maximize its therapeutic benefit. Additionally, if scientists can identify the genetic basis for certain serious side effects, drugs could be prescribed only to people who are not at risk for them. As a result, potentially lifesaving medications, which otherwise might be taken off the market because they pose a risk for some people, could still be available to those who could benefit from them.

Pharmacogenomics Affecting Medical Treatment

Currently, doctors base the majority of their drug prescriptions on clinical factors, such as a patient's age, weight, sex, and liver and kidney function. For a small subset of drugs, researchers have identified genetic variations that influence how people respond. In these cases, doctors can use the pharmacogenomic information to select the best medication and identify people who need an unusually high or low dose.

Use of Pharmacogenomics

One current use of pharmacogenomics involves people infected with the human immunodeficiency virus (HIV). Before prescribing the antiviral drug abacavir (Ziagen), doctors now routinely test HIV-infected patients for a genetic variant that makes them more likely to have a bad reaction to the drug. Another example is the breast cancer drug trastuzumab (Herceptin). This therapy works only for women whose tumours have a particular genetic profile that leads to overproduction of a protein called HER_2. The US Food and Drug Administration also recommends genetic testing before giving the chemotherapy drug mercaptopurine (Purinethol) to patients with acute lymphoblastic leukaemia. Some people have a genetic variant that interferes with their ability to process the drug. This processing problem can cause severe side effects and increase risk of infection, unless the standard dose is adjusted according to the patient's genetic makeup. The FDA also advises doctors to test colon cancer patients for certain genetic variants before administering irinotecan (Camptosar), which is part of a combination chemotherapy regimen. The reasoning is that patients with one particular variant may not be able to clear the drug from their bodies as quickly as others, resulting in severe diarrhoea and increased infection risk. Such patients may need to receive lower doses of the drug.

International HapMap Project

The goal of the International HapMap Project is to determine the common patterns of DNA sequence variation in the human genome and to make this information freely available in the public domain. An international consortium is developing a map of these patterns across the genome by determining the genotypes of one million or more sequence variants, their frequencies and the degree of association between them, in DNA samples from populations with ancestry from parts of Africa, Asia and Europe. The HapMap will allow the discovery of sequence variants that affect common disease, will facilitate development of diagnostic tools, and will enhance our ability to choose targets for therapeutic intervention. The HapMap is a catalogue of common genetic variants that occur in human beings. It describes what these variants are, where they occur in our DNA, and how they are distributed among people within populations and among populations in different parts of the world. The International HapMap Project is not using the information in the HapMap to establish connections between particular genetic variants and diseases. Rather, the project is designed to provide information that other researchers can use to link genetic variants to the risk for specific illnesses, which will lead to new methods of preventing, diagnosing, and treating disease.

Adenine, thymine, cytosine, and guanine, abbreviated A, T, C, and G. More than 6 billion of these chemical bases are strung together in 23 pairs of chromosomes, exist in a human cell. These genetic sequences contain such information that influences our physical traits, our likelihood of suffering from disease, and the responses of our bodies to substances that we encounter in the environment. The genetic sequences of different people are remarkably similar. When the chromosomes of two humans are compared, their DNA sequences can be identical for hundreds of bases. But at about one in every 1,200 bases, on average, the sequences will differ. One person might have an A at that location, while another person has a G, or a person might have extra bases at a given location or a missing segment of DNA. Each distinct 'spelling' of a chromosomal region is called an allele, and a collection of alleles in a person's chromosomes is known as a genotype. Differences in individual bases are by far the most common type of genetic variation. These genetic differences are known as single nucleotide polymorphisms, or SNPs (pronounced 'snips'). By identifying most of the approximately 10 million SNPs estimated to occur commonly in the human genome, the International HapMap Project is identifying the basis for a large fraction of the genetic diversity in the human species.

For geneticists, SNPs act as markers to locate genes in DNA sequences. If a particular SNP is more common among people with hypertension, then SNP could be used as a pointer to locate and identify the gene involved in the disease. However, testing all of the 10 million common SNPs in a person's chromosomes would be extremely expensive. The development of the HapMap will enable geneticists to take advantage of how SNPs and other genetic variants are organized on chromosomes. Genetic variants that are near each other tend to be inherited together. For example, all of the people who have an A rather than a G at a particular location in a chromosome can have identical genetic variants at other SNPs in the chromosomal region surrounding the A. These regions of linked variants are known as haplotypes.

Some pharmacogenomic tests have been acknowledged for a long time and are accepted as routine tests; e.g. it has been known that those patients with glucose-6-phosphate dehydrogenase (G6PD) deficiency should avoid certain drugs because of the risk of haemolysis following their intake. The effect of a drug is traditionally assessed by clinical outcome, which includes laboratory tests and therapeutic drug monitoring (TDM). It has only been in the last 10–15 years that a number of pharmacogenomic tests have been available to supplement the traditional outcome measures and to aid with dose determination and choice of medication.

Bioelectronic Medicines

Two million adverse drug reactions are observed in the US each year. They are the 4th leading cause of death, ahead of pulmonary disease, diabetes, and automobile deaths. Bioelectronic medicine (BEM), which uses neurotechnologies to interface with the nervous system, can offer such opportunities. Neurotechnologies are among the fastest growing segments of the medical device market. Many diseases can be treated, in principle, by precise modulation of the body's nerve signals BEM can revolutionize how we practice medicine, reduce cost and dramatically improve the outcomes of health care. It employs electrical, magnetic, optical, ultrasound, etc. pulses to affect and modify nerve behaviour, which in turn impacts body functions as an alternative or supplement to drug-based interventions. Furthermore, it provides the opportunity for targeted and personalized treatments of diseases and conditions with closed-loop control systems. The purpose of the BEM Technology Roadmap is to capture the high-level work necessary to meaningfully advance neurotechnology-based diagnosis and treatment of diseases at an accelerated rate with intermediate steps defined along the path. It also provides a view of the gaps or misalignments which may need to receive greater research attention and funding support. This Roadmap is intended to provide best estimates of current capabilities, projections of technology needs, research priorities and direction for supporting industries and institutions on necessary collaboration to achieve the expected benefits.

Goals of BEM

In order to meet the goals of advancing bioelectric therapy, the following goals need to be achieved:
- Targeted diseases and conditions must be identified as good candidates for bioelectronic medicine.
- Investigative devices to understand underlying mechanisms are required. For investigative devices, it will be critical to understand what to measure and how to measure it, as well as how it can be integrated in a complete therapy to understand what gaps remain.
- Cross-disciplinary collaborations are needed to efficiently address challenges between biologic/medical/computing disciplines. There is the need to create a synergistic partnership among the scientific researchers, technology developers, and clinical translators.
- The foundation of the work must be built on understanding the biology of the system and the disease.
- System models including biological, chemical, electrical, and mechanical interactions for normal and disease state behaviour are required.
- Disease state focus is required to understand and treat the states of disease relative to the normative state.

BEM Microsystem

An implantable electrode senses biosignals, which are filtered and analyzed. A device reacts to those processed signals via neural interface that stimulates or blocks nerve activity. The resulting data may be stored in the implantable device or communicated externally. Device miniaturization is one of the key success factors of future bioelectronic medicine. Next generation neuromodulation devices are expected to improve the current state of the art in five key areas:

1. **Sensitivity,** i.e. able to sense and decode signals from neurons in a highly sensitive manner against other background interference.
2. **Selectivity,** i.e. able to precisely target specific nuclei in the brain or nerves in the periphery, while avoiding off-target neurons; such targeting should have clear endpoints.
3. **Responsiveness,** i.e. able to capture the neural signatures and to detect biomarkers (a variety of sensors may be needed, both electrical and biochemical, as biomarkers for detection and stimulation effectiveness).
4. **Acceptance,** i.e. miniaturized low-power devices that can be delivered with minimally invasive implantation, thereby reducing patient burden and improving access.
5. **Closing the loop,** i.e. forms a closed-loop system to record and stimulate, block, or more generally neuromodulate to achieve the targeted function consistently.

Telepharmacy

Telepharmacy, analogous to telemedicine, is a more recent concept that refers to pharmaceutical service provision. Strategies to address the barriers to accessing pharmacy services have resulted in the creation of several models of telepharmacy. The National Association of Boards of Pharmacy defines 'telepharmacy' as "the provision of pharmaceutical care through the use of telecommunications and information technologies to patients at a distance". Telepharmacy delivers clinical pharmacy services and the dispensing of a prescription at a remote location without the physical presence of a pharmacist. Typical telepharmacy involves services such as medication order review, dispending and compounding, drug information services, patient counselling, and therapeutic drug monitoring. Hence, telepharmacy uses state-of-the-art technology that allows a qualified pharmacist situated at a central location to supervise a pharmacy assistant or a pharmacy technician situated at a remote site in the dispensing of pharmaceuticals through audio and video computer links. Telepharmacy acts as a potential alternative to around-the-clock on-site pharmacist medication review for remote hospitals. This has been adopted by many health care institutions as an alternative strategy of extending pharmacy coverage areas where 24-hour pharmacy services are not available. The emerging electronic health information systems and related technologies, such as fax, and electronic health records make information more readily available to pharmacist for review before a dose is available for administration to a patient. These technologies are advancing telepharmacy services and enabling pharmacist to contribute efficiently in improving medication use.

Telepharmacy Work

In general, a small rural hospital, pharmacy, or clinic in an isolated area is connected to a commonly utilized service model in larger urban centre that has greater access (often 24 hours) to pharmacist staff. This connection is possible through videophone systems, novel software, and automated dispensing machine. The rural site is usually staffed by either pharmacy technicians or nurses, depending on whether the site is a pharmacy or a clinic. They may communicate the prescriptions (e.g. fax) from patients who report to these sites to the central site, which is then processed by a qualified pharmacist. The central pharmacist reviews the prescription and releases the appropriate items at the rural (e.g. prepackaged medication from the automated dispensing machines) and the label. The pharmacy technician or nurse at the rural sites scans the bar code so that the prescription matches with its label, attaches the label, and supplies it to the patient. The pharmacist at the central end can visually monitor the technician or nurse's work to ensure that the right medications have been filled and dispensed. At the end of the process, the central pharmacist provides a two-way video consultation for the patient to ensure that they understand the intended medication use and administration. This addresses any concerns from the patient's perspectives and enables efficient patient counselling from the central location.

Automated dispensing machines, however, are not always affordable for small rural hospitals or clinics. An alternative was developed by researchers in Fargo, ND, USA, where a technician under the videoconference supervision of a central pharmacist at a distant location prepares medication for dispensing, repackaging, and relabelling. These medications are then directly delivered to the nurse by the pharmacy technician or are dispensed through automated dispensing devices (when available). In another example, to facilitate 24-hour access to the pharmacist by physicians and nurses in the patient care area for face-to-face consultation and communication, a wireless mobile technology cart has been developed for use in remote hospitals.

Types of Telepharmacy Models

1. **Traditional full-service pharmacy:** Like traditional pharmacies, this telepharmacy site encompasses services such as filling prescriptions, medication reviews, and patient counselling. These telepharmacy sites have complete drug inventories that include prescription and over the counter medications along with other health and beauty aids and other general merchandise.
2. **Remote consultation sites:** Prescriptions are prepared at the central pharmacy and are delivered to the rural sites. Audio and video computer links are used to deliver patient counselling and education.
3. **Hospital telepharmacy:** Hospital pharmacist in urban medical centre reviews processes and verifies the prescriptions that are issued and electronically sent from rural hospitals. Automated dispensing machine (ADM) is used to electronically release the prepackage medication. A nurse or pharmacy assistant at rural end double checks the label and medication prior dispenses them to patients. The pharmacist from central (urban) location monitors the verification process and involves in consultation between the patients, nurses, or physicians when required via video conference link.
4. **ADMs:** Pharmacist at a central location upon receiving drug order (electronically or by fax) confirms the patient profile, conducts proper drug utilization review, and finally instructs the ADM to release the medication. With the help of audio and video computer links, patient counselling is then conducted.

Involvement of Pharmacists

In any telepharmacy model, pharmacist can play an active role in the delivery of pharmacy services. The pharmacist involving in telepharmacy models ensures high quality care for the community particularly areas such as medication reviews and patient counselling. A 2013 study of the impact of telepharmacy services has shown that the involvement of pharmacists in the remote review of medication orders when the hospital pharmacy was closed resulted in a decreased number of adverse drug events reported. Adverse drug events and other medication errors contribute to several thousand deaths each year. The annual cost of preventable adverse drug events in the USA alone is estimated at US$2 billion. Similarly, a 2012 US study has shown that adverse patient outcomes including prolonged hospitalization and potential death may have been prevented using telepharmacy services as potential alternatives to around-the-clock on-site pharmacist medication review for rural hospitals. With the growing population of patients with chronic medical conditions, all around the world, involvement of pharmacists in telepharmacy models to improve monitoring and encourage medication compliance can decrease the risk of medication errors, adverse drug events, decreased medication cost, and the chances for treatment failure. This means that we need to be cautious of some of the telepharmacy models that often exclude active pharmacist involvement including internet pharmacies, vending machine models, mail-order pharmacies, and models that shift pharmacist's roles to other health care professionals such as doctors and nurses. Despite the differences in health care system between countries, telepharmacy models involving the active role of pharmacists are successful in several states of the USA and in Australia.

Clinical Benefits and Challenges of Telepharmacy

Advantages

1. *Access to health care services:* The primary advantage of telepharmacy is the easy access to health care services in remote and rural locations. Routine access to prescription medication and access to pharmacists are recognized as fundamental aspects to the delivery of patient-centred health care in remote and rural communities. Pharmacist can provide high-level pharmaceutical care services in remote areas that have lost or are losing access to health care services. Approximately half of the 410 small rural hospitals in the USA reported on-site pharmacist availability (<5 h wk), and 90% of the hospitals reported that nurses were responsible for medication dispensing and administering. Development of several models of telepharmacy addressed this scenario by enabling full-services operation that encompasses active role of remote and central pharmacists, medication utilization review, patient counselling, and patient education to the remote site using various technologies.

2. *Economic benefits:* Telepharmacy has several economic benefits. It is reported that starting a new pharmacy store is much expensive than the cost involved in the equipment and recruitment of pharmacy technician for telepharmacy. One skilled pharmacist can provide service to multiple sites. Hence, considering the rising pay scale for pharmacist and further expenses in hiring additional pharmacists for rural sites, costs are minimized. A telepharmacy model targeted to low-income population showed that >60% of patients would have faced difficulties in affording their medications, if the telepharmacy model did not exist.

   Health care providers receive telepharmacy as an ideal alternative to treatment delays when pharmacists are not present on site. Travel time and other costs associated with the travel are avoided when patients are not referred to other sites.

3. *Patient satisfaction:* Medication access and information in rural areas via telehealth has an advantage of patient satisfaction. One of the prominent barriers in the clinic used to be with the elderly patients missing their appointments because they did not want to go out of their homes. This remote technology has allowed pharmacists to review patient's medications without them having to travel. This has increased patient trust and satisfaction with the service. A US study to identify the underlying factors determining patient satisfaction depending upon health care delivery mode or community-specific factors reported that rural community patients value receiving pharmacy services locally via telepharmacy services rather than having to travel outside of their community. Similar study in the USA aiming to evaluate the telepharmacy program reported that >75% of the patients involved in the study were satisfied with the service and communication with pharmacist via video conference.

4. *Effective patient counselling:* Telepharmacy ensures greater satisfaction of patients with regard to the pharmacist counselling and time required obtaining medication. A study on telepharmacy-related services and outcomes in the USA reported that pharmacists recommend using the webcam-enabled telepharmacy services because they provide better privacy and longer counselling duration. Effectiveness of telepharmacy counselling was also illustrated by another study that used compressed video to explain the metered-dose inhaler techniques instead of using traditional package insert instructions. The ability of students to provide effective patient consultation via telepharmacy and examined any differences of students to counsel patients via telepharmacy and face-to-face consultation. They reported that students can successfully provide patient consultation without having prior practice with telepharmacy equipment. However, the study also highlighted that students performed better during the face-to-face consultation, suggesting that additional training and practices with telepharmacy consultation are warranted.

Disadvantages

1. *Pharmacy regulation laws:* Despite the widespread potential of telepharmacy, the laws and policies that govern pharmacy operations do not adequately address the growing industry. A number of policy issues, such as the physical location of pharmacists that provide telepharmacy services, minimum amount of time that pharmacist must be on site, the types of technology used, and the roles of pharmacists, pharmacy technicians, nurses, or other health care providers in medication distribution systems, need to be addressed. The regulations govern not only the system that ensures safe medication handling but also the operation of comprehensive medication use system, defining what role telepharmacy plays in this broader scope of pharmacy services in acute-care settings. Telepharmacy is still a novel concept, and there is a delay in the implementation of new laws, although professional and technological innovations are being used. In places nowhere telepharmacy laws exist, there is a lack of uniformity among various jurisdictions. Execution and implementation of comprehensive and uniform telepharmacy law is still a challenge.

2. *Operational difficulties:* Telepharmacy undoubtedly is a great concept, but it is sometimes challenging to put into practice. The rural hospitals and clinics with telepharmacy services experience operational and resource challenges. Telepharmacy services experience operational and resource challenges. Telepharmacy services may

only be possible with more complex and sophisticated equipment with high-speed digital connection (e.g. Integrated Service Digital Network), which are often limited in rural areas. Organizational cultures can also play significant roles as barriers for incorporating and embedding telepharmacy technologies into existing health care systems. Face-to-face versus remote workflow might often be overwhelming and less spontaneous for both patients and health care providers. A study on normalization (the routine integration of program in everyday practice) of telehealth care suggested that successful normalization of telehealthcare services was dependent upon a positive link with a policy level sponsor, involvement of organized, cohesive groups, development of supportive organizational structure, and the expansion of new procedures by professionals.

3. *More time, effort, and money:* The start-up of telepharmacy (hardware, software, connectivity, and operational cost) involves considerable time, effort, and money. The North Dakota telepharmacy project estimated tentative cost (drug store fixtures: US$20,000, drug inventory: Between US$60,000 and US$80,000, the digital subscriber lines: US$800/month, hardware: US$2,000, pharmacy operation software: US$5,000–7,000, video conference setup: US$6,500, video conference equipment: US$3,500–15,000, transmission/connectivity: US$250/month, firewall security systems: US$1,200, and other miscellaneous costs) for the operation of successful telepharmacy model. This cost estimation, however, is based on a 2004 study. The actual cost today is expected to increase several folds. Moreover, the integration of telepharmacy systems to the traditional health care systems has not been implemented in countries that use telepharmacy services. This makes private as well as government health care programs reluctant in funding telepharmacy expenditures. For example, individuals currently paying their health insurance will get funded only from the traditional health care expenditure, while their telepharmacy expenditures will not be covered.

4. *Reluctance to use technology:* Other disadvantage of telepharmacy involves reluctance or inability to use the technology. This is predominant in elderly people who are suspicious about technology. When face-to-face interaction is not present, the pharmacist's ability to fully access patient's condition might be hindered.

Continuity of Care

In circumstances where face-to-face contact is not possible, the pharmacist should provide an ethical indirect supply service that adheres with the regulations of quality use of medicines. Ensuring continuity of care and compliance with good dispensing practice becomes more complex on remote sites. Pharmacy technicians must rely upon the pharmacist in all aspects of pharmacy practice. Despite pharmacy technician being monitored or supervised by pharmacists from central location, risk of violation of regulations is difficult to avoid. Unlike regular pharmacies, the use of unauthorized medications or dispensing medications without proper prescription is hard to control.

3D Printing of Pharmaceuticals

The 3D printing technology has caught the attention of medical devices industry and pharmaceutical industry due to its applications on various platform in health care industry. Even though this technology exists for a long time, it is of public interest highly now due to the approval of 3D-printed tablet and other medical devices and also with the advent of USFDA's guidance on technical considerations specific to devices using additive manufacturing which encompasses three-dimensional (3D) printing has triggered many thoughts about this technology which needs to be considered for successful delivery of intended product. 3D printing can play a important role in multiple active ingredient dosage forms, where the formulation may be as a single blend or multilayer-printed tablets with sustained release properties. This decreases the frequency and number of dosage form units consumed by the patient on a daily routine. 3D printing technology has high potential in individualized dosage form concept called the polypill concept. This brings about the possibility of all the drugs required for the therapy into a single dosage form unit. Three-dimensional printing technology is a novel rapid prototyping technique in which solid objects are constructed by depositing several layers in sequence. The rapid prototyping involves the construction of physical models using computer-aided design in three dimensions. It is also known as additive manufacturing and solid free form fabrication. 3D printing technology has enabled unprecedented flexibility in the design and manufacturing of complex objects, which may be utilized in personalized and programmable medicine.

Regulatory expectations US FDA, 2017 issued guidance on technical considerations for additive manufactured medical devices, this guidance outlines various requirements, like design and manufacturing process considerations, device testing considerations and labelling. It also suggests the validation of the processes involved to provide high degree of assurance according to the established procedures. In addition, documentation must be done to conform to the existing guidelines in the quality system regulation for device validation. Process validation must be performed to ensure and maintain quality for all devices and components built in a single build cycle, between build cycles, and between machines, where the results of a process (i.e. output specifications) cannot be fully verified by subsequent inspection and test. Software also should be validated for its intended use according to an established protocol.

The following examples are suggested in the guidance with respect to powder bed fusion technologies.

- In-process monitoring of parameters such as: Temperature at the beam focus, melt pool data, build-space environmental conditions (e.g. temperature, pressure, humidity)
- Power of the energy delivery system (e.g. laser, electron beam, extruder)
- Status of mechanical elements of the printing system (e.g. recoater, gantry)
- Manual or automated visual inspection with defined acceptance criteria
- Non-destructive evaluation
- Test coupon evaluation

Steps involved in a 3D Printed Dosage Form

Pharmaceutical product is designed in three dimensions with computer aided design. Design is converted to a machine-readable format which describes the external surface of the 3D dosage form. The computer programme then slices this surface into several distinct printable layers and transfers that layer-by-layer to the machine.

Advantages of a 3D Printed Drug Delivery

- High drug loading ability when compared to conventional dosage forms.
- Accurate and precise dosing of potent drugs which are administered at small doses.

- Reduces cost of production due to lesser material wastage.
- Suitable drug delivery for difficult to formulate active ingredients like poor water solubility, drugs with narrow therapeutic window.
- Medication can be tailored to a patient in particular based on genetic variations, ethnic differences, age, gender and environment.
- In case of multidrug therapy with multiple dosing regimens, treatment can be customized to improve patient adherence.
- As immediate and controlled release layers can be incorporated due to the flexible design and manufacture of this dosage form, it helps in choosing the best therapeutic regime for an individual.
- Avoids batch-to-batch variations seen in bulk manufacturing of conventional dosage forms.
- 3D printers occupy minimal space and are affordable.
- Manufacture of small batch is feasible and the process can be completed in a single run.

Integration of Personalized Medicine with Health care Network

As 3D printers perform as computerized fabricators that manufacture 3D objects based on command generated by computer software, it has an immense possibility of integrating the 3D printers with the health care network. This concept uses sensor technology which will enable sensors to be placed on patients. These sensors generate clinical data feed that eventually gets stored in health care network. The health care professional may manufacture the next dose according to the patient's physiological changes reflected in the clinical data transmitted. Hence, such a dispensing system offers a clear advantage of shortening the time of a clinical response to patient's needs and improving patient's compliance.

To incorporate the practical application of 3D-printed dosage form into the dispensing scenario existing today, further research and development in the clinical scenario is essential. First of all, the software technology used can be further optimized and improved. Secondly, excipients need to be developed for optimum application in 3D formulations. Thirdly, manufacturing process has to be developed and optimized for a wide range of drug products. Fourthly, efficacy, safety and stability of new 3D-based formulations have to be studied further because the built in flexibility should not become a liability on safety. The principle employed in 3D printing drug delivery systems is the construction and stacking of layers of 3D-printed objects. The name of the technology is usually related to the technique involved in layer formation. 3D printing is repeated and co-ordinated two-dimensional printing.

SPRITAM®—FDA Approved First 3D-Printed Pill

SPRITAM utilizes aprecia's proprietary ZipDose® technology platform, a groundbreaking advance that uses three-dimensional printing to produce a porous formulation that rapidly disintegrates with a sip of liquid. ZipDose® technology enables the delivery of a high drug load, up to 1,000 mg in a single dose. SPRITAM enhances the patient experience-administration of even the largest strengths of levetiracetam with just a sip of liquid. Aprecia developed its ZipDose® technology platform using the 3DP technology that originated at Massachusetts Institute of Technology. The ZipDose® technique is based on layer-by-layer powder bed fusion system. The first layer consists of the active pharmaceutical ingredient and excipients required for the matrix tablet. Subsequently, a binder liquid is deposited for perfect integration and aggregation between all of the successive and identical layers.

Polypill Concept

The concept of 'polypill' refers to a single tablet that includes the combination of several drugs. This concept is highly beneficial for geriatric population, as patients of this age category are prone to multiple disorders and hence multiple therapy. As per published research data, five different active pharmaceutical ingredients with different release profiles have been formulated in a single 3D dosage form. Three drugs (pravastatin, atenolol, and ramipril) are printed in the extended release compartment. The drugs are physically separated by a permeable membrane of hydrophobic cellulose acetate. An immediate release compartment containing aspirin and hydrochlorothiazide is deposited on top of the extended release compartment three-dimensional (3D) extrusion-based printing is used to manufacture the 'polypill' to demonstrate that complex medication regimes may be combined in a single tablet and that it is viable to formulate and 'dial up' this single tablet for the particular needs of an individual. The tablets are used to illustrate this concept incorporate an osmotic pump with the drug captopril and sustained release compartments with the drugs nifedipine and glipizide. This combination of medicines should potentially be used to treat diabetics suffering from hypertension. The room temperature extrusion process is used to print the formulations used excipients commonly employed in the pharmaceutical industry (Fig. 6.1).

Powder-Based 3D Printing

This technique uses powder jetting or powder bed to spread thin layers of powder and simultaneously applying liquid binder drops with the help of inkjet printers. The ink (binders and APIs or binder solutions) is sprinkled over a powder bed in two beginning the procedure, until the manufacture of the 3D product is finished in a layer-by-layer way. Here thickness of the cured layers depends upon the energy of the UV light to which resin is exposed. The resin should be FDA approved for human use with the ability to solidify upon exposure to laser beam.

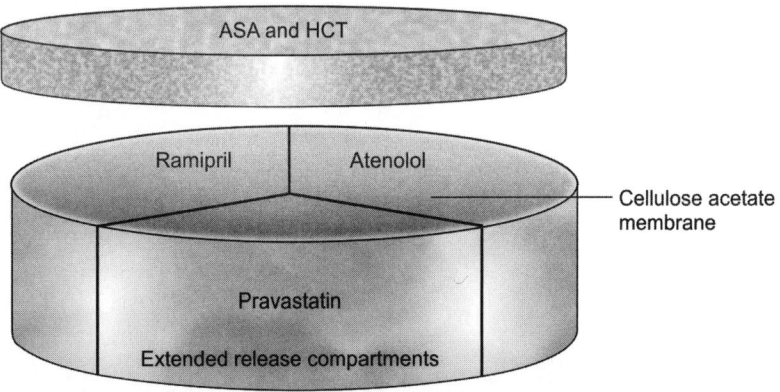

Fig 6.1: 3D-printed polypill

QUESTIONS

A. Short Answer Type Questions

1. Discuss about regulatory aspects of cosmeceuticals.
2. What do you mean by 3D printing of pharmaceuticals?
3. Discuss on International HapMap Project.
4. Write the uses of pharmacogenomics.
5. Define bioelectric medicine.
6. What are clinical benefits of telepharmacy?

B. Long Answer Type Questions

1. Write different pharmacogenomics factors which affect drug design.
2. Describe in detail about the nanoparticles which uses in cosmeceuticals.
3. What is customized drug delivery system? Explain in detail.
4. Mention the major classes of nanocosmeceuticals.
5. Discuss in detail about telepharmacy.

Protein and Peptide Delivery and Vaccine Delivery Systems

PROTEIN AND PEPTIDE DELIVERY SYSTEMS

Introduction

Proteins are the most abundant macromolecules in the living cells, occurring in all cells and all parts of cells. Cells can produce proteins that have strikingly different properties and activities, by joining same 20 amino acids in different combinations and sequences. Proteins are the large organic compounds made of amino acids arranged in a linear chain and joined together by peptide bonds. Peptides are short polymers formed from the linking, in a defined order of amino acids. The term protein is used for molecules composed of over 50 amino acids, and peptide for molecules composed of less than 50 amino acids. Scientific advances in molecular and cell biology have resulted in the development of two new biotechnologies. The first utilizes recombinant DNA to produce protein products. The second technology is hybridoma technology. Various protein and peptide drugs are epidermal growth factor, tissue plasminogen activator.

Structure of Protein

There are four types:
1. *Primary structure:* The amino acid sequence.
2. *Secondary structure:* Regularly repeating local structures stabilized by hydrogen bond.
3. *Tertiary structure:* Three-dimensional structure of polypeptide.
4. *Quaternary structure:* The structure formed by several protein molecules (polypeptide chains).

Types of Proteins and Peptides

Depending on the number of amino acids, they are classified as follows:
- Polypeptides
- Oligopeptides
- Fibrous proteins
- Globular proteins
- Oligomeric proteins

Importance of Protein and Peptide Drugs

- The proteins and peptides are very important in biological cells.
- Management of illness through medication is entering a new era in which a growing number of biotechnologically produced peptide and protein drugs are available for therapeutic use.
- Ailments that can be treated effectively by this new class of therapeutic agents include cancers, memory impairment, mental disorders, and hypertension.
- Lack of proteins and peptides causes diseases like diabetes mellitus.
- Diabetes mellitus is caused due to the lack of protein called insulin.
- Nowadays, R-DNA technology and hybridoma techniques also used in protein and peptide-based pharmaceuticals.

Advantages of Protein and Peptide Drugs

- The protein tissue plasminogen activator is used for heart attack, and stroke.
- Oxytocin is used in management of labour pain.
- Erythropoietin is mainly used for production of RBC.
- Bradykinin increases the peripheral circulation.
- Somatostatin decreases bleeding in gastric ulcer.
- Gonadotropin induces ovulation.
- Insulin maintains blood sugar level.

Functions of Protein and Peptide Drugs

- Mechanical support from fibrous protein.
- Generation and transmission of nerve impulses.
- Transport and storage of small and biological molecules.
- Enzymatic catalysis in biochemical reactions.
- Coordinated motion via muscle contraction.
- Immune protection through antibodies.
- Control of growth and differentiation via hormones.

Disadvantages of Protein and Peptide Drugs

- Very large and unstable molecules.
- Structure is held together by weak non-covalent forces.
- Easily destroyed by relatively mild storage conditions and gastric juices.
- Hard to obtain in large quantities.

Problems with Proteins (*in vivo*—in the body)

- Elimination by B and T cells.
- Proteolysis by endo-/exo-peptidases.
- Small proteins filtered out by the kidneys very quickly.
- Unwanted allergic reactions may develop (even toxicity).
- Loss due to insolubility/adsorption

Stability Problems and Causes

Physical Stability

It involves transformations in the secondary, tertiary, or quaternary structure of the molecule.

1. Denaturation

Any non-proteolytic modification of the unique structure of a native protein that affects definite changes in physical, chemical, and biological properties. Peptides and proteins are comprised both polar amino residues and non-polar amino acid residues.

Factors that favour denaturation

- When solvent changes from an aqueous to organic solvents or to a mixed solvent.
- pH changes alter the ionization of the carboxylic acid and amino acids and thereby the charges carried by the molecules.
- Alteration in the ionic strength
- Temperature rise
- Denaturation may be reversible or irreversible
- Denaturation may lead to decrease in solubility, alteration in surface tension, loss of crystallizing ability, changes in constituent group reactivity and molecular profile, vulnerability to enzymatic degradation, loss or alteration of antigenicity and loss of specific biological activity.

Methods to prevent denaturation

- Denatured protein is restored on removal of denaturants.
- Maintaining pH
- Maintaining ionic strength
- Maintaining temperature

2. Adsorption

- Peptides and proteins are amphiphilic in nature; hence they tend to adsorb at interfaces such as air-water and air-solid, e.g. insulin.
- Conformational rearrangement leading to denaturation can be induced by their interfacial adsorption.
- After adsorption, they form some short-range bonds (van der Waals, hydrophobic, electrostatic, hydrogen, ion-pair bonds) with the surface resulting into further denaturation of polypeptide moieties.
- Adsorption of peptides and proteins at the interfaces are rapid, but the rates of conformational changes are relatively slower.
- On adsorption, there may be a loss or change in biological activity as the molecular structure is rearranged.
- If peptide and protein drug entities are adsorbed at interfaces, there may be a reduction in the concentration of drug available to elicit its function. Such loss of proteinaceous drug(s) may occur during purification, formulation, storage and/or delivery.

Methods to prevent adsorption

- Insulin adsorption may be minimized by the addition of 0.1 to 1% albumin.
- Excess agitation should prevent during production.
- The headspace within the confines of the container should be small.
- Use of surfactants to reduce adsorption.
- Smooth glass walls best to reduce adsorption or precipitation.

3. Aggregation and Precipitation

- The denatured, unfolded protein may rearrange in such a manner that hydrophobic amino acid residue of various molecules associate together to form the aggregates.
- If the aggregation is on a macroscopic scale, precipitation occurs. Interfacial adsorption may be followed by aggregation and precipitation. The extent to which aggregation and precipitation occurs is defined by the relative hydrophilicity of the surfaces in contact with the polypeptide/protein solution.

Causes
- The presence of large air-water interface generally accelerates this process.
- Presence of large headspace within the confines of the container also accelerates the course of precipitation. Insulin forms finely divided precipitates on the walls of the containers, referred to as frosting. The presence of large air-water interface generally accelerates this process.
- Increase in thermal motion of the molecules due to agitation. Solvent composition, solvent dielectric profile, ionic strength.

To prevent aggregation and precipitation
- Organic solvent such as 10–15% propylene glycol can suppress the formation of peptide liquid crystals.
- Excess agitation should prevent during production.
- The headspace within the confines of the container should be small.
- The ionic strength, solvent composition, solvent dielectric profile and pH should be carefully controlled at every step in production.
- Use of surfactants to reduce aggregation.

Chemical Instability

- Involves alteration in the molecular structure producing a new chemical entity, by bond formation or cleavage.
- The stability of peptide and proteins against a chemical reagent is decided by temperature, length of exposure, and the amino acid composition, sequence and conformation of the peptide/protein.

1. Deamidation

- This reaction involves the hydrolysis of the side chain amide linkage of an amino acid residue leading to the formation of a free carboxylic acid.
- Asparagine glutamine leading to conversion of a neutral residue to a negatively charged residue and primary sequence isomerization.
- In vivo deamidation is observed with human growth hormone, bovine growth hormone, prolactin, adrenocorticotropic hormone, insulin, lysozyme and secretin.

Factors
- pH
- Temperature
- Ionic strength
- The deamidation of Asn residues is accelerated at neutral and alkaline pH.
- The tertiary structure of the protein also affects its stability, as observed with trypsin in which the tertiary structure prevents deamidation.

Methods to prevent deamidation
- The use of genetic engineering and by recombinant DNA technology.
- The asparagine residues can be selectively eliminated and replaced by other residues, provided conformations and bioactivity of protein can be maintained.

2. Oxidation and Reduction

Oxidation commonly occurs during isolation, synthesis and storage of proteins.

Factors
- The oxidative degradation reactions can even occur in atmospheric oxygen under mild conditions (autoxidation).
- Temperature.
- pH, trace amounts of metal ions and buffers influence these reactions.
- Oxidation may take place involving side chains of histidine (his), lysine (lys), tryptophan (trp), and thyronine (tye) residues in proteins.
- The thioether group of methionine (met) is particularly susceptible to oxidation. Under acidic conditions, met residues can be oxidized by atmospheric oxygen.
- Oxidizing agents like hydrogen peroxide, dimethylsulphoxide and iodine can oxidize met-to-met sulphoxides.
- The thiol group of cysteine can be oxidized to sulphonic acid; oxidation by iodine and hydrogen peroxide is catalyzed by metal ions and may occur spontaneously by atmospheric oxygen. Usually the oxidation of amino acid residues is followed by a significant loss of biological activity as observed after oxidation of met residues in calcitonin, corticotrophin and gastrin. Glucagon is an exception as it retains biological activity even after oxidation.

Methods to prevent oxidation and reduction
- Oxidation scavengers may block these acid or base catalyzed oxidations, e.g. phenolic compounds, propyl gallate.
- Reducing agents—ascorbic acid, sodium sulphate, thioglycerol and thioglycolic acid.
- Chelating agents—EDTA, citric acid nitrogen flush, refrigeration, protection from light and adjustment of pH.
- Avoiding vigorous stirring and exclusion of air by degassing solvents can prevent air initiated oxidation

3. Proteolysis

The hydrolysis of peptide bonds within the polypeptide or protein destroys or at least reduces its activity.

Factors that favour proteolysis and prevention
- Exposing the proteins to harsh conditions (extremes of pH or high temperature or proteolytic enzymes)
- Bacterial contamination
- Proteases may also gain access during the isolation, purification and recovery of recombinant proteins from cell extracts or culture fluid.
- This problem can be minimized by the manipulation of the solution conditions during the stage of purification and/or by addition of protease inhibitors. Some proteins even have autoproteolytic activity. This property aids in controlling the level or function of protein *in vivo*.

4. Disulphide Exchange

Thiol-disulphide exchange showing the linear intermediate in which the charge is shared among the three sulphur atoms. The thiolate group attacks a sulphur atom of the disulphide bond, displacing the other sulphur atom and forming a new disulphide bond. This results in an alteration in the three-dimensional structure followed by a resultant change in biological activity. This reaction occurs in neutral or alkaline medium and accelerates by thiols which are generated by disulphide exchange.

Methods to prevent disulphide exchange: By thiol scavengers such as *p*-mercuribenzoate, copper ions.

5. Racemization

It is the alteration of l-amino acids to d, l-mixtures. With the exception of gly, all the mammalian amino acids are chiral at the carbon-bearing chain and are susceptible to base-catalyzed racemization. Racemization may form peptide bonds that are sensitive to proteolytic enzymes. This reaction can be catalyzed in neutral and alkaline media by thiols, which may arise as a result of hydrolytic cleavage of disulphides.

Methods to prevent racemization

The thiolated ions carry out nucleophilic attack on a sulphur atom of the disulphide. Addition of thiol scavengers, such as *p*-mercuribenzoate, N-ethylmaleimide and copper ions, may prevent susceptible sulphur and disulphide.

6. Beta-Elimination

The mechanism involved in the beta-elimination is similar to the racemization, i.e. it proceeds through a carbanion intermediate. Higher elimination rate prevails under alkaline conditions which ultimately lead to loss of biological activity. Protein residues susceptible to beta-elimination under alkaline conditions include cys, lys, ser.

Barriers to Oral Absorption

- Age-related development of macromolecule permeability barrier
- Physical barrier: Size, charge, solubility
- Chemical barriers: pH solubility profile
- Enzyme barriers

Age-Related Development of Macromolecule Permeability Barrier

It is found out that permeability of the neonate's intestine is good for the macromolecules and as the age increases the permeability reduces for macromolecule and increases for small molecules.

Physical Barrier

- Size, charge and solubility is in our hand to change by formulation and chemistry change.
- For example, sustained release human insulin by attaching with lipophilic molecule.

Surface adsorption

- Glass and plastic surfaces adsorb proteins and peptides.
- To avoid surface adsorption, albumin, gelatin, sodium chloride can be used.

Aggregation behaviour: To prevent aggregation, additives are used such as urea, glycerol, EDTA, lysine, poloxamer.

Chemical Barriers

pH

- Solution pH is important for stability purpose. For simple peptides, pH of minimum degradation should be identified. Peptides are usually formulated at slightly acidic pH (3–5). For proteins, pH is set away from isoelectric pH to avoid aggregation.
- Insulin is more stable at pH 5.4. However, for solubility reasons, insulin injection pH are 2.5–3.5 or 7–7.8.

Enzyme Barriers/Protein Instabilities

The degradation of proteins and peptides can be divided into two main categories:
1. Those that involve a covalent bond.
2. Those involving a conformational change. This process is often referred to as denaturation.

Control of Barrier for Protein and Peptide Drug Delivery

Because of the difficulties encountered by peptides and proteins in crossing mucosal membranes, penetration enhancers are generally needed to facilitate the absorption of peptides and proteins in pharmacologically active amounts. Penetration enhancers are typically compounds of low molecular weight and are of four major types:
1. *Chelators:* EDTA, citric acid, salicylates, N-acyl derivatives of collagen, and enamines (N-amino acyl-derivatives).
2. *Synthetic surfactants:* Sodium lauryl sulphate, polyoxyethylene-9-1aurylether, and polyoxyethylene-20-cetylether.
3. *Natural and semisynthetic surfactants:* Bile salts (sodium deoxycholate, sodium glycocholate, and sodium taurocholate) and derivatives of fusidic acid.
4. *Fatty acids and their derivatives:* Sodium caprylate, sodium caprate, sodium laurate, oleic acid, monoolein and acylcarnitines.

Clearly, in order to promote the absorption of peptides and proteins from the mucosal routes, the many components of the enzymatic barrier must be controlled. This can be achieved to some extent by modifying the peptide or protein structure, through co-administering protease inhibitors, or by using the formulation approach.

Drug Delivery Classification

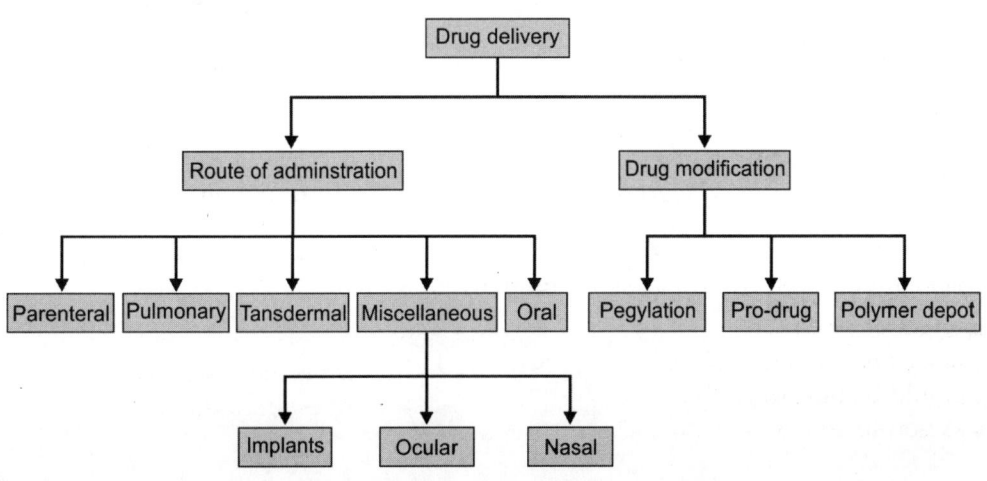

Parenteral Routes of Administration

- Parenteral route is most efficient way for systemic delivery of proteins and peptides.
- This is the best choice to achieve therapeutic activity.
- Mainly three routes of administration:
  - Intravascular
  - Intramuscular
  - Subcutaneous

Advantages

- Route of delivery for 95% of proteins
- Allows rapid and complete absorption
- Avoids first pass metabolism

Disadvantages

- Problems with overdosing, necrosis
- Local tissue reactions/hypersensitivity
- Everyone hates getting a needle

Intravenous Route

Excessively metabolized and tissue drug bound at the site of IM can be administered by this route, e.g. insulin, interferon.

Disadvantages: Causes pain, tissue necrosis and thrombocytopenia.

Advantages: Antibiotics can be administered.

Intramuscular Route

- Gamma globulins given by this route are proved to have long-term protection from hepatic infection.
- Some drugs given by this route include long-acting insulin, GH.

Disadvantages: Not used for all protein and peptide drugs because of metabolism of drugs at the site of injection.

Subcutaneous Route

- Controlled release is obtained from implantable polymeric devices.
- These are prepared from cross-linked polymers which are biocompatible and biodegradable, e.g. polylactic acid.
- Release of insulin, bovine serum albumin, LH was prolonged by this route.

Parenteral Drug Delivery System

- Polymer-based drug delivery system
- Liposome-based drug delivery system
- Hydrogel-based drug delivery system
- Emulsion-based drug delivery system

Polymer-Based Drug Delivery System

Polymers are used as carriers in this drug delivery system.

Characters of polymers

- It should be biodegradable.
- It should be biocompatible.
- And non-toxic.

Two types of polymers are used widely:
1. **Natural polymers:** Collagen, haemoglobin and gelatin.
2. **Synthetic polymers:** Mainly poly esters like PLA and PGA are used widely.

Liposome-Based Drug Delivery System

- Spherical vesicles with a phospholipid bilayer
- Liposomes are microscopic vesicles composed of one or more aqueous compartments.

Liposomes in proteins delivery: Example: Lecithin used in controlled drug release.

Liposomes in peptide drug delivery: Bleomycin: A peptide with anti-tumour activity, reduces normal tissue toxicity. Negatively charged liposomes produce a prolonged hypoglycaemic effect in diabetic drugs, which are injected by subcutaneous injection.

Advantages of liposome drug delivery

- Soluble in both organic and aqueous media.
- Liposomes are important for targeting drugs directly to the liver, and brain. Liposomes easily crosses blood–brain barrier, e.g. dopamine converted to L-dopa.
- Used as a vehicle for vaccines.

Disadvantages

- Less stable, easily susceptible to oxidation.
- Hence liposomes are replaced by noisome an alternate for liposomes.

Hydrogel-Based DDS

Hydrogels are three-dimensional networks of hydrophilic polymers that are insoluble with hydrogels are polymers which have the ability to swell in water. Biodegradable hydrogels are used due to its biocompatibility. Examples: Hydroxymethylacrylate used to minimize mechanical irritation to surrounding tissue.

Emulsion-Based DDS

Emulsions can be used for parenteral drug delivery of proteins and peptides used to prolong the release of drug, e.g. subcutaneous administration of muramyl dipeptide in a W/O emulsion. It is used to potentiate immune system.

Cellular Carriers

Proteins and peptides can be incorporated in erythrocytes to achieve the prolong release or targeting. Resealed erythrocytes as delivery system for C-reactive protein, and mainly used to target liver and spleen.

Pumps

Types of Pumps

1. **Implantable pumps:** Drug is implanted subcutaneously, and delivered by IV infusion. Pumps are filled with drug through a septum with a needle. Pumps deliver drugs to central vein for 7–14 days a constant rate.
2. **Mechanical pumps:** Easily manipulated to deliver protein and peptide drugs. Example: Insulin has been successfully delivered by portable syringe.

Non-Parenteral Routes of Administration

Parenteral route is not properly achievable, hence other routes are preferred.

1. Oral route
2. Rectal route
3. Nasal route
4. Pulmonary route
5. Buccal route
6. Transdermal route
7. Ocular route

1. Oral Route

Encapsulated peptides or proteins in amino acids with microsphere of approximately 10 μ in diameter, used for oral delivery, e.g. insulin and heparin. Orally administered insulin produces hypoglycemic effect.

Disadvantages
- Acid catalyzed degradation in stomach.
- Proteolysis in GIT.

2. Rectal Route

- Rectum is highly vascularized body cavity.
- Rectal mucosa is devoid of villi.
- Drugs are in form of suppositories, gel, dry powders, e.g. insulin, calcitonin.

Advantages
- Reduced proteolytic degradation.
- Improved systemic bioavailability with co-administration of absorption enhancers, e.g. surfactants.
- Large dose can be administered.

3. Nasal Route

The nasal route has been employed for producing local action on the mucosa which is more permeable compared to oral mucosa. Nasal absorption is through passive diffusion, e.g. insulin, human growth hormone.

Advantages
- Rapid onset of action
- First pass metabolism can be avoided.
- Better drug absorption

Disadvantages
- Long-term usage causes toxicity.
- Size of proteins and peptide drugs reduces systemic bioavailability.

4. Pulmonary Route

Lungs are attractive site for systemic delivery of proteins and peptides because of their enormous surface area (70 sq. m). Alveoli and lungs are the absorption sites. Drugs are absorbed through lungs by simple diffusion, carrier-mediated transport.

Advantages
- Decrease in dose requirement
- Fast absorption
- Increased patient compliance

Disadvantages
- Inflammation may be observed in lungs.
- Degree of bioavailability was less due to hydrolytic enzymes present in lungs.

5. Buccal Route

Mucoadhesive dosage forms can be used for buccal route. Adsorption enhancers like salicylates or a surfactant is used for protein and peptide delivery through buccal route.

Example: Oxytocin, vasopressin, insulin are reported to be absorbed through buccal mucosa. And adhesive gel, patches, tablets are used. Insulin is absorbed through buccal mucosa in the presence of sodium glycolate. The drugs are absorbed through oral mucosa mainly through the non-keratinized regions.

Advantages
- It can be attached or removed without any discomfort and pain.
- Well acceptability by patients.
- Drugs are absorbed rapidly.

Disadvantages
- Administration time is limited.
- Drug loss by accidental swallowing.

6. Transdermal Route

This is topical medication. Drug is absorbed through the skin, e.g. insulin, vasopressin.

Advantages
- Controlled administration of drug is possible.
- Improved patient compliance.
- Drugs with short half-lives can be administered.

Disadvantages
- High intra- and inter-patient variability.
- Low permeation because of high molecular weight.
- Hydrophilicity and lipophilicity of stratum corneum.

A number of approaches are available for effective protein and peptide drug delivery. They are:
- Iontophoresis
- Phonophoresis
- Penetration enhancers
- Prodrug (chemical modification)

Iontophoresis: Used for local and systemic delivery of proteins and peptides. In this, an electric current is used to drive the molecules across the skin surface, e.g. transport of insulin using iontophoresis.

Phonophoresis: The absorption is enhanced by thermal effect of ultrasonic waves and subsequent alteration of physical structure of skin surface.

Penetration enhancers: Penetration enhancers are usually required to facilitate the absorption of peptides and proteins in pharmacologically active amounts.

Prodrug (chemical modification): The chemical modification of protein and peptide drug delivery system of drugs is important to improve the enzymatic stability as well as membrane permeations. It is applicable for the reducing the immunogenicity.

7. Ocular Route

In this route, enkephalins, thyrotropin-releasing hormones, luteinizing hormones, glucagon and insulin are administered.

Protein and peptide-based pharmaceuticals are rapidly becoming a very important class of therapeutic agents and are likely to replace many existing organic-based pharmaceuticals in the very near future. Peptide and protein drugs will be produced on a large scale by biotechnology processes and will become commercially available for therapeutic use. Their need in the clinical and therapeutic regions has intensified the investigation for their convenient and effective delivery through non-invasive system.

VACCINE DELIVERY SYSTEMS

Introduction

Vaccines are biological product which acts by reinforcing the immunological defense of the body against foreign agencies or their toxins. The agent or product through which immunization is active is called immunization agents. Active immunization is process of increasing resistance to infection where microorganisms or product of their activity act as an antigen and stimulate certain body cells produce an antibody with specific protective capacity. Passive immunization results in intermediate protection of short duration are achieved by antibodies administration. Vaccines may be single component or mixed component vaccines.

Advantages

- Virosomes technology is approved by the FDA for use in humans, and has a high safety profile.
- Virosomes are biodegradable, biocompatible, and non-toxic.
- No disease-transmission risk.
- No autoimmunogenic or anaphylaxis.
- Broadly applicable with almost all important drugs (anticancer drugs, proteins, peptides, nucleic acids, antibiotics, fungicides)
- Enables drug delivery into the cytoplasm of target cell.
- Promotes fusion activity in the endolysosomal pathway.
- Protects drugs against degradation.

Disadvantages

- Shelf-life is too short.
- Scale up related problems.
- Poor quality of raw material.

- Pay-load is too slow.
- Absence on any data on safety of these carrier systems on chronic use.
- But in recent years, several solutions have been worked upon to overcome above.

How do Vaccines Work?

When inactivated or weakened disease-causing microorganisms enter the body, they initiate an immune response. This response mimics the body's natural response to infection. But unlike disease-causing organisms, vaccines are made of components that have limited ability, or are completely unable to cause disease.

Uptake of Antigens

The components of the disease-causing organisms or the vaccine components that trigger the immune response are known as "antigens". These antigens trigger the production of "antibodies" by the immune system. Antibodies bind to corresponding antigens and induce their destruction by other immune cells. The induced immune response to either a disease-causing organism or to a vaccine configures the body's immune cells to be capable of quickly recognizing, reacting to, and subduing the relevant disease-causing organism. When the body's immune system is subsequently exposed to a same disease-causing organism, the immune system will contain and eliminate the infection before it can cause harm to the body. Antigen is any substance which introduce parenterally in body simulates the production of an antibody with it specifically and an observable manner. Most antigens are either proteins or large polysaccharides. The complete antigen is able to induce antibody formation and produce a specific and observable reaction with the antibody so produced. The smallest unit of antigenicity is known as the antigenic determinant or epitope. The epitopic is that small area on the antigen usually consisting of four or five amino acids or monosaccharide reduce possessing specific chemical structure electrical charge and steric configuration capable of sensitizing an immunocyte and of reacting with its complementary site on the specific antibody or T cell receptor. The combining area on the antibody molecules corresponding to epitope is called paratope.

Antigens generated by endogenous and exogenous antigen processing activate different effector functions.

Exogenous Pathogens

Eliminated by: Antibodies and phagocyte activation by T helper cells that use antigens generated by exogenous processing.

Stages of exogenous antigen uptake (Fig. 7.1)
- *Uptake:* Access of native pathogens to intracellular pathways of degradation
- *Degradation:* Limited proteolysis of antigens to peptides
- *Antigen-MHC complex formation:* Loading of peptides on MHC molecules
- *Antigen presentation:* Transport and expression of peptide-MHC complexes on the surfaces of cells for reorganization by T cells.

Endogenous Pathogens

Eliminated by: Killing of infected cells by CTL that use antigens generated by endogenous processing.

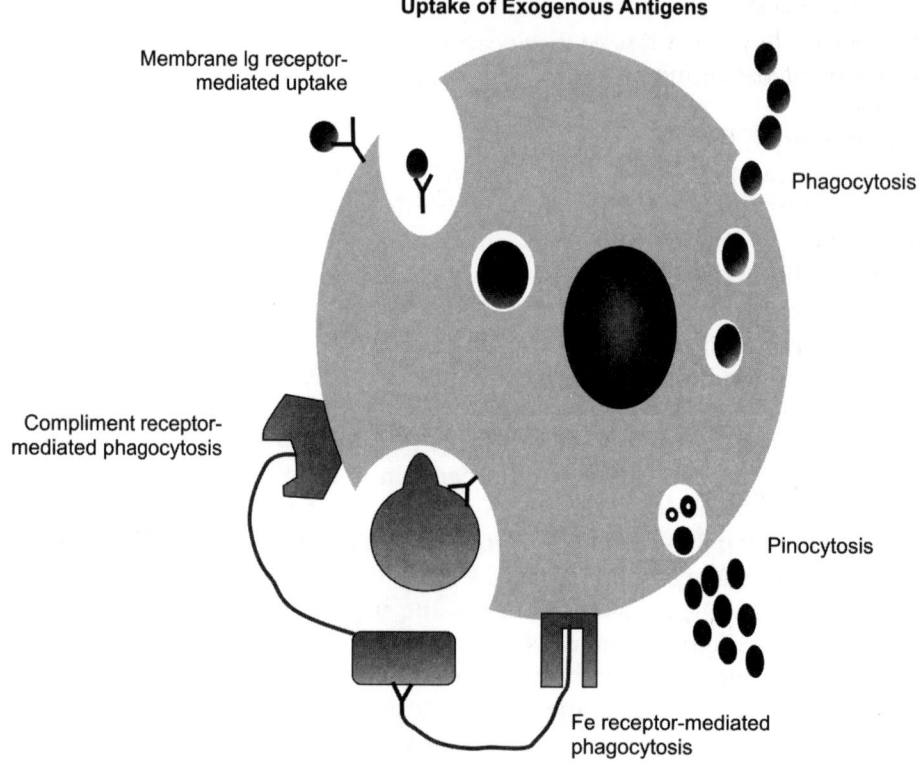

Uptake of Exogenous Antigens

Membrane Ig receptor-mediated uptake

Phagocytosis

Compliment receptor-mediated phagocytosis

Pinocytosis

Fe receptor-mediated phagocytosis

Uptake mechanisms direct antigen into intracellular vesicles for exogenous antigen processing

Fig. 7.1: Exogenous pathway

Stages of endogenous antigen uptake

- *Uptake:* Antigens/pathogens already present in the cells
- *Degradation:* Antigens synthesized in cytoplasm undergo limited proteolytic degradation in the cytoplasm.
- *Antigen-MHC complex formation:* Loading of peptide antigens onto MHC Class 1 molecules is different to the loading on MHC Class-2 molecules.
- *Presentation:* Transport and expression of antigen-MHC complex on the surface of cells for reorganization by T cells.

Antibodies

Antibodies are globulin proteins (a protein family with compact globular form), therefore, the term immunoglobulins (Ig) for antibodies are used. Antibodies are made in response to an antigen and can recognize and bind to the antigen. A bacterium or virus may have several epitopes that causes the production of antibodies. Each antibody has at least two identical sites that bind to epitopes known as antigen-binding site. The number of antigen-binding site on an antibody is called the valence of that antibody. Most human antibodies are bivalent.

Antigen–Antibody Reaction

Antigens and antibodies combine with each other specifically and in an observable manner.

These reactions serve several purposes:

- In the body, they form the basis of antibody-mediated immunity in infection diseases or of tissue injury in some types of hypersensitive and autoimmune diseases.
- In the laboratory, they help in the diagnosis of infections.
- In the identification of infectious agents and of non-infectious antigens.
- These reactions can be used for the detection and quantization of either antigen or antibodies.
- Antigen-antibody reactions *in vitro* are known as serological reactions.

Both participate in the formation of agglutinate and precipitates. Antigens and antibodies can combine in varying proportion unlike chemical with fixed valences. Both antigens and antibodies are multivalent. Antibodies are generally bivalent though IgM molecule may have five or ten combining site. Antigens may have valance up to hundreds.

Single Shot Vaccines

The single shot vaccine is combination product of a prime component antigen with an appropriate adjuvant and a microsphere component that encapsulates antigen and provides the booster immunization by delayed release of the antigen. Many aspects need to be taken into consideration when developing such controlled released technology-based vaccine.

Important Determinants for Single Shot Vaccine Development

- Biodegradable technology
- Encapsulation efficiency
- Particle size distribution
- Preservation of bioactivity during formulation and release
- Scalable production processes
- Effects of combination with various adjuvants
- Effects of different administration routes

Formulation and Manufacturing of Single Shot Vaccines

Important factors in the manufacture of a microsphere-based vaccine are high encapsulation efficiency and a consistent particle production process. Several formulation parameters play an important role in obtaining a robust process. Below we discuss the process and equipment used to manufacture several formulations (Fig. 7.2).

- Several factors are critical parameters for the formulation of consisting microsphere:
  - *First:* The size distribution of the microsphere can be controlled by the shear force applied during the emulsification step in the bioreactor vessels. Factors that have been identified to influence this shear force are the mechanical stirring speed in the bioreactor vessels and the viscosity of PEG solution which is determined by concentration and molecular weight of the PEG.
  - *Second:* The presence of excipients in the starting composition can influence the matrix density and encapsulation efficiency to the microsphere product either by direct effect on the microsphere formation or on the protein characteristic. Finally, polymerization condition such as KPS concentration, pH, and temperature, can influence the strength of the form hydrogel matrix.

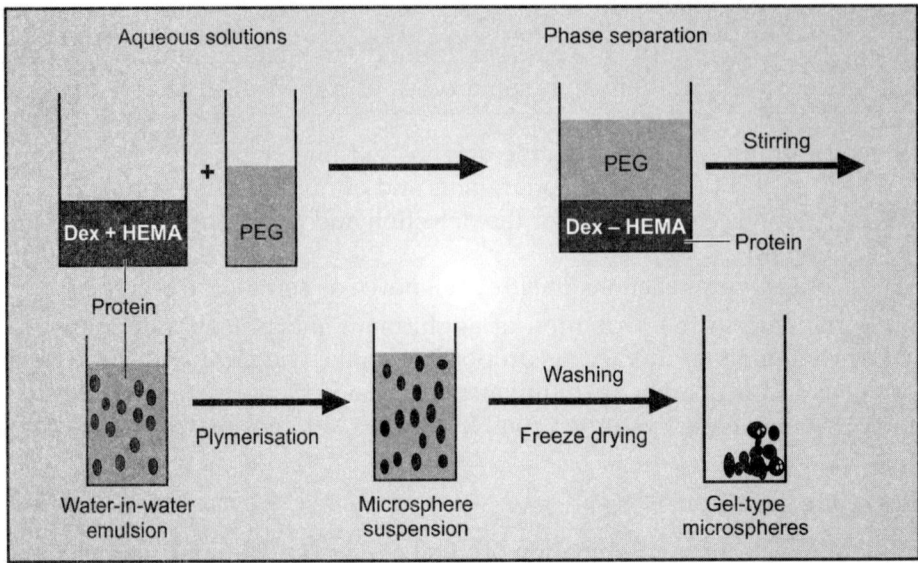

Fig. 7.2: Formulation of single shot vaccine

- Controlling particle size during process scale-up.
- The dextran microsphere preparation method described by researcher Steinke's et al was initially performed on a 5 g scale (containing 120 mg of microsphere), and used vortexing as a means to emulsify the dex-HEMA phase in a continuous PEG phase. However, vortexing is not practically at a large scale. Therefore, we evaluate the feasibility of stirring, a process that is relatively scale-up as a means of emulsification ultimately at 500 g scale.

Transdermal Delivery Vaccine

The skin is the largest and most accessible organ of the body. Vaccine administration to skin offers many advantages include ease of access disease a potential for generation of both systemic and mucosal immune responses. The skin is a site of vaccine delivery. It approaches to overcome these barriers are cover included formulation approaches such as liposome, electroporation, and technologies that creates micron size pores in the skin. The World Health Organization estimates that 32% of hepatitis B virus infections, 40% of hepatitis C and 5% of human immunodeficiency virus infection in developing country are attributable to unsafe injection practice. The development of needle-free immunization method has thus become an important goal in global health care. Dermal vaccination or transcutaneous immunization is a needle-free method of vaccine delivery which has the potential to reduce the risk of needle burn disease, access to vaccination by simplifying procedure (trained personnel and use of sterile equipment not required) and assist in the implementation of multiple boosting and multivalent vaccine regimes.

Skin as a Site for Vaccine Delivery

The skin has multiple barrier properties to minimize water loss from the body and prevents the permeation of environmental contaminants into the body. These barriers can be considered as physical, enzymatic and immunological. They range from formulation approaches such as liposomes to minimally invasive technology that creates channel in the skin such as micro-needle. All methods aim to overcome the stratum corneum barrier and target vaccines to immune responsive cell such as Langerhans cell.

Immunization by dermal route for primary delivery method under investigation and development as follows:

a. Liquid jet
b. Epidermal powder immunization
c. Topical application of vaccines to the epidermis via
   • Hair follicles
   • Tap stripping to remove the stratum corneum
   • Thermal or radiowave-mediated ablation of the stratum corneum
   • Colloidal carriers such as microemulsion and liposome's increase dermal absorption
   • Low frequency ultrasound as an adjuvant and to increase skin penetration
   • Topically applied adjuvant to induce a potent immune responses
   • Electroporation of the stratum corneum
   • Shallow microneedles that penetrate into the epidermis

Application of Transdermal Delivery Vaccine

• Application of liquid-jet injector focused on delivery of macromolecules that do not passively permeate the skin.
• For administration of insulin and human growth hormone.

Delivery Systems Used to Promote Uptake

Absorption Enhancers

Absorption enhancement is the technology aimed at enabling non-injection delivery of poorly membrane permeable compounds. The term absorption enhancer usually refers to an agent whose function is to increase absorption by enhancing membrane permeation, rather than increasing solubility, so such agents are sometimes more specifically termed as permeation enhancers. Absorption enhancers are functional excipients included in formulations to improve the absorption of a pharmacologically active drug.

Liposomal Delivery Systems

Liposomes are composed of phospholipid bilayers capable of entrapping hydrophilic moieties in the aqueous compartment and hydrophobic moieties in the lipid bilayers with cholesterol imparting rigidity to the bilayer. Viruses, proteins, glycoproteins, nucleic acids, carbohydrates, and lipids can be entrapped and targeted at cellular and subcellular level for evoking immune responses. As vaccine adjuvants, these systems exert immunomodulatory effects by virtue of their particulate nature and their ability to bind with cell surface lipid receptors such as CD1a. There are many methods of preparation of liposome vaccine formulations for entrapment of antigenic peptides and antigen encoding plasmid DNAs. Liposomes are versatile and robust delivery systems for systems for induction of antibody and T lymphocyte responses to associated subunit antigens. Liposomal vaccines based on viral membrane proteins (virosomes) have been approved as products in Europe for hepatitis A and influenza.

Controlled Release Microparticles for Vaccine Delivery

PLGA (polylactide co-glycolic acid) is used as a biodegradable microparticle for vaccine delivery due to the abundance of data and information on its properties, uses, and role in ongoing studies. A particularly interesting area is the use of biodegradable microparticles to deliver DNA vaccines. DNA vaccines, or so-called third generation vaccines, "involve the deliberate introduction into tissues of a DNA plasmid carrying an antigen-coding gene that transfers cells in vivo and results in an immune response". Biodegradable microparticles, in particular PLGA and PLA, are good devices for DNA vaccine delivery because the DNA is protected from enzymatic degradation. Malaria is a mosquito-borne disease caused by a parasite. People with malaria often experience fever, chills, and flu-like illness. Left untreated, the disease can be lethal. Annually, 350–500 million cases of malaria occur worldwide. Researchers effectively encapsulated a subunit malaria antigen, SPf66, in PLGA-mixture microspheres and demonstrated high antibody levels in mice and monkeys. The purpose of their work was to provide a minimal dose vaccine with a clinically relevant antigen, SPf66 (Phase III trials), and the data propose that PLGA is a promising vehicle for delivery. The microparticles (1.3 μm average diameters) appear smooth and spherical under electron microscopy. Scanning electron microscopy of PLGA formulation.

Single Dose Vaccine Delivery Systems Using Biodegradable Polymers

Biodegradable polymers are defined as polymers comprised monomers linked to one another through functional groups and have unstable links in the backbone. Broken down into biologically acceptable molecules that are metabolized and removed from the body via normal metabolic pathways. There are two types of biodegradable polymers.

1. **Natural biodegradable polymers:** Albumin, collagen, gelatin, etc.
2. **Synthetic biodegradable polymers:** Aliphatic poly (esters), polyanhydride, polyphosphazene, pseudo poly amino acid, poly (orthoesters), etc.

Biodegradable Polymers as Adjuvants

We need adjuvants to increase the therapeutic efficiency. They form depot of antigen at the site of inoculation with slow release of antigens. It can improve the performance of vaccines by targeting the antigen to APC. Biodegradable polymers such as poly (lactide co-glycolic acids) is most commonly used for vaccine delivery. This polymer is mainly required for controlled release of the drug from polymer matrix. Targeting to appropriate cell types to generate optimum response. Development of formulation that can be used as non-invasive.

Single Dose Vaccine Delivery Using Prefilled Syringes

There are over 20 pharmaceutical companies manufacturing prefilled syringes for at least 50 injectable drugs and vaccines, e.g. heat-stable vaccines, seasonal influenza vaccine, polio vaccine, etc. A prefilled syringe is a single dose packet of parenteral drug to which a needle has been fixed. Prefilled syringes are ready to use disposable syringes contains premeasured dosage, reduce dosing errors and increase patient compliance.

Knowledge of Peptide-Based Vaccines

A peptide vaccine is a type of subunit vaccine in which a peptide of the original pathogen is used to immunize an organism. These types of vaccine are usually rapidly degraded once injected into the body, unless they are bound to a carrier molecule such as a fusion protein. The role of a therapeutic cancer vaccine essentially involves activating the soldiers, namely

- Dendritic cells,
- Macrophages,
- Cytotoxic T cells, and
- Natural killer cells to act against the tumour cells.

Dendritic cells and macrophages are the professional antigen presenting cells (APCs) of the immune system. In simple terms, they eat any foreign substance encountered by them, and display antigens derived from it onto their surface. Such APCs then interact with and activate the helper and cytotoxic T cells, as well as educate them to recognize the cancerous cells.

Role of a Cancer Vaccine

The vast majority of published pre-clinical studies have demonstrated the requirement of T lymphocytes for the eradication of solid tumours. Cytotoxic T lymphocytes (CTLs) or CD8+ T cells represent the primary effector cells involved in tumour-specific immune-mediated destruction of cancer cells. Peptides are efficient tools for stimulation of antigen-specific CD8 T cell. A variety of cancer associated antigens has been identified, and is being studied for immune system activation. They may be peptides present on the surface of cancer cells, certain enzymes that aid a vital cancer-promoting process, receptors for certain growth factors, etc. These antigens are classified as tumour-associated antigens (TAA) and tumour-specific antigens (TSA). The peptide vaccine thus prepared is injected into the patient. The APCs (antigen-presenting cells) of the patient's immune system engulf these peptides, and present them on the surface in order to educate the other immune cells. The educated immune cells, when encounter the same antigen on a cancerous cell, bring about the destruction of that cell.

Knowledge of Nucleic Acid-Based Vaccines

Effective use of 'naked' nucleic acids as vaccines would undoubtedly be one of the most important advances in the history of vaccinology. While nucleic acids show much promise for use as vaccine vectors in experimental animals, not a single naked nucleic acid vector has been approved for use in humans. Nucleic acid vaccines have not been clearly demonstrated to have any convincing efficacy in the prevention or treatment of infectious diseases or cancer.

How do nucleic acid vaccines work?

It has been a decade since workers found that injection of 'naked' plasmid DNA, that is DNA without any associated lipid, protein or carbohydrate, could elicit an immune response. While the earliest studies were done using DNA, some subsequent studies have explored the use of RNA vaccines. Hence, they are collectively referred as nucleic acid vaccine. They are relatively simple to generate and safe to administer. In contrast to vaccines that employ recombinant bacteria or viruses, genetic vaccines consist only of DNA or RNA, which is taken up and translated into protein by host cells. Unfortunately, immunization with naked nucleic acid is relatively inefficient and virus vectors generally induce far greater immune responses than DNA vaccines. A most recent improvement upon plasmid nucleic acid vectors was the incorporation of alpha virus replicons. 'Self-replicating' or replicon-based genetic vaccines were designed to overcome the poor efficacy of some current DNA-based and RNA-based genetic vaccines. There are many DNA vaccines in clinical and pre-clinical trials, including vaccines for HIV, herpes, hepatitis and influenza. The DNA vaccine is composed of a plasmid DNA that contains the genetic code for a TSA or TAA. When this DNA plasmid is injected into the skin or muscle, it is engulfed and internalized by the surrounding cells as well as APCs. Here, the genetic information is decoded; the peptide antigen is synthesized and displayed onto the surface, and cross-presented to the APCs. The APCs then educate other cells, and initiate an immune response against the tumour cells. The efficiency of DNA vaccine can be increased by addition of certain pathogenic sequences adjacent to the antigen sequence or by use of modern delivery systems like nanoparticles.

Mucosal Delivery of Vaccines

Mucosal surface area is major portal of entry for many human pathogens that are the cause of infectious disease worldwide. Immunization by mucosal routes may be more effective at inducing protective immunity against mucosal pathogens at their sites of entry. Efforts have focused on efficient delivery of vaccine antigens to mucosal sites that facilitate uptake by local antigen-presenting cells to generate protective mucosal immune responses. The adult human mucosa lines the surfaces of the digestive, respiratory and genitourinary tracts, covering an immense surface area (400 m^2) that is 200 times greater than that of the skin. Mucosal surfaces are typically categorized as Type-1 and Type-2 mucosa. Type-1 mucosa include surface of the lung and gut, whereas Type-2 mucosa include surfaces of the mouth, oesophagus and cornea.

Mucosal vaccination offers protection against microorganisms which gain access to body via mucosal membranes. Patient compliance, ease of administration, reduction in possibility of needle-borne injections, and stimulation of both systemic and mucosal immunity are some of the advantages. Co-administration of antigens with adjuvants like aluminium hydroxide, complete Freund's adjuvant, incomplete Freund's adjuvant, cholera toxin, heat labile enterotoxin of *E. coli*, etc., potentiated immune response of antigen. For example, Freund's adjuvant when administered subcutaneously to neonatal mice-induced mixed T helper 1 and 2 responses with interferon component against *Helicobacter pylori* infection. Delivery systems like PLG microspheres, PLGA microparticles carrying immunogenic agents, etc. are taken up by Peyer's patches. Particles of <5 µm further move into lymph nodes and spleen-stimulating-specific IgG, IgM responses. Chitosan, a bioadhesive polysaccharide discussed earlier is suitable for mucosal vaccination due to its ability to open up tight junctions and promote paracellular transport of antigen across mucosa.

Nasal Mucosa Delivery

Nasal mucosa is the first contact site for antigens being inhaled, systemic and local immunity can be stimulated by activation of T cells, B cells, and dendritic cells present in nasal associated lymphoid tissue located beneath nasal epithelium in the form of

IgG and secretory IgA. Hence, nasal delivery of vaccines can be used to treat upper respiratory tract infections and also to produce systemic immunity. Intranasal vaccines include those against influenza A and B virus, proteasome-influenza, adenovirus-vectored influenza, group B meningococcal native, attenuated respiratory syncytial virus and parainfluenza virus.

Vaccines are one of the most effective health interventions ever developed. Although various vaccines have been successfully developed for several diseases, research is still in progress to develop vaccines for life-threatening diseases like cancer, AIDS, etc. Understanding the mechanism of absorption enhancement may be very useful toward registration. However, it seems reasonable that once a delivery technology is proven to be successful for one particular drug, that technology might be readily adapted to improving the delivery of other poorly absorbed drugs. As the vaccines have a lot of benefits, they do carry some harmful effects too.

QUESTIONS

A. Short Answer Type Questions

1. Mention the different barriers for protein drug delivery system.
2. Write a short note on single shot vaccines.
3. Give the significance of protein and peptide drug delivery system.
4. Write the functions of protein and peptide drug delivery system.
5. What are the pharmaceutical approaches used in protein drug delivery system?
6. What do you mean by vaccine delivery system?

B. Long Answer Type Questions

1. Write about the different properties and barriers for protein drug delivery system.
2. Discuss in detail about protein and peptide drug delivery systems and their applications.
3. What is vaccine? Discuss on different uptakes of antigens in vaccine delivery system.
4. Describe on protein drug delivery system and their merits in detail.

8

Biotechnology in Drug Delivery System and Nucleic Acid-Based Therapeutic Delivery System

BIOTECHNOLOGY IN DRUG DELIVERY SYSTEM

Introduction

Drug delivery is becoming a whole interdisciplinary and independent field of research and is gaining the attention of pharmaceutical makers, medical doctors and industry. A targeted and safe drug delivery could improve the performance of some classical medicines already on the market and, moreover, will have implications for the development and success of new therapeutic strategies, such as peptide and protein delivery, glycoprotein administration, gene therapy and RNA interference. Many innovative technologies for effective drug delivery have been developed, including implants, nanotechnology, cell and peptide encapsulation, microfabrication, chemical modification and others. On the long way from the clinic to market, however, several issues will have to be addressed, including suitable scientific development, specific financial support as a result of altered scientific policy, government regulations and market forces.

Recombinant DNA Technology

DNA is the keeper of all the information needed to recreate an organism. All DNA is made up of a base consisting of sugar, phosphate and one nitrogen base. There are four nitrogen bases: Adenine (A), thymine (T), guanine (G), and cytosine (C). The nitrogen bases are found in pairs, with A and T and G and C paired together. The sequence of the nitrogen bases can be arranged in an infinite way, and their structure is known as the famous 'double helix'. The sugar used in DNA is deoxyribose. The four nitrogen bases are the same for all organisms. The sequence and number of bases is what creates diversity. DNA does not actually make the organism; it only makes proteins.

The DNA is transcribed into mRNA and mRNA is translated into protein, and the protein then forms the organism. By changing the DNA sequence, the way in which the protein is formed changes. This leads to either a different protein, or an inactive protein. Now that we know what DNA is, this is where the recombinant comes in. Recombinant DNA is the general name for taking a piece of one DNA, and combining it with another strand of DNA. Thus, the name recombinant! Recombinant DNA is also sometimes referred to as 'chimera'. By combining two or more different strands of DNA, scientists are able to create a new strand of DNA. The most common recombinant process involves combining the DNA of two different organisms.

Formation of Recombinant DNA

There are three different methods by which recombinant DNA is made. They are transformation, phage introduction, and non-bacterial transformation. Each are described separately below.

1. **Transformation:** The first step in transformation is to select a piece of DNA to be inserted into a vector. The second step is to cut that piece of DNA with a restriction enzyme and then ligate the DNA insert into the vector with DNA ligase. The insert contains a selectable marker which allows for identification of recombinant molecules. An antibiotic marker is often used so a host cell without a vector dies when exposed to a certain antibiotic, and the host with the vector will live because it is resistant. The vector is inserted into a host cell, in a process called transformation. One example of a possible host cell is *E. coli*. The host cells must be specially prepared to take up the foreign DNA. Selectable markers can be for antibiotic resistance, colour changes, or any other characteristic which can distinguish transformed hosts from untransformed hosts. Different vectors have different properties to make them suitable to different applications. Some properties can include symmetrical cloning sites, size, and high copy number.

2. **Non-bacterial transformation:** This is a process very similar to transformation, which was described above. The only difference between the two is that non-bacterial does not use bacteria such as *E. coli* for the host. In microinjection, the DNA is injected directly into the nucleus of the cell being transformed. In biolistics, the host cells are bombarded with high velocity microprojectiles, such as particles of gold or tungsten that is coated with DNA.

3. **Phage introduction:** Phage introduction is the process of transfection, which is equivalent to transformation, except a phage is used instead of bacteria. *In vitro* packaging of a vector is used. This uses lambda or MI3 phages to produce phage plaques which contain recombinants. The recombinants that are created may be identified by differences in the recombinants and non-recombinants using several selection methods.

Working of rDNA

Recombinant DNA works when the host cell expresses protein from the recombinant genes. A significant amount of recombinant protein will not be produced by the host unless expression factors are added. Protein expression depends upon the gene being surrounded by a collection of signals which provide instructions for the transcription and translation of the gene by the cell. These signals include the promoter, the ribosome, binding site, and the terminator. Expression vectors, in which the foreign DNA is inserted, contain these signals. Signals are species specific. In the case of *E. coli*, these signals must be *E. coli* signals as *E. coli* is unlikely to understand the signals of human promoters and terminators. Problems are encountered, if the gene contains introns or contains signals which act as terminators to a bacterial host. This results in premature termination, and the recombinant protein may not be processed correctly, be folded correctly, or may even be degraded. Production of recombinant proteins in eukaryotic systems generally takes place in yeast and filamentous fungi. The use of animal cells is difficult due to the fact that many need a solid support surface, unlike bacteria, and has complex growth needs. However, some proteins are too complex to be produced in bacterium, so eukaryotic cells must be used.

Importance of rDNA

Recombinant DNA has been gaining importance over the last few years, and recombinant DNA will only become more important in the 21st century as genetic diseases become more prevalent and agricultural area is reduced. Below are some of the areas where recombinant DNA will have an impact.
- Better crops (drought and heat resistance)
- Recombinant vaccines (hepatitis B)
- Prevention and cure of sickle cell anaemia
- Prevention and cure of cystic fibrosis
- Production of clotting factors
- Production of insulin
- Production of recombinant pharmaceuticals
- Plants that produce their own insecticides
- Germ line and somatic gene therapy

Monoclonal Antibodies

Monoclonal antibodies (mAbs) are defined as "laboratory-produced molecules engineered to serve as substitute antibodies that can restore, enhance, or mimic the immune system's attack on cancer cells" by binding to antigens found on the surface of cancer cells. Experiments to create this type of treatment have existed for more than a century. In the 18th century, it was discovered by Dr Edward Jenner that "fluid obtained from a smallpox pustule when injected into a recipient provided immunity from acquiring the disease. The earliest antibodies were traditionally created by "immunizing experimental animals with an antigen with subsequent purification of the serum to isolate the antibody fraction".

The initial mAbs were generated utilizing murine (from mice) protein and were not well tolerated for long periods of time by humans. Therefore, the production mechanisms were forced to be re-evaluated and eventually changed by the development of technology, allowing for fully humanized antibodies. The first monoclonal antibody to be approved by the US Food and Drug Administration was muromonab-CD3, which was used as an anti-rejection medication. The first monoclonal antibody that was found successful in the treatment of solid tumours was trastuzumab (Fig. 8.1).

Classification and Types of mAbs

There are four classifications of mAbs: Murine, chimeric, humanized, and human.

Murine: The first mAb to be discovered and reproduced was the murine monoclonal antibody. This type of mAb arises from harvesting B lymphocytes from the spleen of a mice and then fused with an immortal myeloma cell line lacking the hypoxanthine-guanine-phosphoribosyltransferase (HPTR) gene. All of these mAbs are identified with a name that ends in -omab (i.e. muromonab-CD3, blinatumomab, capromab). Allergic reactions are common when used in humans and often result in the induction of anti-drug antibodies. Murine mAbs also have a short half-life when used in humans because

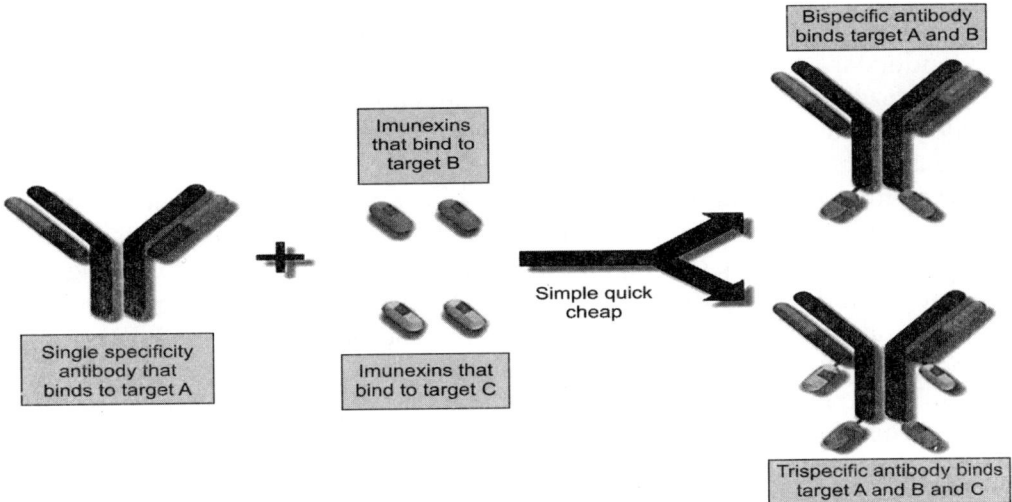

Fig 8.1: Structure of monoclonal antibody

of a relatively weak binding to the human FcRn. For oncology, these mAbs may not be the most beneficial as they are "relatively poor recruiters of effector function, antibody-dependent cellular cytotoxicity, and complement-dependent cytotoxicity, essential functions needed for tumour destruction.

Chimeric: Chimeric mAbs utilize the murine antigen-specific variable region, but the remaining heavy and light chains are human. This was accomplished using genetic engineering techniques, which resulted in mAbs that are approximately 65% human and 35% murine. The chimeric mAbs are identified with names ending in -ximab (i.e. rituximab, infliximab, cetuximab). Compared with their murine counterparts, these mAbs "show an extended half-life in man and exhibit decreased immunogenicity, but nevertheless, the propensity of chimeric mAbs to induce anti-drug antibodies is still considerable".

Humanized: Humanized mAbs are created by grating the murine hypervariable regions of the light and heavy chains onto a human Ab framework. This results in molecules that are approximately 95% human. This resulted in decreased production of anti-drug antibodies. However, the process to create these molecules is arduous and has limitations. These mAbs are identified with names ending in -zumab (i.e. trastuzumab, alemtuzumab, bevacizumab).

Human: With the development of new technology, fully human mAbs are able to be created. These are created utilizing animals carrying human Ig genes. These transgenes include parts of the variable regions, which enable the recombination of the human antibodies. The animal's own endogenous Ig genes have been inactivated, enabling the generation of fully human mAbs. These mAbs are less antigenic and better tolerated compared with the other classes of mAbs. Additionally, they appear to remain present in the human body's circulation compared with the other classes. These mAbs are identified with names ending in -umab (i.e. ofatumumab, daratumumab, denosumab). There are three types of mAbs that are dependent upon how they are administered or used: Unconjugated or naked, conjugated, and bispecific.

Mechanism of Action

The understanding of how these antibodies target cancer cells has helped to revolutionize the methods used to treat cancer and resulted in a more tolerable toxicity profile than standard chemotherapy. When utilizing mAbs in oncology, several mechanisms of action exist to destroy the cancer cells. These mechanisms include impeding tumour cell survival cascades, inhibiting tumour growth by interfering with tumour angiogenesis, eluding programmed cell death, and evading immune checkpoints. Some of the different mechanisms of action include the following.

1. **Direct tumour cell killing:** This action is stimulated by receptor agonist activity, such as an antibody binding to a tumour cell surface receptor and activating it, leading to cell death. It can also be stimulated by receptor antagonist activity "such as an antibody binding to a cell surface receptor and blocking dimerization, kinase activation, and downstream signaling, leading to reduced proliferation and apoptosis". An mAb binding to an enzyme can lead to neutralization and apoptosis, while conjugated antibodies can be used to deliver a payload, such as a drug, to the tumour cell.

2. **Immune-mediated tumour cell killing:** In this setting, the immune system will seek out cancer cells and destroy them. This type of cell death may be carried out by the initiation of one of several mechanisms. These mechanisms include:
   a. Phagocytosis
   b. Complement activation
   c. Antibody-dependent cellular cytotoxicity (ADCC)
   d. Genetically modified T cells being targeted to the tumour by single-chain variable fragment
   e. T cells being activated by antibody-mediated cross-presentation of antigen to dendritic cells
   f. Inhibition of T cell inhibitory receptors.

3. **Vascular and stromal cell ablation:** This action is also initiated by one of many options. These include:
   a. Vasculature receptor antagonism or ligand trapping;
   b. Stromal cell inhibition;
   c. Delivery of a toxin to stromal cells; or
   d. Delivery of a toxin to the vasculature.

Applications

1. **Diagnostic tests:** Once monoclonal antibodies for a given substance have been produced, they can be used to detect the presence of this substance. Proteins can be detected using the Western blot and immune-dot blot tests. In immune histochemistry, monoclonal antibodies can be used to detect antigens in fixed tissue sections, and similarly, immune fluorescence can be used to detect a substance in either frozen tissue section or live cells.

2. **Analytic and chemical uses:** Antibodies can also be used to purify their target compounds from mixtures, using the method of immune precipitation.

3. **Therapeutic uses:** Therapeutic monoclonal antibodies act through multiple mechanisms, such as blocking of targeted molecule functions, inducing apoptosis in cells which express the target, or by modulating signaling pathways.

4. **Cancer treatment:** One possible treatment for cancer involves monoclonal antibodies that bind only to cancer cell-specific antigens and induce an immune response against the target cancer cell. Such mAbs can be modified for delivery of a toxin, radioisotope, cytokine or other active conjugate or to design bispecific antibodies that can bind with their Fab regions both to target antigen and to a conjugate or effector cell. MAbs approved by the FDA (for cancer) as of 2005 include: Alemtuzumab, bevacizumab, cetuximab, gemtuzumab ozogamicin, ipilimumab, ofatumumab, panitumumab, pembrolizumab, ranibizumab, rituximab, trastuzumab, etc.

5. **Autoimmune diseases:** Monoclonal antibodies used for autoimmune diseases include infliximab and adalimumab, which are effective in rheumatoid arthritis, Crohn's disease, ulcerative colitis and ankylosing spondylitis by their ability to bind to and inhibit TNF-α. Basiliximab and daclizumab inhibit IL-2 on activated T cells and thereby help prevent acute rejection of kidney transplants. Omalizumab inhibits human immunoglobulin E (IgE) and is useful in treating moderate-to-severe allergic asthma.

NUCLEIC ACID-BASED THERAPEUTIC DELIVERY SYSTEM

Introduction

Nucleic acids have changed biomedical research and become essential research tools. Nucleic acid molecules are useful in a variety of biochemical, diagnostic, and therapeutic applications. Gene therapy is a technique used to correct defective genes which are responsible for disease development. Gene therapy involves the transference of new genetic material to the cell for obtaining a therapeutic benefit, which offers new option for the treatment of various diseases. Nucleic acid-based molecules (deoxyribonucleic acid, complementary deoxyribonucleic acid, complete genes, ribonucleic acid, and oligonucleotides) are used as research tools within the gene therapy and in molecular medicine.

A nucleic acid is a complex, high molecular weight biochemical macromolecule which is composed of nucleotide chains that transfers genetic information. Nucleic acid molecules are useful in a variety of biochemical, diagnostic, and therapeutic application for a wide range of human disorders. The physicochemical properties of nucleic acids are associated with molecular weights that range from 7 kDa for antisense oligonucleotides to over 1 MDa for plasmid DNA, and strong negative charge.

Delivery of Nucleic Acid

Nucleic acids have transformed the biomedical research and have become useful research tools. Nucleic acid delivery systems are based on viral or non-viral methods. Non-viral carrier (synthetic vector) delivery systems have several advantages that include improved biosafety and flexibility. They are simple to manufacture and modify as compared with viral vectors. The discovery of lipofection has increased the use of cationic lipids for nucleic acid delivery *in vitro* and *in vivo*, and they are also used in clinical trials of human gene therapy.

Cationic lipids form cationic liposomes which bind electrostatically to anionic nucleic acids and form complexes that are taken by endocytosis into the cell. Cationic lipids may fuse to the cell membranes and are toxic in some cases. They easily undergo

DNA-induced fusion and yield larger particles (>100 nm) that are less likely for endocytosis and show poor vascular mobility. Cationic polymers are small and narrow sized, they show high resistance to nucleases, and their physical properties (e.g. hydrophilicity and charge) are easily controlled by copolymerization.

Cationic polymers are used to induce DNA condensation due to the formation of strongly charged complexes with the anionic phosphate groups which are present on the DNA backbone. The so formed complexes have colloidal dimensions, and can protect nucleic acids from enzymatic degradation, and also facilitate cellular entry. These cationic complexes regulate DNA transcription via the following mechanism:

1. The complex adheres to the cell surface by electrostatic interactions.
2. Cellular endocytosis transfers the carrier-DNA complex into endosomes.
3. The complex translocates from the endosomes to the cytoplasm by lipid fusion (buffering effect).
4. The complex or DNA released from the complex moves into the nucleus, and allows transcription to start.

Nanoparticles as Drug Carriers

Nanoparticulate carriers are preferred over their viral carriers for nucleic acid delivery due to the safety affects. They can also be formulated to modify the level and duration of gene expression as per the targeted disease condition. Nucleic acid delivery is done by employing cationic nanoparticles so as to condense the previous formed due to electrostatic interactions. These carriers have the potential to leave the endolysosomal compartment because of the charged interaction with endolysosomal membrane. This gives protection to the corresponding nucleic acid molecules. Cationic agents also interact with the anionic cell membranes for an efficient delivery. Polymeric nanoparticles, which are produced by using PLGA/PLA, are embedded within the polymer. So nucleic acid remains associated with the polymer for weeks before being released. Other than polymeric nanoparticles, nanoparticulate systems based on 1,2-dioleoyl-3- dimethylammonium propane (DODAP), an ionizable amino lipid, are also developed for large quantities of nucleic acid molecules. This technology has been applied to include other nucleic acids, like DNA, siRNA and aptamers, to form stable nucleic acid-lipid particles.

Synthetic Nucleic Acid Delivery

Synthetic nucleic acid delivery systems are prepared particularly by synthetic organic chemistry for the functional delivery of therapeutic nucleic acids by *in vitro*, *ex vivo* and *in vivo* into the cells. Cationic liposomes and polymers are prepared and then combined with therapeutic nucleic acids to form lipid-based nanoparticles (LNPs) or polymer-based nanoparticles (PNPs). The previously formed PNPs and LNPs are difficult for clinical studies due to cytotoxicity and poor biocompatibility.

Self-assembled synthetic gene delivery systems represent the bottom-up approach to gene delivery and gene silencing, novel cationic and procationic amphiphiles are developing so that nucleic acids can be delivered and transported to various targets in the body in a controlled manner. These supramolecular assemblies are safer than viruses, but they are lagging behind them in efficiency.

Drug Delivery Based on Nucleic Acid Nanostructures

The field of DNA nanotechnology has progressed rapidly in recent years and hence a large variety of 1D-, 2D- and 3D-DNA nanostructures with various sizes, geometries and shapes is readily accessible. Two methods were developed to obtain well-defined and structurally stable DNA nano-objects. The first one involves DNA tiles that utilize the helical turn of DNA to form crossovers between two or more double strands within its structure. This design principle yields more rigid building blocks of high structural integrity that can be used for the construction of larger crystals of DNA. Later this method is greatly expanded and generalized to allow the assembly of DNA into any desired shape like squares, triangles, star shapes using a single viral DNA strand (Fig. 8.2).

The second method to obtain rigid DNA nano-objects relies on the tensegrity principle. The squares considered earlier were unstable due to flexible junctions. DNA triangles, however, do not face this shortcoming of this principle to construct a large number of DNA nanocages resistant to deformation like tetrahedra, octahedra, dodecahedra and icosahedra.

Gene Therapy

Gene therapy can be broadly defined as the transfer of genetic material to cure a disease or at least to improve the clinical status of a patient. One of the basic concepts of gene therapy is to transform viruses into genetic shuttles, which will deliver the gene of interest into the target cells. Safe methods have been devised to do this, using several viral and non-viral vectors. Two main approaches emerged: *In vivo* modification and *ex vivo* modification. Retrovirus, adenovirus, and adeno-associated virus are suitable for gene therapeutic approaches which are based on permanent expression of the therapeutic gene. Non-viral vectors are far less efficient than viral vectors, but they have advantages due to their low immunogenicity and their large capacity for therapeutic DNA. To improve the function of non-viral vectors, the addition of viral functions such as receptor-mediated uptake and nuclear translocation of DNA may finally lead to the development of an artificial virus. Gene transfer protocols have been approved for human use in inherited diseases, cancers and acquired disorders. Although the available vector systems are able to deliver genes *in vivo* into cells, the

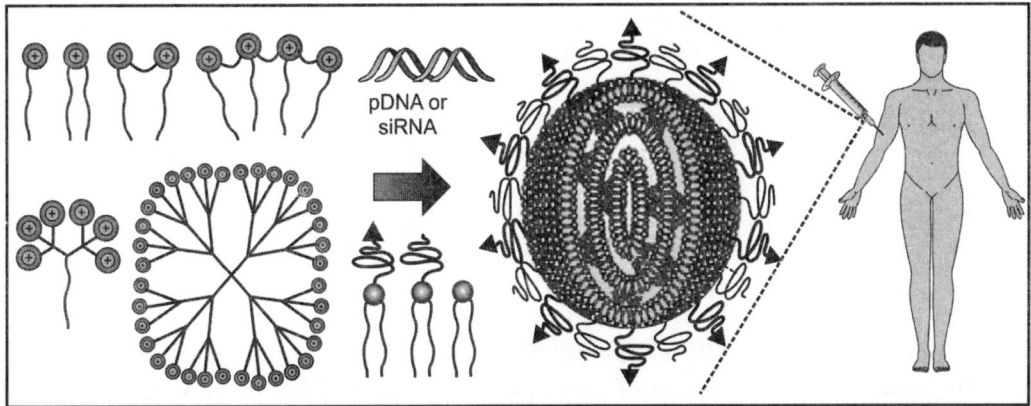

Fig 8.2: Nucleic acid nanostructures

ideal delivery vehicle has not been found. Thus, the present viral vectors should be used only with great caution in human beings and further progress in vector development is necessary.

Gene Therapy Technologies

The transfer of genetic material can be accomplished *in vivo* through local or systemic inoculation or *ex vivo* where the target of interest is collected and modified outside of the organism before return to the host. Transfer of synthetic DNA can be accomplished by transduction or transfection. Such methods of transfer include either direct injection of DNA into the recipient cells, or utilizing methods to induce membranes permeation, receptor-mediated uptake or endocytosis. Transduction utilizes recombinant virus as a vector for gene transfer. Entry of these vectors is mediated by cell-surface receptors. Concerns regarding the immunogenicity of viral vector systems due to activation of memory responses against constituent viral proteins or a primary response to neoantigens have spawned the evolution of synthetic gene delivery systems which exploit transfection, the transfer of DNA via physical, chemical or electrical methods. Benefits of non-viral methods for DNA transfer include a reduction of risks associated with viruses (immune response, insertional mutagenesis) and limitations to gene delivery (such as length of the transgene cassette).

Physical Methods to Enhance Delivery

1. **Electroporation:** Electroporation is a method that uses short pulses of high voltage to carry DNA across the cell membrane. This shock is thought to cause temporary formation of pores in the cell membrane, allowing DNA molecules to pass through. Electroporation is generally efficient and works across a broad range of cell types. However, a high rate of cell death following electroporation has limited its use, including clinical applications.
2. **Gene gun:** The use of particle bombardment, or the gene gun, is another physical method of DNA transfection. In this technique, DNA is coated with gold particles and loaded into a device which generates a force to achieve penetration of DNA/gold into the cells. For example, if the DNA is integrated in the wrong place in the genome, e.g. in a tumour suppressor gene, it could induce a tumour. This has occurred in clinical trials for X-linked severe combined immunodeficiency (X-SCID) patients, in which haematopoietic stem cells were transduced with a corrective transgene using a retrovirus, and this led to the development of T cell leukaemia in 3 of 20 patients.
3. **Sonoporation:** Sonoporation uses ultrasonic frequencies to deliver DNA into cells. The process of acoustic cavitation is thought to disrupt the cell membrane and allow DNA to move into cells.
4. **Magnetofection:** In a method termed magnetofection, DNA is complexed to a magnetic particle and a magnet is placed underneath the tissue culture dish to bring DNA complexes into contact with a cell monolayer.

Chemical Methods to Enhance Delivery

1. **Oligonucleotides:** The use of synthetic oligonucleotides in gene therapy is to inactivate the genes involved in the disease process. There are several methods by which this is achieved. One strategy uses antisense specific to the target gene to

disrupt the transcription of the faulty gene. Another uses small molecules of RNA called siRNA to signal the cell to cleave specific unique sequences in the mRNA transcript of the faulty gene, disrupting translation of the faulty mRNA and, therefore, expression of the gene.

2. **Lipoplexes and polyplexes:** To improve the delivery of the new DNA into the cell, the DNA must be protected from damage and positively charged. Initially, anionic and neutral lipids are used for the construction of lipoplexes for synthetic vectors.

3. **Dendrimers:** A dendrimer is a highly branched macromolecule with a spherical shape. The surface of the particle may be functionalized in many ways and many of the properties of the resulting construct are determined by its surface. In particular, it is possible to construct a cationic dendrimer, i.e. one with a positive surface charge. When in the presence of genetic material such as DNA or RNA, charge complimentarily leads to a temporary association of the nucleic acid with the cationic dendrimer. On reaching its destination, the dendrimer–nucleic acid complex is then taken into the cell via endocytosis.

4. **Hybrid methods:** Due to every method of gene transfer having shortcomings, there have been some hybrid methods developed that combine two or more techniques. Virosomes are one example; they combine liposomes with an inactivated HIV or influenza virus. This has been shown to have more efficient gene transfer in respiratory epithelial cells than either viral or liposomal methods alone. Other methods involve mixing other viral vectors with cationic lipids or hybridizing viruses.

Electrical Methods

Electrotransfer is more well-established. Applying an electrical field to cells alters the resting transmembrane potential, which can induce permeability though the formation of reversible structural membrane changes (electropores). A large number of animal studies have been performed across on a range of tissues, with the main application being immunotherapy. Therapeutic levels of gene expression have been achieved, as well the co-transfer of multiple plasmids. Although more efficient than chemical or physical methods, the efficiency of electrotransfer is still less than that seen with viral vectors.

Diseases that can be treated by gene therapy are classified as either genetic or acquired. Gene therapy is a novel therapeutic approach, which is defined as the treatment of disease by replacing, altering, or supplementing a gene that is absent or whose absence or abnormality is responsible for disease. Gene therapy is a novel treatment method which utilizes genes or short oligonucleotide sequences as therapeutic molecules. This technique is used to treat defective genes which contribute to disease development. Gene therapy involves one or more foreign genes into an organism to treat hereditary or acquired genetic defects. In gene therapy, the therapeutic protein which is encoded by DNA is packaged within a vector, which transports the DNA inside cells. Genetic diseases are mainly caused by the mutation or deletion of a single cell. A single gene is not the sole cause of acquired diseases. The expression of a single cell is delivered directly to the cells by a gene delivery system so as to potentially eliminate a disease. Gene therapy utilizes the transfer of genetic information for modification of a phenotype for therapeutic purposes.

Gene Therapy Approaches

Classical gene therapy: It involves therapeutic gene delivery and their optimum expression inside the target cell. The foreign genes carry out following functions.

- Produce a product (protein) that the patient lacks.
- Produces toxin so that diseased cell is killed.
- Activate cells of the immune system so as to help in killing of diseased cells.

Non-classical gene therapy: It involves the inhibition of gene's expression associated with the pathogenesis, or corrects a genetic defect and restores the normal gene expression.

Methods of Gene Therapy

There are mainly two approaches for the transfer of genes in gene therapy:
1. Transfer of genes into patient cells outside the body (*ex vivo* gene therapy)
2. Transfer of genes directly to cells inside the body (*in vivo*)

Ex vivo gene therapy

- In this mode, genes are transferred to the cells grown in culture, transformed cells are selected, multiplied and then introduced into the patient.
- The use of autologous cells avoids immune system rejection of the introduced cells.
- The cells are sourced initially from the patient to be treated and grown in culture before being reintroduced into the same individual.
- This approach is to the tissues like haematopoietic cells and skin cells which can be removed from the body, genetically corrected outside the body and reintroduced into the patient body and survive for a long period of time.

In vivo gene therapy

- It involves the transfer of cloned genes directly into the tissues of the patient.
- This is done in those tissues whose individual cells cannot be cultured *in vitro* in sufficient numbers (like brain cells) and where re-implantation of the cultured cells is not efficient.
- Liposomes and certain viral vectors are employed for this purpose because of lack of any other mode of selection.
- In case of viral vectors, such type of cultured cells was often used which have been infected with the recombinant retrovirus *in vitro* to produce modified viral vectors regularly. These cultured cells will be called vector-producing cells (VPCs). The VPCs transfer the gene to surrounding disease cells.
- The efficiency of gene transfer and expression determines the success of this approach, because of the lack of any way for selection and amplification of cells which take up and express the foreign gene.

Target Sites for Gene Therapy

Targeting gene defects include single mutation, multiple mutations in several genes, or even show missing or extra copies in a particular disease. A defect in one specific gene may impair the normal function of the corresponding expressed protein (Table 8.1).

Table 8.1: Target sites for gene therapy

Disease	Target cells
Cancer	Tumour cells, antigen presenting cells (APCs), blood progenitor cells, T cells, fibroblasts, muscle cells
Inherited monogenic disease	Lung epithelial cells, macrophages, T cells, blood progenitor cells, hepatocytes, muscle cells
Infectious disease	T cells, blood progenitor cells, antigen presenting cells (APCs), muscle cells
Cardiovascular disease	Endothelial cells, muscle cells
Rheumatoid arthritis	Synovial lining cells
Cubital tunnel syndrome	Nerve cells

Targeted killing of specific cells (Fig. 8.3): It involves genes encoding toxic compounds (suicide genes), or prodrugs to kill the transformed cells. This is popular in cancer gene therapies.

Thymidine kinase (TK) phosphorylates is introduced in a prodrug ganciclovir which is further phosphorylated by endokinases to form ganciclovir triphosphate. Ganciclovir triphosphate causes chain termination when incorporated into DNA.

Targeted inhibition of gene expression (Fig. 8.4): This is to block the expression of any diseased gene or a new gene indicating a protein which is harmful for a cell. This is for treating infectious diseases and some cancers.

Targeted gene mutation correction: It is used to correct a defective gene to restore its function which is done by homologous recombination at genetic level or by using therapeutic ribozymes or therapeutic RNA editing at mRNA level.

Vectors for Gene Therapy

Vectors for gene therapy can be classified into two types:
1. Viral vectors
2. Non-viral

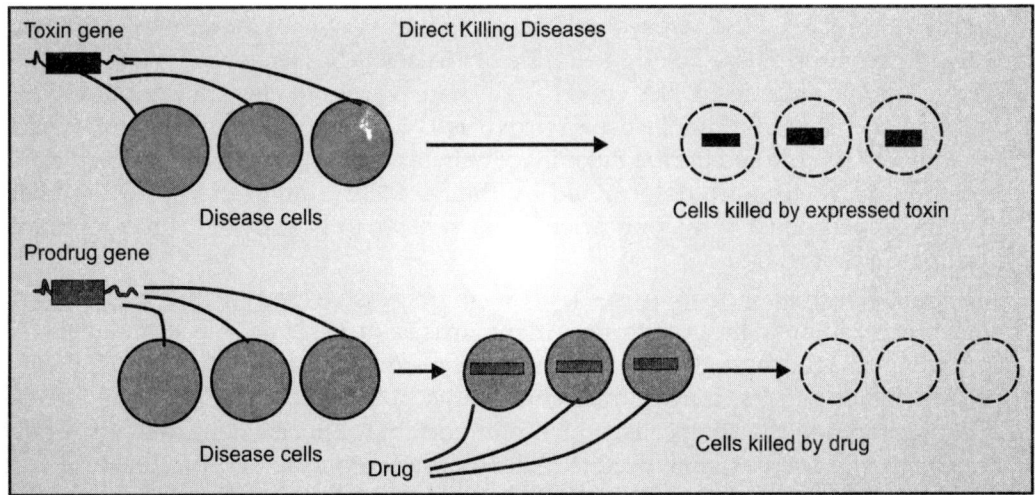

Fig 8.3: Targeted killing of specific cells

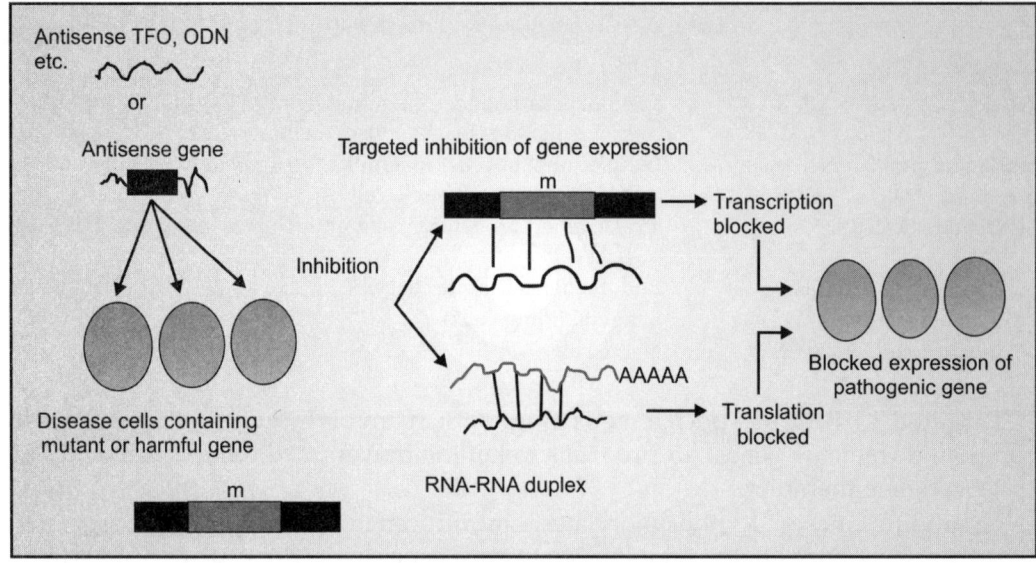

Fig 8.4: Targeted inhibition of gene expression

Viral vectors: Viral gene delivery systems consist of viruses that are modified to be replication-deficient which were made unable to replicate and can deliver the genes to the cells to provide expression. Viral systems have advantages such as constant expression and expression of therapeutic genes. Adenoviruses, retroviruses, lentiviruses, etc. are used for viral gene delivery.

There are some limitations that restrict the use of these systems, which includes the use of viruses in production, immunogenicity, toxicity and lack of optimization in large-scale production. Viruses have appropriate mechanisms for transfer of genetic material to the target cell; it involves the use of viral vectors that provide high transduction effectiveness and advanced level of gene expression. The optimal design of a viral vector depends on the types of virus to be used.

1. *Retroviral vectors:* First viruses used as vectors in this gene therapy experiments were retroviruses. These belong to a class of viruses (RNA as genetic material) that creates double stranded DNA copies with the enzyme reverse transcriptase. The first and the most commonly used retrovirus is Moloney murine leukemia virus (M-MuLV). It is cultured *in vitro* but is inactive in *in vivo* experiments. The advantages of retroviral vectors are determined by their stability integration into the host genome, generation of viral for efficient gene transfer, infectivity of the recombinant viral particles (Fig. 8.5).

2. *Adenoviral vectors:* Adenoviruses (Ad) were first discovered in 1953 by isolation from human adenoid tissue cultures. Adenovirus has a 36 kb, double-stranded DNA genome packaged in a 100 nm icosahedral capsid. Wild-type adenovirus infects cells in the upper respiratory tract and results in mild cold. Adenovirus infects dividing and non-dividing cells, which is important for *in vivo* gene delivery. They are commonly used as gene vectors. Adenoviruses replicate and produce virions, which contain the nucleus of the infected cell. Adenoviral particles do not contain lipid or membrane and are, therefore, stable in solvents such as ether or ethanol.

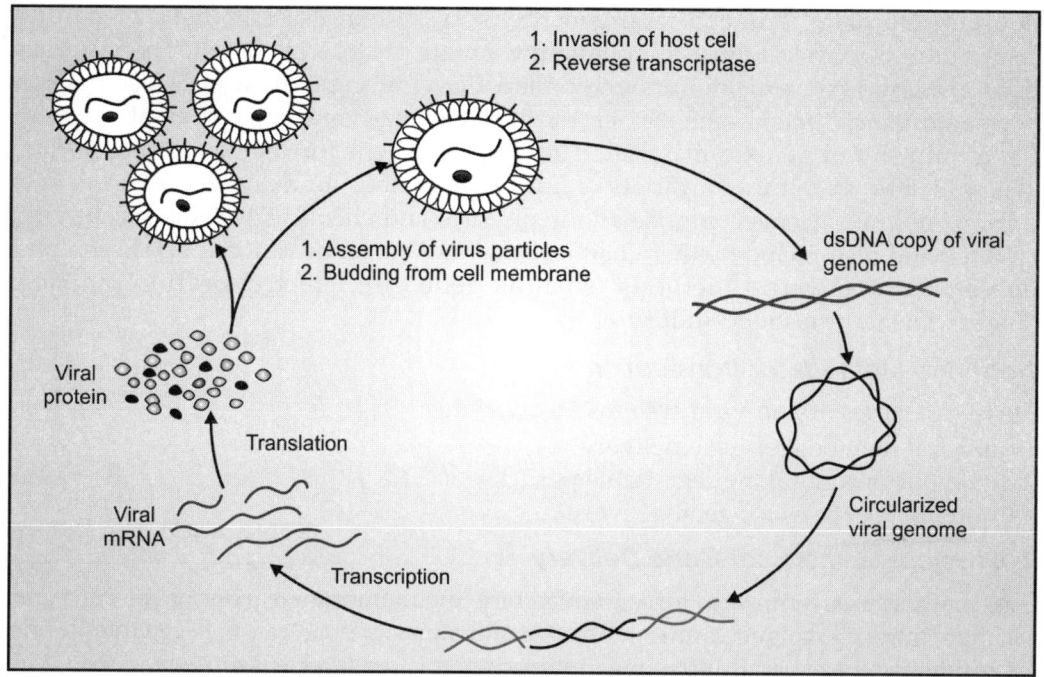

Fig 8.5: Viral genome integrated into host DNA

Adenoviruses are one of the largest and most complex viruses, whose Ad structure is analyzed with cryoelectron microscopy and X-ray diffractometry. Crystal structures of single Ad protein contain fibre knob, shaft, domains, penton base, hexon, and cysteine protease. Ad capsid consists of 252 subunits called capsomeres, which contain 240 hexon proteins and 12 of the penton bases.

3. *Baculovirus:* Baculoviruses are a diverse group of DNA viruses which is capable of infecting more than 500 insect species. Among them *Autographa californica* baculovirus which is multiple nucleopolyhedrovirus (AcMNPV) contains a circular double-stranded DNA genome of ≈134 kb and is the most widely used. Budded AcMNPV is highly infectious to cultured insect cells, thus recombinant baculoviruses are engineered for carrying exogenous genes to infect insect cells for the production of numerous recombinant proteins. Baculovirus neither replicates nor is toxic inside the transduced mammalian cells. Baculovirus DNA degrades in the cells over time and there is no evidence of baculoviral DNA integration into host chromosomes unless selective pressure is applied.

4. *Lentiviral systems:* Lentivirals are viral systems without small retrovirus-like viral proteins and have no capacity for replication. They provide gene delivery to non-dividing cells. This application is used in targeting post-mitotic and highly differentiated cells. The most important advantage of lentiviruses is their ability for gene transfer to non-dividing cells. They contain accessory genes which regulate viral gene expression, control combination of infectious particles and modulate viral replication in infected cells. For example, HIV-1 is one of the most widely used lentiviral vectors, and contains six accessory genes.

Non-viral gene delivery systems: It develops gene expression to specific cells for treatment of human diseases or for transfer of genetic material to inhibit the production of a target protein. The non-viral gene delivery system uses synthetic or natural compounds or physical forces for delivering a piece of DNA into a cell. The materials used are less toxic and immunogenic than the viral gene. Non-viral vectors can overcome the cell membrane barrier and intracytoplasmic compartmentalization of the administered genetic material. These are efficient for increasing membrane penetration *in vitro*. It uses a variety of lipid formulations for delivering DNA to host cells. Non-viral systems comprise all the physical and chemical systems except viral systems and also include either chemical methods (such as cationic liposomes and polymers) or physical methods (such as gene gun, electroporation, particle bombardment, ultrasound utilization).

Non-Viral Methods for Transfection

Three categories of non-viral systems are available:
1. Physical methods for gene delivery
2. Synthetic or natural biodegradable particles
3. Inorganic particles for gene delivery

1. Physical Methods for Gene Delivery

This method uses a physical force to overcome the membrane barrier of the cells and facilitate intracellular gene transfer. These make transient penetration in cell membrane by mechanical, electrical, ultrasonic, hydrodynamic, or laser-based energy for DNA entry into the targeted cells. These methods include the following.

a. **Needle and jet injection:** Needle injections are localized injection of naked DNA which were first demonstrated intramuscularly in 1990 and then in several other tissues, including liver, skin, and brain. DNA uptake is mostly localized in the area where needle track is applied. Physical damage induced by needle insertion is responsible for the uptake of DNA. Different agents such as transferrin, water-immiscible solvents, non-ionic polymers, surfactants, or nuclease inhibitors have been tested to enhance the overall gene expression by this procedure. The jet injection was first come in 1947 as a needle-free drug delivery method. Jet injection is done through a high-speed, ultrafine stream of DNA solution driven by a pressurized gas, usually CO_2. The injection generates pores on membranes of target cells and allows intracellular gene transfer. The jet injection-based gene transfer is ideal for DNA-based vaccine development and for topical immunization purpose. This method has been used to directly transfect skin cancer cells to facilitate conventional chemotherapy.

b. **Hydroporation:** Hydroporation, also called hydrodynamic gene delivery method, is used for gene delivery to hepatocytes in rodents. Hydrodynamic gene delivery is based on the principle of characteristics and structure of capillaries and the fluids passing through blood veins. The hydrodynamic method employs the high pressure as a driving force for gene transfer. Hydrodynamic gene delivery uses the hydrodynamic pressure created by the injection of the large volume of DNA solution with blood pressure inside veins and then the permeability of the capillary endothelium increases and pore forms in the plasma membrane of parenchyma cells.

c. **Gene gun:** Delivery with gene gun method is also called ballistic DNA delivery or DNA-coated particle bombardment. It was first used for gene transfer to plants in 1987. This method depends on the impact of heavy metal particles on target tissues and delivery of coated DNA on particles in passing. The particles are accelerated to sufficient velocity by highly pressurized inert gas, usually helium. Macroparticles made of gold, tungsten or silver have been used for gene delivery through gene gun. Gene gun-based gene transfer has been extensively tested for intramuscular, intradermal and intratumour genetic immunization. This method has been used in vaccination against the influenza virus and in gene therapy for treatment of ovarian cancer.

d. **Electroporation:** Electroporation includes controlled electric application to increase cell permeability. Electroporation was first developed in 1960s, with studies on the degradation of cell membrane with electric induction. It is by generating pores on a cell membrane through electric pulses. The efficiency is determined by the intensity of the pulses, frequency and duration. Electroporation is temporary destabilization of the cell membrane targeted tissue by insertion of a pair of electrodes into it so that DNA molecules in the surrounding media of the destabilized membrane would be able to penetrate into cytoplasm and nucleoplasm of the cell.

e. **Ultrasound:** Ultrasound has many clinical advantages as a gene delivery system, due to its easy and reliable procedure. Microbubbles applied by ultrasound increased gene expression. Microbubbles or ultrasound contrast agents decrease cavitation threshold with ultrasound energy. The microbubbles were modified with plasmid DNA before the injection and then ultrasound was applied.

f. **Magnetofection:** Magnetofection is a simple and efficient transfection method that has the advantages of the non-viral biochemical and physical transfection systems. In this method, the magnetic fields are used to concentrate particles containing nucleic acid into the target cells. DNA is complexed with magnetic nanoparticles which is made of iron oxide and coated with cationic lipids or polymers through electrostatic interaction. The magnetic particles are then concentrated on the target cells by the influence of an external magnetic field.

2. Synthetic or Natural Biodegradable Particles

Synthetic or natural biocompatible particles may be composed by cationic polymers, cationic lipids or cationic peptides, and also the combination of these components. The potential advantages of biodegradable carriers are their reduced toxicity and avoidance of accumulation of the polymer in the cells.

3. Inorganic Particles for Gene Delivery

In many publications, inorganic nanoparticles such as gold nanoparticles, iron oxide nanoparticles, and quantum dots, have been reported as alternative gene delivery vehicles. This is suggested on account of their unique intracellular behaviour with powerful cellular imaging capacities. There are three general strategies to modify inorganic nanoparticles for gene delivery. The first strategy involves the use of positively charged inorganic nanoparticles to form a complex with the negatively charged gene material. The second strategy involves the direct conjugation of genetic material onto the inorganic nanoparticle with a responsive linker. The third strategy involves the use of cationic amphiphilic polymer grown from the nanoparticle to aid in the complex formation between the inorganic nanoparticle and genetic material.

Polymer-Based Non-Viral Vectors

Polymers are long-chained structures composed of small spliced molecules called monomers. Polymers that are composed of a repeated monomer are called homopolymers, while those composed of two monomers are called copolymers. Natural and synthetic polymers are used in drug delivery systems. Biodegradable and non-biodegradable polymers are used according to the type of controlled release mechanism. Biodegradable polymers are non-water soluble, and undergo chemical or physical change in biologic environments.

Polyamides, dextran, and chitosan are examples of biodegradable polymers. Non-biodegradable polymers are not degraded in biological environments. Hydrophilic polymers are hydrogels, which are non-water soluble and swell in water, while hydrophobic polymers are non-water soluble and do not swell. Examples of hydrophilic hydrogel polymers include polyvinyl alcohol, polyvinyl acetate, polyethyleneglycol, polyacrylic acid, polyhydroxyethyl methacrylate, and polymethacrylic acid.

Examples of hydrophobic polymers include silicones, and polyethylene vinyl acetate.

For successful delivery, polymers should package DNA in small sizes. So the extracellular and intracellular stability of DNA is increased; cellular uptake by endocytosis is enabled; and, by transporting it to the nucleus, the active form of DNA can be released within the nucleus.

A synthetic gene delivery system:
1. Should protect the negatively-charged phosphate DNA skeleton against anionic cell surface from load repulsion.
2. Should be condensed to suitable length intervals of DNA with a macromolecular structure for cellular internalization.
3. Should protect DNA from all extracellular and intracellular nuclease degradations.

Liposomal Gene Delivery Systems

Liposomes have been explored as a delivery system for DNA as early as in 1979. The encapsulation of plasmid DNA into liposomes and the introduction of poliovirus RNA and SV40 DNA into cells via liposomes were reported between 1979 and 1980. These are vesicles that can easily merge with the cell membrane. Since, they both are made up of phospholipid bilayers, and these are surrounded by the molecule to be transported and promote its transport after fusing with the cell membrane. The technique which is used to inject the genetic material into a cell by means of liposomes is known as "lipofection or liposome transfection or lipoplex". Lipoplexes are non-viral synthetic nucleic acid carriers utilizing cationic phosphate lipid mixtures to condense and protect the nucleic acid.

Principle: Lipofection generally uses a positively charged (cationic) lipid to form a structure with the negatively charged (anionic) genetic material. Fusion of the liposome/nucleic acid transfection complex with the negatively charged cell membrane takes place. The transfection complex is then entering into the cell through endocytosis. Once enter inside the cell, the complex must escape the endosomal pathway, diffuse through the cytoplasm and enter the nucleus for gene expression. For example, animal cells, plant cells, bacteria, and yeast protoplast are susceptible to lipofection method.

Characteristics: Liposomes are generally formed by the self-assembly of dissolved lipid molecules, each of which contains a hydrophilic head group and hydrophobic tails and these can exhibit a range of sizes and morphologies upon the assembly of pure lipids or lipid mixtures suspended in an aqueous medium. During the compaction of polynucleotides into liposomes assemblies, a number of structures have been known to appear. Each structure is formed in the most energetically favourable conformation based upon the specific lipids used in the system. A dependent term known as "structure packing parameter" which can be used to suggest what shape the amphiphile will take depending on the ratio of size variables.

Based on the charge on head group in lipoplex, these lipids are categorized into three types.

Classification of Lipids

1. Cationic lipids (monovalent Cl and multivalent Cl)
2. Neutral lipids
3. Anionic lipids

1. Cationic Lipids

- Its idea is to neutralize charge of plasmid with positively charged lipids to capture plasmid more efficiently and to deliver DNA into cells.
- The basic structure of cationic lipids mimics the chemical and physical attributes of biological lipids.
- Here, lipoplex is formed by combining the cationic lipids, neutral lipids and genetic material.
- Cationic lipids should be chemically stable, biodegradable and protect against degradation of DNA by cell.

Cationic lipids are divided into two types:

a. **Monovalent cationic lipids:**
  i. *DOTMA:*
    - It was one of the first synthesized cationic lipid.
    - Its structure consists of two unsaturated oleoyl chains (c18; $\Delta 9$) bond to an ether bond to the 3-carbon skeleton of a glycerol with a quaternary amine as cationic head group. DOTMA proved to facilitate up to 100-fold more efficient gene expression then the use of DEAE-dextran co-ppt or Ca_2PO_4.
    - Liposomal sensitivity is 25–30%.

  Procedure:
    - Mix cationic lipids + neutral lipids + DNA to cell results in the formation of aggregation composed of DNA and cationic lipids.
    - DOTMA either alone or in combination with other neutral lipids spontaneously form MLV which may be further sonicated to form SUV.
    - DOTMA (lipofective TM) can reduce cytotoxicity.

  ii. *DOTAP:*
    - It was first synthesized by "Leventis and Silvius" in 1990.
    - Its structure consists of a quaternary amine head group coupled to glycerol backbone with 2-oleoyl chains.
    - Differences between DOTMA and DOTAP are that ester bonds link the chains to the backbone rather than ether bonds.
    - Liposomal sensitivity is 25–30%.
    - But DOTAP is completely protonated at pH (7.4). So, that more energy is required to separate the DNA from the lipoplex for successful transfection.
    - Thus, for DOTAP to be more effective in gene delivery, it should be combined with a helper lipid as seen in most cationic lipid formulation.
    - In this, high temperature and long incubation time have been used to create lipoplex that exhibit resistance to serum interaction.

   iii. *DC-CHOL:*
- It was first synthesized by "Gao and Huang" in 1991.
- It contains a cholesterol moiety attached by an ester bond to a hydrolysable dimethyl ethylene diamine.
- Cholesterol is chosen for its biocompatibility and stability and it imparts to lipid membrane.

b. **Multivalent cationic lipids:**
   i. *DOSPA:*
- It is similar to DOTMA except for a spermine group which is bound via a peptide bond to a hydrophobic chain.
- This cationic lipid, used with a neutral helper lipid DOPE in a 3:1 ratio which is commercially available as the transfection regent "Lipofectamine".

   ii. *DOGS:*
- Its structure is similar to DOSPA as both molecules have a multivalent spermine head group and two 18 carbon alkyl chains.
- However, the chains in DOGS are saturated and are linked to the head group through a peptide bond and lack a quaternary amine.
- DOGS is commercially available under the name "Transfectam".
- This lipid has been used to transfect many cell lines, with transgene expression levels more than 10-fold greater than those seen in calcium phosphate transfections.
- In addition, "researcher showed that not only DOGS is very effective in delivering the CAT reporter plasmid, but it is also associated with no noticeable cytotoxicity".

2. Neutral Lipids
- Most liposomal formulations used for gene delivery consist of a combination of charged lipids and neutral helper lipids.
- The neutral helper lipids used are often dioleoylphosphatidylethanolamine (DOPE), which is the most widely used neutral helper lipid, or dioleoylphosphatidylcholine (DOPC).
- Neutral lipids stabilize the complex in serum and reduce toxicity.
- Results have shown that the use of DOPE versus DOPC as the helper lipid yields higher transfection efficiencies in many cell types.

3. Anionic Lipids
- In general, gene delivery by anionic lipids is not very efficient.
- The negatively charged head group prevents efficient DNA compaction due to repulsive electrostatic forces that occur between the phosphate backbone of DNA and the anionic head groups of the lipids.
- However, due to the fact that cationic liposomes can be inactivated in the presence of serum, are unstable upon storage, and exhibit some cytotoxicity both *in vitro* and *in vivo*.
- Commonly used lipids in this category are phospholipids that can be found naturally in cellular membranes such as phosphatidic acid, phosphatidylglycerol, and phosphatidylserine. Little toxicity, compaction with body fluids, complicated and time-consuming process.
- DNA entrapment in anionic liposomes is still inefficient, and cytotoxicity data remain inadequate.

- Sometimes, the DNA molecules get entrapped within the aqueous interior of these liposomes.
- Then, divalent cations are used (e.g. Ca^{2+}, Mg^{2+}, Mn^{2+}, and Ba^{2+}) which can neutralize the mutual electrostatic repulsion.
- They are termed as pH sensitive due to destabilization at low pH.
- Due to reduced toxicity and interference from serum proteins, pH-sensitive liposomes are considered as potential gene delivery vehicles than the cationic liposomes.

Advantages
- Simplicity
- Non-infectious
- Long-term stability
- Low degree of toxicity
- Protection of nucleic acid from degradation
- Easy to manipulate and use
- Easier to prepare than viral vectors
- Lack of immunogenic response
- Low cost, economical
- Provides nuclease protection and target ability.
- Efficient delivery of nucleic acids to cells in a culture dish.
- It has no constraints on the size of the gene that has to be delivered.

Disadvantages
- Targeting is not specific.
- Low transfection efficiency.
- Only transient expression.
- Difficult *in vivo* application.
- Not applicable to all types of cell.

Uses
- Liposomes composed of DOPE/OLEIC ACID/CHOL are capable of transfecting mouse LLK-cells (cells lacking thymidine kinase with exogenous Tk gene).
- Cationic lipids prepared from DOPE and DC-CHOL are reported to be significantly enhance the growth inhibitory effect of antisense oligodeoxynucleotides (ASODN) against the human telomerase transcriptase on human cervical adenocarcinoma cell both *in vitro* and *in vivo*.
- Cationic liposomes are used to deliver CDNA of cystic fibrosis transmembrane conductance regulator (CFTR) to epithelial tissue of respiratory system which is currently in clinical trials.

Nucleic Acids as Therapeutic Agents

Many human disorders often result from the overproduction of a normal protein. Single-stranded oligonucleotides could be used to hybridize to genes (antigene) or mRNAs (antisense) to reduce transcription or translation thereby reducing protein production. Synthetic RNA/DNA molecules called aptamers bind to proteins and prevent them from functioning.

Aptamers in Therapeutics

Aptamers are single-stranded DNA or RNA molecules, selected by an iterative process known as systematic evolution of ligands by exponential enrichment. Various advantages of aptamers such as high temperature stability, animal free, cost-effective production and its high affinity and selectivity for its target. Two aptamers—one targeting nucleolin and a second targeting CXCL12 are currently undergoing clinical trials for treating cancer patients. DNA aptamers are double-stranded nucleic acid segments that can directly interact with proteins. Aptamers interfere with the molecular functions of disease-implicated proteins. Aptamers are preferred over antibodies in protein inhibition owing to their specificity, non-immunogenicity, and stability of pharmaceutical formulation. DNA aptamers have demonstrated promise in intervention of pathogenic protein biosynthesis against HIV-1 integrase enzyme. RNA aptamers are single-stranded nucleic acid segments that can directly interact with proteins. Aptamers recognize their targets on the basis of shape complementarity. Their binding specificity and affinity for the target are extremely high and similar to monoclonal antibodies. RNA aptamers are efficient pathogenic protein biosynthesis against HIV-1 transcriptase.

Aptamer Stabilization

Nucleic acid-based therapeutics, particularly RNA-based treatments, overcome specific cell targeting, delivery and stabilization and inhibitor RNA molecules, mainly due to the highly abundant cytoplasmic and serum ribonucleases. This is done by the development of modified nucleotides, which can be incorporated at precise positions during the chemical synthesis with minimal interference in the desired activity. Besides preventing degradation by exo- and endonucleases, chemical modifications may improve pharmacokinetic and pharmacodynamic properties of the nucleic acid, while reducing the immunogenicity. Thus, most of the aptamers with potential clinical application have been subjected to these chemical substitutions.

Antiviral Aptamers

Targeting viral factors have become one of the most popular aptamer therapeutic uses, since they can interfere at any stage of the viral cycle, including entry, translation, replication, packaging and budding. The first viral target chosen for the aptamer isolation was the viral polymerase, largely due to its innate ability for interacting with nucleic acids.

1. **Virus entry:** HIV targets helper T cells by glycoprotein 120. The use of gp120 as protein target for aptamers allows, not only for the inhibition of viral entry, but also for the specific delivery of other antiviral compounds.

2. **Replication:** Viral RNA-dependent RNA polymerases have been a common target for the identification of aptamers. These proteins usually share classical reverse transcriptase features with unique conformational and functional properties.

3. **Protein synthesis and maturation:** Many viruses have developed alternative translational mechanisms to that employed by the cellular cap-mRNAs, thus rendering a candidate target for virus inhibition.

4. **Encapsidation:** The isolation of aptamers targeting viral core proteins is an interesting strategy for the investigation of the packaging process and the signals that govern it. For example, RNA aptamers against the nucleocapsid protein were isolated by different groups and proved efficient inhibition of the HIV genomic RNA packaging stage in cell culture.

Anticoagulant Aptamers

Anticoagulants are a major class of pharmaceutical agents that can be used to prevent clotting events during certain clinical situations or for the treatment of cardiovascular diseases. The most commonly used reagent, heparin, may unleash serious secondary effects, such as haemorrhages, decrease in the platelet number and even allergies. Thrombin protein is a preferred target for the development of anticoagulant compounds. This factor is a serine protease with a key role in haemostasis by the activation of procoagulant factors, which greatly amplify the coagulation reaction. Aptamers are able to control this with the isolation of DNA aptamer that interfere with the proteolytic activity of thrombin.

Oligonucleotide Therapies

The scope of the oligonucleotide therapeutics field has expanded substantially over the last few years. One of the most exciting developments is the realization that thousands of non-coding RNAs play important roles in cellular function and that these entities can be readily manipulated using oligonucleotides. Antisense oligonucleotides are synthetic genetic materials that interact with natural genetic material and modulate them in a systematic way. Antisense oligonucleotides as a form of molecular medicine to modulate gene function was first acknowledged in the late 1970s. This therapy involves blocking translation, thereby inhibiting protein formation. An antisense oligonucleotide (ASO) refers to a short synthetic strand of deoxyribonucleotide analogue that hybridizes with the complementary mRNA. Antisense oligonucleotides have been used to modify the expression of specific genes. They are not only useful in the study of loss-of-gene function and target validation, but also act as a novel therapeutic strategy to treat any disease that is linked to dysregulated gene expression. Antisense oligonucleotides can also manipulate alternative splicing, thus can be used to modulate the ratio of different splice variants or correct splicing defects.

Mechanism of Action

ASO is taken up by cellular endocytosis, hybridize with the target mRNA resulting in the formation of ASO-mRNA heteroduplex leading in majority of times to: Either activation of RNase H or steric hindrance of ribosomal subunit binding. Both these mechanisms result in selective degradation of bound mRNA and ultimately target protein knockout. RNase H-dependent oligonucleotides can induce the degradation of mRNA when targeted to any region of the mRNA. The steric-blocker oligonucleotides physically avert the progression of splicing only when targeted to the 5'-cap or AUG initiation codon region. Other mechanisms by which ASO can act is by entering the nucleus directly and altering maturation of mRNA, splicing activation, 5'-cap formation inhibition, arrest of translation and double-stranded RNase activation. RNA interference (RNAi) is a fundamental endogenous mechanism for control of gene expression. It can involve selective message degradation, translation arrest or modulation of transcription.

First Generation ASOs—Phosphorothioate

First generation ASOs are those in which one of the non-bridging oxygen atoms in the phosphodiester bond is replaced by a sulphur atom which introduces chirality at phosphorus. The phosphorothioates are the most widely studied oligonucleotides.

The disadvantages of this modification are slight reduction in the affinity of the ASO for its mRNA target because of decrease in the melting temperature of the ASO-mRNA heteroduplex approximately by 0.50C per nucleotide and production of non-specific effects by interactions with cell surface and intracellular proteins.

Second Generation ASOs

Second generation ASOs with O-alkyl modifications are developed to further enhance nuclease resistance and increase binding affinity for target mRNA.

Third Generation ASOs

The third generations ASOs are developed to further enhance target affinity, nuclease resistance, biostability and pharmacokinetics. Peptide nucleic acid (PNA), locked nucleic acid (LNA) and phosphorodiamidate morpholino oligomer (PMO) are the three most studied third-generation ASOs.

Delivery of oligonucleotide: ASOs penetrate into the targeted cells through active transport which in turn depends on temperature and concentration and structure of the oligonucleotide. Oligonucleotides endocytosis has shown to be mediated by the nucleic acid specific receptors. Naked oligonucleotides are internalized poorly by cells.

Cationic liposomes, such as lipofectin and transfectam have been used to protect ASOs and to ease their entry into the cell. These liposomes have high affinity for negatively charged cell membranes and are delivered by endosomal pathway into cells.

Antisense Technologies

Antisense technologies are techniques that form a very powerful weapon for studying gene function and for discovering new specific treatments of diseases in humans, animals, and plants. In antisense technology, synthetically produced molecules seek out and bind to messenger RNA (mRNA), blocks the final step of protein production. mRNA is the nucleic acid molecule that carries genetic information from the DNA to the other cellular machinery involved in the protein production. By binding to mRNA, the antisense drugs interrupt and inhibit the production of specific disease-related proteins. Sense refers to the original sequence of the DNA or RNA molecule. Antisense refers to the complementary sequence of the DNA or RNA molecules.

Inserting Antisense into Cells

- *Endocytosis:* One of the simplest methods to get nucleotide in the cell, it relies on the cells natural process of receptor-mediated endocytosis. The drawbacks to this method are the long amount of time for any accumulation to occur, the unreliable result, and the inefficiency.
- *Microinfection:* As the name implies, the antisense molecule would be injected into the cell. The yield of this method is very high, but because of the precision needed to inject a very small cell with smaller molecules, only about 100 cells can be injected per day.
- *Liposome encapsulation:* This is the most effective method, but also a very expensive one. Liposome encapsulation can be achieved by using products such as lipofect ACE to create a cationic phospholipids bilayer that will surround the nucleotide sequence. The resulting liposome can merge with the cell membrane allowing the antisense to enter the cell.

- *Electroporation:* The conventional method of adding a nucleotide sequence to a cell can also be used. The antisense molecule should transverse the cell membrane offers a shock is applied to the cells.

Antisense technology suppresses the gene for the protein that makes tomatoes: Poil flavor saur tomatoes are transgenic tomatoes constructed to have artificial DNA that coded for aRNA that is complementary to the RNA that coded for the protein that caused spoiling.

Steps involved in the generation of antisense sequences as drug candidates:

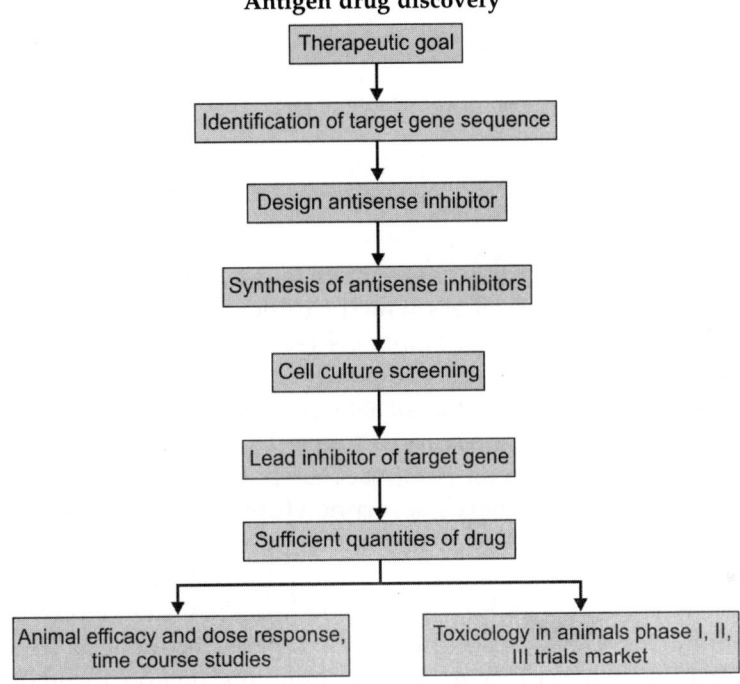

A. **Short Answer Type Questions**

1. Give a short note on monoclonal antibodies.
2. Write a short note on gene therapy.
3. What do you mean by aptamers?
4. What is recombinant DNA technology?
5. Write the significance of recombinant DNA.
6. Mention the application of monoclonal antibodies.

B. **Long Answer Type Questions**

1. Discuss about nucleic acid-based therapeutic delivery system. Give their advantages and disadvantages.
2. Describe liposomal gene delivery systems in detail.
3. Write the method of preparation of recombinant DNA technology and its working principle.
4. Write the important monoclonal antibodies in drug delivery. Discuss their different types.

Nanogels and Hydrogels as Novel Drug Delivery Systems

NANOGELS

Introduction

Nanogels may be defined as highly cross-linked nano-sized hydrogel systems that are either co-polymerized or monomers which can be ionic or non-ionic. The size of nanogels ranges from 20–200 nm. Nanogels (NGs) are currently under extensive investigation due to their unique properties, such as small particle size, high encapsulation efficiency and protection of active agents from degradation, which make them ideal candidates as drug delivery systems (DDS). Stimuli-responsive NGs are cross-linked nanoparticles (NPs), composed of polymers, natural, synthetic, or a combination there of that can swell by absorption (uptake) of large amounts of solvent, but not dissolve due to the constituent structure of the polymeric network. NGs can undergo change from a polymeric solution (swell form) to a hard particle (collapsed form) in response to:

- Physical stimuli such as temperature, ionic strength, magnetic or electric fields;
- Chemical stimuli such as pH, ions, specific molecules, or
- Biochemical stimuli such as enzymatic substrates or affinity ligands.

The interest in NGs comes from their multi-stimuli nature involving reversible phase transitions in response to changes in the external media in a faster way than macroscopic gels or hydrogels due to their nanometric size. NGs have a porous structure able to encapsulate small molecules such as drugs and genes, then releasing them by changing their volume when external stimuli are applied. They can be administered through various routes, including oral, pulmonary, nasal, parenteral, intraocular, etc.

Properties of Nanogels

Biocompatibility and Degradability

Nanogel is made up of either natural or synthetic polymers. They are highly biocompatible and biodegradable thereby avoiding its accumulation in the organs. Chitosan, ethyl cellulose, methyl cellulose and various polysaccharide-based polymers like dextran, pullulan and dextrin can be used to prepare the nanogel. Polysaccharides are mostly carbohydrate-based polymers, formed of repeating monosaccharide units linked by glycosidic bonds. These polymers are stable, non-toxic, hydrophilic and biodegradable in nature.

Swelling Property in Aqueous Media

Due to the fact that nanogels are very small, soft materials, they have the ability to swelling presence of an aqueous medium. It is considered to be the fundamental property influencing the mechanism of action followed by this drug delivery system. It depends on:

- The structure of nanogels: This includes the polymer chain's chemical nature as well as cross-linking degree and in case of polyelectrolyte gels; the charge density.
- Environmental parameters which are related to the variables of the aqueous medium. For instance, in polyelectrolyte gels, pH as well as ionic strength and ions' chemical nature are influencing factors. Likewise, temperature is a trigger of swelling in case of thermoresponsive gels. Providing appropriate circumstances allow rapid swelling/deswelling. Regardless of the trigger, swelling takes place only when the osmotic pressure exerted by medium ions and the polymer's network swelling pressure are imbalanced.

Higher Drug Loading Capacity

Just like any other nanodelivery system, nanogels are expected to have greater loading capacity compared to conventional dosage forms. This is mainly due to the swelling property which allows the formulation to absorb large quality of water. Thus, upon incorporation and loading the water will provide cargo space sufficient to contain salts and biomaterials. Loading takes place through three methods:

1. *Physical entrapment:* It can refer to the linkage between hydrophilic chains and hydrophobic regions of the polymer or to dissolving hydrophobic molecules in hydrophilic vehicle.
2. *Covalent attachment of bioactive molecules:* It leads to the formation of dense drug-loaded core.
3. *Controlled self-assembly:* It is generally for polyelectrolyte-based nanogel. The high loading efficiency is attributed to interaction between oppositely charged electrolytes.

Other factors also contribute to the high loading capacity, such as the composition, molecular weight, the possible interaction between the drug and the employed polymer and the different functional groups in each polymeric unit.

Permeability and Particle Size

What distinguishes nanodelivery system is that tiny manipulation in particle size, surface charge and hydrophobicity can remarkably improve permeability. In spite of the fact that nanoparticles are capable of permeation by diffusion through tissues or compromised areas of endothelium and in some cases through a particular transport system, they created a challenge crossing blood–brain barrier (BBB). So, in order to overcome such dilemma, nanogels were formulated in a way where they possess a diameter of 20–200 nm. It is small enough to cross BBB and in the same time avoid rapid clearance mechanisms.

Non-Immunologic Response

Any agent that enters systemic circulation is rapidly eliminated by the mononuclear phagocyte system through opsonization and phagocytosis. Opsonization is nothing but marking foreign agents and make them visible to phagocytes. Opsonins bind on the surface of nanoparticle and facilitate the attachment of phagocytes. A few methods are adopted to help nanoparticle flee recognition and remain longer in bloodstream. All of which are based on minimizing protein binding. For example, hydrophilic polymers can act as a shield that hinders or delays binding with opsonins rendering them unnoticeable by immune system and its defenses.

Colloidal Stability

When handling nanoparticle there is always a propensity of aggregation that compromises the colloidal stability. Formulators tend to alter the surface charge to avoid the formation of aggregates in bloodstream and further complication. It can be achieved through increasing zeta potential (minimum of ±30 mV) that results in larger repulsive forces between particles that electrostatically stabilize them. Other techniques involve the incorporation of a surface modifier like PEG that produce steric effect and hydration forces to give a stable nanosuspension. If we compare polymeric micellar nanogel systems and surfactant micelles on basis of stability, we will find that the former exhibits better stability, lower critical micelle concentration decrease in dissolution rates, and longer retention of loaded drugs. They also have a high water content that assures good dispersion stability.

Advantages of Nanogels

Nanogels are considered advantageous over other drug delivery systems for a number of reasons, including:

1. High biocompatibility which makes nanogels a very promising approach to drug delivery systems.
2. High biodegradability, which is crucial to avoid accumulation of nanogel material in the bodily organs, thereby leading to toxicity and adverse system.
3. Nanogels are inert in the bloodstream and the internal aqueous environment, meaning that they do not induce any immunological responses in the body.
4. Extremely small size, which induces a number of effects such as:
   - Enhanced permeation capability.
   - Avoidance of rapid renal exclusion. Escaping renal clearance leads to prolonged serum half-life.
   - Avoidance of clearance by phagocyte cells and the uptake by reticuloendothelial system, which permits both passive and active drug targeting.
   - Capability to cross the blood-brain barrier.
   - Enhanced penetration of endothelium in pathological sites like solid tumours, inflammation tissues and infracted areas. Since tumour tissues have a high capillary permeability, more nanoparticle permeate into the tumour tissues and accumulate there, which increases the amount of drug delivered and the selectivity of the drug delivery.
   - Improved ability to access areas that is not accessible by hydrogels, upon intravenous administration.
   - Safe delivery of drug carrying nanogel particle into the cytoplasm of target cells, therefore, making them ideal for intracellular drug delivery.
   - Rapid responsiveness to environmental changes such as pH and temperature.
5. Nanogels are administered via a variety of routes including oral, pulmonary, nasal, parenteral, intraocular and topical routes.

6. Nanogels are suitable to administer both hydrophilic and hydrophobic drugs, as well as charged solutes and other diagnostic agents. This property is highly influenced by the type of functional groups present in the network of polymer chains, the crosslinking density and the type of crosslinking agent incorporated in the polymeric network.

7. Nanogels have a high affinity to aqueous solution resulting in their ability to swell or de-swell, imbibing water when placed in an aqueous medium. This is the most beneficial characteristics of nanogels as it makes them ideal candidates for the uptake and delivery of proteins, peptide, bio-macromolecules as well as bulky drugs.

8. Drug loading in nanogels is relatively high when compared to other nanocarriers and drug delivery systems. This is due to the effect of the functional groups present in the polymeric network. By forming hydrogen bonds or other weak linkages within the polymeric network and interacting with drug or protein molecules at the interface, functional groups on the polymeric network tremendously increase the drug loading capacity of nanogels.

9. Incorporating drug into the nanogels is easy, spontaneous, and does not necessarily require any chemical reaction. This makes the process of preparing nanogels efficient since the drug is not needed in the initial steps of the manufacturing process and can be introduced to the nanogel network in subsequent steps when the nanogel swell with water or aqueous biological fluid.

10. Nanogels are prepared to be capable of releasing drug in a controlled and sustained pattern at the target site, thereby enhancing the therapeutic efficiency of the drug and avoiding its adverse reaction.

11. Targeted drug delivery is possible in nanogels due to the presence of functional groups that conjugate with antibodies and/or drugs, resulting in high selectivity and preventing the accumulation of drug in non-target tissues like muscular and adipose tissues. Moreover, the chemical modification of nanogels to incorporate ligands leads to targeted drug delivery and triggered drug release.

12. The synthesis of nanogels is generally a stress-free process since mechanical energy is not employed and harsh conditions like sonication or homogenization are not involved. Also, there is no introduction of organic solvents to the process in any of its steps. Hence, the drug can be easily loaded without being exposed to any sort of vigorous condition throughout the preparation process.

13. Nanogel dispersions are known to have and exceptionally large surface area which is essential for a variety of *in vivo* application.

14. Bio-macromolecules as well as delicate compounds with low or high molecular weights can be successfully and efficiently encapsulated in the nanogels for the purpose of prolonging the activity of these molecules in the biological environment.

15. Nanogels can be formulated in the form of polymeric micellar nanogel systems that exhibit slower rates of dissociation stability over the surfactant micelles, lower critical micelle concentration and, most importantly, longer retention of loaded drug.

Drug Release Mechanism of the Nanogels

There are multiple mechanisms to which the release of the drug or the biomolecule is attributed to including: Simple diffusion, degradation of nanogel structure, pH and temperature changes, counterion displacement or induced due to external energy source.

pH Responsive Mechanism

As the name indicates, drug release responds to pH changes in the surrounding environment. In other words, the release of drug can take place in different physiological environments that acquire different pH values. The most release will take place in the appropriate pH which means that the release is mainly achieved in a targeted area of the body that possesses that pH. This mechanism is based on the fact that polymers employed in the synthesis of a nanogel contain pH-sensitive functional groups that deionize in the polymeric network. The deprotonation results in increase in osmotic pressure, swelling and porosity of the polymer which triggers the release of the electrostatically bound molecules.

Thermosensitive and Volume Transition Mechanism

Some nanogels are reactive to a specific temperature known as volume phase transition temperature (VPTT) which means they display a change in volume according to the temperature. If the surrounding medium is below VPTT, the polymer becomes quenched and hydrated which makes it swell and release the drug loaded. Above VPTT, the opposite occurs and the nanogel shrinks abruptly and the content flows out. Previously, the thermoresponsive nanogels used to rupture cellular network when they expand and increase in volume. So, some alterations were applied on thermosensitive drug-containing nanogels like changing the polymers ratio to achieve lower critical solution temperature. A good example is the biocompatible magnetic field targetability of poly (N-isopropylacrylamide) and chitosan nanogel which is quiet employed in hyperthermic cancer treatment.

Photochemical Internalization and Photoisomerization

Photoisomerization refers to a process in which a bond of restricted rotation undergoes some conformational changes due to exposure to light. Double bond containing molecules are good example; they isomerize usually from a *trans* orientation to *cis* orientation upon light irradiation. When photosensitizer-loaded nanogels are excited, they produce two species of oxygen (singlet and reactive) which can result in oxidation in the cellular compartment walls that highly influence the release of therapeutic agents into the cytoplasm. Azodextran nanogel loaded with aspirin was a subject of release studies. The observations showed that *cis–trans* isomerization of azobenzene by photoregulation causes the formation of E-configuration of azo group.

Classification of Nanogels

Nanogels are classified according to two bases:

1. Based on their Behaviour Towards a Specific Stimulus

Non-responsive nanogels: When non-responsive nanogels come in contact with water, they absorb it, resulting in swelling of the nanogel.

Stimuli-responsive nanogels: Environmental conditions, such as temperature, pH, magnetic field, and ionic strength, control whether swelling will occur or not and the extent of swelling or deswelling of the nanogels. Any changes in any of these environmental factors, which act as stimuli, will lead to alteration in the behaviour of the nanogels as a response, hence the term stimuli-responsive nanogels. Nanogels that are responsive to more than one environmental stimulus, are termed as multi-responsive nanogels.

2. Based on the Type of Linkages Present in the Network Chains of Polymeric Gel Structure

Physically cross-linked nanogels: Physically cross-linked nanogels, which are also called pseudo-gels, depend greatly on the characteristics of the polymer used in their production including polymer composition, temperature, concentration of the polymer, type of cross-linking agent, and the ionic strength of the medium. Weak linkages like van der Waals forces, hydrogen bonding or hydrophobic, electrostatic interactions are the forces that form this type of nanogels. Physically cross-linked nanogels can be produced within a short time via a number of simple methods. These methods involve a variety of processes such as association of amphiphilic blocks, self-assembly, aggregation of polymeric chains as well as complexation of oppositely charged polymeric chains.

Liposome-modified nanogels: Liposome-modified nanogels are physically cross-linked, stimuli-responsive nanogels, which are being studied as transdermal drug delivery devices, due to their unique properties. These nanogels involve the incorporation of poly [N-isopropyl-acrylamide] co-polymeric groups into the liposomes, resulting in a high degree of responsiveness to both pH and temperature. In addition, succinylated poly[glycidol]s are infused to the liposomes, under pH of less than 5.5, in order to create nanogels that effectively and efficiently deliver Calcein to the cytoplasm of target cells.

Micellar nanogels: Micellar nanogels are produced by supramolecular self-assembly of both hydrophilic and hydrophobic blocks or by graft copolymers in an aqueous solution. Micellar nanogels consist of a hydrophilic shell (corona), made of polymer blocks, surrounding a hydrophobic core, and stabilizing the whole micelle. The purpose of this conformation is to provide sufficient space to contain drugs or biological macromolecules just by physically entrapping these particles inside the borders of the shell, thereby acting as a drug delivery system. As the micelle enters the body, the hydrophilic shell interacts with the aqueous media by forming hydrogen bonds in order to protect the hydrophobic core that is carrying the drug to its target cells. This process protects the drug molecules from being hydrolyzed or degraded by enzymes.

Hybrid nanogels: When particles of a nanogel are dispersed in organic or inorganic medium, it is known as a hybrid nanogel. Self-assembly and aggregation of amphiphilic polymers, such as pullulan-PNIPAM, hydrophobized polysaccharides, and hydrophobized pullulan, were the processes used for the formation of nanogels in aqueous medium. Specifically, cholesterol-bearing pullulan (CHP) nanogels were investigated. These are stable monodispersed nanogels formed by the self-aggregation of CHP molecules (formed of pullulan backbone and cholesterol branches) with hydrophobic groups providing physical crosslinking points. CHP nanogels were found to have the unique abilities to not only complex with molecules like DNA, proteins and various drugs but also to coat solid surfaces like liposomes, particles and even cells. Hybrid nanogels have significance, particularly, as drug delivery systems for insulin and anticancer drugs.

Chemically cross-linked nanogels: Where physically cross-linked nanogels are linked by weak forces, chemically cross-linked nanogels are formed by networks of strong covalent bonds and other permanent chemical linkages. The strength of the linkage is highly dependent on the type of functional groups present in the molecules of the nanogel network. In order to synthesize this type of nanogels, polymeric chains are cross-linked at specific points, called the cross-linking points, which are determined by the multifunctional cross-linking agent present. Using different polymers and different chemical linking strategies leads to the production of nanogels with a variety of properties for a number of applications. In addition, the physiochemical properties of the nanogel can be modified depending on the type of cross-linking agent used to produce the polymer and the position of cross-linking points. Hydrophilic polymers or amphiphilic copolymers, produced by polymerization of vinyl monomers, are usually used to produce chemically cross-linked nanogels. For example, a nanogel ranging in size from 20 to 200 nm, in which polymeric chains containing pendant thiol groups were cross-linked by an environment friendly chemical method, was produced.

Synthesis of Nanogels

Photolithographic Techniques

Photolithographic techniques, photochemical reaction for activation and subsequent reaction, have been explored in strive of producing 3D hydrogel particles and nanogels for drug delivery. In this method, stamps or replica moulds are treated to give the surface-specific properties that allow the moulded gels to release the incorporated agents. Microfabrication of such gels follow the general strategy where poly (dimethylsiloxane) (PDMS) stamps are utilized to mould, release, and stack gels into three-dimensional structures. Surface modification enhances the release or adhesion of moulded gels to a substrate. The most known techniques to modify PDMS stamps are usually achieved by hexa (ethylene glycol)-terminated self-assembled monolayers (SAMs), or by adsorbed monolayers of bovine serum albumin (BSA).

Modified Pullulan Technique

The example that can be given for this category is self-assembled hydrophobized pullulan nanogel. The pullulans are modified in two stages; initially methacrylates are used, then with hydrophobic 1-hexadecanethiol. The end product is an amphiphilic material that upon addition of water starts to assemble itself by hydrophobic interaction among alkyl chains. Another example is cholesterol-based pullulan nanogel. Here, pullulan was substituted with 1.4 cholesterol and the nanogel is fabricated by simply reacting cholesterol isocynate in dimethyl sulfoxide and pyridine. This mixture is freeze dried and in aqueous phase it formed nanogel which further formed a complex with W-9 peptide, a TNF-alpha and RANKL antagonist for delivery of osteological disorder. Cholesteryl pullulan (CHP) bearing methacrylol is formulated by the reaction of CHP with glycidyl methacrylate. The degree of substitution is 6.2 per 100 glucose unit (CHPMA6). CHPMA6 is formed nanogel in water self-assembly.

Emulsion Polymerization Technique

l-proline functionalized PMMA [poly (methyl methacrylate)] nanogel with a range of catalyst functionalization (0.5–15 wt%) and cross-linking densities (0–50 wt%) are prepared by the emulsion polymerization technique. In emulsion polymerization technique, monomer droplets are formed by mechanical stirring.

Reverse Microemulsion Polymerization Technique

Lithium-loaded polyacrylic acid (PAA) nanogels are formulated by reverse microemulsion polymerization technique. 3.43 g span 80 and 2.62 g span 80 are added to 100 ml hexane that is oil phase and kept for stirring using magnetic stirrer. Aqueous phase is prepared by adding 1.5 ml of 10% (w/w) LiOH in water to 500 μl acrylic acid. Add 214 μl of 5% (w/v) N,N'-methylenebisacrylamide (MBA) suspension, 500 μl of 2% (w/v) potassium persulfate and 40 μl of 20% (w/v) N,N,N',N'-tetramethylene-diamine (TEMED) to aqueous phase. Microemulsion is formed by adding aqueous phase drop-wise into oil phase. Emulsion is transferred to 60°C water bath and stirred at 400 rpm using magnetic stirrer, kept overnight at room temperature. Supernatants are decanted and pellets are collected. Microemulsion is thermodynamically stable.

Free Radical Crosslinking Polymerization Technique

Photocrosslinked biodegradable photoluminescent polymers (PBPLPs) nanogel is prepared by free radical crosslinking of a vinyl-containing fluorescent prepolymer for drug delivery and cell imaging. Development of PBPLPs nanogel shows a new era to develop nanobiomaterials in theranostic nanomedicine for drug delivery and cell imaging.

Inverse Mini-Emulsion Polymerization Technique

Fluorescent dye Rhodamine B or fluorescein-labeled nanogels are prepared by activators generated electron transfer atom transfer radical polymerization (AGET ATRP) of oligo (ethylene oxide) monomethyl ether methacrylate (OEO300MA) by inverse mini-emulsion polymerization of water/cyclohexane at ambient temperature. Hydroxyl containing ATRP initiator is used to control polymerization to produce functional HO-POEO300MA nanogels. Cell adhesive nanogels are synthesized using ACRL-PEO-GRGDS as a co-monomer during the polymerization. In O/W mini-emulsion technique, monomer droplets are formed by applying high shear stress by ultrasonication or high-pressure homogenizer. Mini-emulsion is kinetically stable.

Applications of Nanogel

1. Cancer: Cancer treatment involves targeted delivery of drugs with expected low toxicities to surrounding tissues and high therapeutic efficacy.
2. Autoimmune disease
3. Ophthalmic
4. Diabetics: An injectable nano-network that responds to glucose and releases insulin has been developed. It contains a mixture of oppositely charged nanoparticles that attract each other. Glucose molecules can easily enter and diffuse through the gel. Thus, when levels are high, lots of glucose passes through the gel and triggers release of the enzyme that converts it to gluconic acid. This increases acidity, which triggers the release of the insulin.
5. Neurodegenerative: Nanogel is a promising system for delivery of oligonucleotides (ODN) to the brain. Nanogels bound or encapsulated with spontaneously negatively charged ODN results in formation of stable aqueous dispersion of polyelectrolyte complex with particle sizes less than 100 nm which can effectively transported across the BBB.
6. In stopping bleeding: A nanogel composed of protein molecules in solution has been used to stop bleeding.
7. Anti-inflammatory action

Present Status of Nanogels

- Nanogels are promising and innovative drug delivery system that can play a vital role by addressing the problems associated with old and modern therapeutics such as non-specific effects and poor stability.
- Nanogels appear to be excellent candidates for brain delivery.
- One future goal of research in this area should be the improved design of microgels/nanogels with specific targeting residues to enable highly selective uptake into particular cells.
- This will be especially important for the targeting of cancer cells, thereby reducing non-specific uptake into healthy cells.

HYDROGELS

Hydrogels are three-dimensional network of hydrophilic cross-linked polymer that do not dissolve but can swell in water or can respond to the fluctuations of the environmental stimuli. Hydrogels are highly absorbent (they can contain over 90% water) natural or synthetic polymeric networks. Hydrogels also possess a degree of flexibility very similar to natural tissue, due to their significant water content.

Properties

- Both solid-like and liquid-like properties
- High biocompatibility
- Can trap large quantity of water in the network structure ("hydro")
- Shrink when dried
- Environmental stimuli respondent

Various Criteria for the Classification of Hydrogels

- On the basis of preparation:
  - Homopolymer
  - Copolymer
  - Semi-interpenetrating network
  - Interpenetrating network
- On the basis of crosslinking:
  - Chemical hydrogels
  - Physical hydrogels

Homopolymer

- Homopolymers are referred to polymer networks derived from single species of monomer.
- It is the basic structural unit and comprising any polymer network.
- Homopolymers may have cross-linked skeletal structure depending on the nature of the monomer and polymerization technique.
- Cross-linked homopolymers are used in drug delivery system and in contact lenses.
- Polyethylene glycol (PEG) based hydrogels are responsive towards external stimuli and hence these smart hydrogels are widely used in drug delivery system.

Copolymeric Hydrogel

- Copolymeric hydrogels are composed of two types of monomer in which at least one is hydrophilic in nature.

- Synthesized the biodegradable triblock poly (ethylene glycol)-poly (caprolactone)-poly (ethylene glycol) (PEG) copolymeric hydrogel for the development of drug delivery system.
- The mechanism involve here is the ring-opening copolymerization of caprolactone (nylon 6).

Semi-Interpenetrating Network (Semi-IPN)

- If one polymer is linear and penetrates another cross-linked network without any other chemical bonds between them, it is called a semi-interpenetrating network.
- Semi-IPNs can more effectively preserve rapid kinetic response rates to pH or temperature due to the absence of restricting interpenetrating elastic network.
- While still providing the benefits like modified pore size and slow drug release, etc.
- This pH sensitive semi-IPN was synthesized by copolymerization in the presence of N,N'-methylene bisacrylamide as a cross-linking agent.
- The network contained both covalent and ionic bonds.
- The covalent bonds retained the three-dimensional structure of hydrogel and the ionic bonds imparted the hydrogel with higher mechanical strength and pH responsive reversibility.

Interpenetrating Network (IPN)

- IPNs are conventionally defined as intimate combination of two polymers, at least one of which is synthesized or cross-linked in the immediate presence of the other.
- This is typically done by immersing a prepolymerized hydrogel into a solution of monomers and a polymerization initiator.
- IPN method can overcome thermodynamic incompatibility occurs due to the permanent interlocking of network segments and limited phase separation can be obtained.
- The main advantages of IPNs are relatively dense hydrogel matrices can be produced which feature stiffer and tougher mechanical properties, controllable physical properties and more efficient drug loading compared to other hydrogels.

Hydrogel Fabrication

- Chemical hydrogels
  - Covalently cross-linked
  - Volume phase transition
  - Thermoset hydrogels
  - Reliable shape stability and memory
- Physical hydrogels
  - Hydrogen bonding
  - Hydrophobic interaction
  - Stereo complex formation
  - Ionic complexation
  - Noncovalently crosslinked
  - Thermoplastic hydrogels
  - Sol–gel phase transition
  - Limited shape stability and memory

Properties of Hydrogels

Mechanical Properties

Mechanical properties of hydrogels are very important for pharmaceutical applications. For example, property of maintaining its physical texture during the application of drug delivery.

Changing the degree of crosslinking has been utilized to achieve the desired mechanical property of the hydrogel.

Biocompatible Properties

It is important for the hydrogels to be biocompatible and non-toxic in order to make it applicable in biomedical field.

Cell culture methods, also known as cytotoxicity tests, can be used to evaluate the toxicity of hydrogels.

Environment-Sensitive Hydrogel

- Respond to environmental change: Temperature, pH, specific molecule
- Reversible volume phase transition or sol-gel phase transition
- "Intelligent" or "smart" hydrogel

Applications of Hydrogels

- Hydrogels will provide new and improved methods of regenerative medicine, biotechnology, pharmacology, and biosensors in the near future.
- Hydrogels can influence cell behaviour by mimicking the extracellular matrix
- Hydrogels can influence the cell behaviour and its biochemical and biophysical processes.
- Polymer chains that are typically hydrophilic, usually highly absorbent and very flexible.
- Hold potential in biomedical field due to water-carrying capacity.
- Can hold up to 600× their weight in water!
- Can hold many times their weight and flexible!
- Can be used in contact lenses.

Applications of Hydrogels in Drug Delivery

- Benefits of controlled drug delivery
- More effective therapies with reduced side effects
- The maintenance of effective drug concentration levels in the blood
- Patient's convenience as medicines hence increased patient compliance
- Hydrogels that are responsive to specific molecules, such as glucose or antigens, can be used as biosensors as well as drug delivery systems.
- Sensitive hydrogels like temperature, pH sensitive, which are used for the targeted delivery of proteins to colon, and chemotherapeutic agents to tumours.

Advantages of Hydrogels

- Hydrogels possess a degree of flexibility very similar to natural tissue, due to their significant water content.
- Entrapment of microbial cells within hydrogel beads has the advantage of low toxicity.

- Environmentally sensitive hydrogels have the ability to sense changes of pH, temperature, or the concentration of metabolite and release their load as result of such a change.
- Timed release of growth factors and other nutrients to ensure proper tissue growth.
- Hydrogels have good transport properties.
- Hydrogels are biocompatible.
- Hydrogels can be injected.
- Hydrogels are easy to modify.

Disadvantages of Hydrogels

- Hydrogels are expensive.
- Hydrogels cause sensation felt by movement of the maggots.
- The surgical risk associated with the device implantation and retrieval.
- Hydrogels are non-adherent; they may need to be secured by a secondary dressing.
- Hydrogels used as contact lenses cause lens deposition, hypoxia, dehydration and red eye reactions.
- Hydrogels have low mechanical strength.
- Difficulty in handling
- Difficulty in loading

QUESTIONS

A. Short Answer Type Questions

1. What is hydrogel?
2. Write a short note on hydrogels.
3. Write the application of nanogels.
4. What is nanogel?
5. Write the classification of nanogels.
6. Mention different properties for nanogels.
7. Give the application of hydrogels.

B. Long Answer Type Questions

1. Discuss about nanogels in detail.
2. Describe drug release mechanism from nanogel in detail.
3. Write different methods for synthesis of nanogels.
4. Write about application of hydrogels in controlled drug delivery system.
5. Give a detail note on present status of nanogels.

Parenteral Controlled Drug Delivery Systems

INTRODUCTION

Parenteral drug delivery systems are the preparations that are given other than oral route. Parenteral drug delivery systems are most preferred drug delivery systems as they meet many benefits over other dosage forms in many cases such as unconsciousness, nausea, in emergency clinical episodes. The parenteral administration route is the most common and efficient for delivery of active drug substances with poor bioavailability and the drugs with a narrow therapeutic index. But parenteral route offers rapid onset of action with rapid declines of systemic drug level. For the sake of effective treatment, it is often desirable to maintain systemic drug levels within the therapeutically effective concentration range for as long as treatment calls for. It requires frequent injection, which ultimately leads to patient discomfort. For this reason, drug delivery system which can reduce total number of injection throughout the effective treatment, improve patient compliance as well as pharmacoeconomic. These biodegradable injectable drug delivery systems offer attractive opportunities for protein delivery and could possibly extend patent life of protein drugs. Parenteral drug delivery system seeks to optimize therapeutic index by providing immediate drug to the systemic pool in required quantity to treat—cardiac attacks, respiratory attacks. The parenteral administration route is the most effective and common form of delivery of active drug substances for which the bioavailability is limited by high first pass metabolism effect and for drugs with a narrow therapeutic index. For this reason, whatever drug delivery technology that can reduce the total number of injection throughout the drug therapy period will be truly advantageous not only in terms of compliance, but also for potential to improve the quality of the therapy. Such reduction in frequency of drug dosing is achieved, in practice, by the use of specific formulation technologies that guarantee that the release of the active drug substance happens in a slow and predictable manner.

Objectives
- Site-specific delivery
- Reduced side effects
- Increased bioavailability
- Increased therapeutic effectiveness

Advantages Over Conventional Drug Delivery System

- Improved patient convenience and compliance.
- Reduction in fluctuation in steady-state levels.
- Increased safety margin of high potency drugs.
- Maximum utilization of drug.
- Reduction in health care costs through improved therapy, shorter treatment period, less frequency of dosing

Disadvantages of Controlled Release Dosage Forms

- Decreased systemic availability
- Poor *in vitro–in vivo* correlation
- Possibility of dose dumping
- Retrieval of drug is difficult in case of toxicity, poisoning or hypersensitivity reactions.
- Reduced potential for dosage adjustments.
- Higher cost of formulations.

Routes of Administration

- Intravascular
- Intramuscular
- Subcutaneous
- Intradermal
- Intra-articular
- Intraspinal
- Intrathecal
- Intracardiac
- Intrasynovial
- Intravaginal

Characteristics

- Free from living microbes
- Free from microbial products such as pyrogens
- Should match the osmotic nature of the blood
- Free from chemical contaminants

Additives Used during Formulation of Parenterals

- Vehicles
- Stabilizers
- Buffering agents
- Tonicity factors
- Solubilizers
- Wetting, suspending, emulsifying agents
- Antimicrobial compounds

Approaches for Formulations

- Use of viscous, water-miscible vehicles, such as an aqueous solution of gelatin or polyvinylpyrrolidone.

- Utilization of water-immiscible vehicles, such as vegetable oils, plus water-repelling agent, such as aluminium monostearate.
- Formation of thixotropic suspensions
- Preparation of water-insoluble drug derivatives, such as salts, complexes, and esters.
- Dispersion in polymeric microspheres or microcapsules, such as lactide-glycolide homopolymers or copolymers.
- Co-administration of vasoconstrictors

Type of Formulation

- Dissolution-controlled depot formulations
- Adsorption-type depot preparations
- Encapsulation-type depot preparations
- Esterification-type depot preparations

CLASSIFICATION

- Injectable
- Implants
- Infusible devices

Injectable

- Solutions
- Suspensions
- Emulsions
- Microspheres
- Microcapsules
- Nanoparticles
- Niosomes
- Liposomes
- Resealed erythrocytes

Solutions

Aqueous solutions
- High viscosity solutions
- For compound with molecular weight more than 750
- For water solution drugs
- Gelling agents or viscosity enhancers are used.
- Complex formulations
- Drug forms dissociable complex with macromolecule
- Fixed amount of drug gets complexed
- Given by IM route

Oil solutions
- Drug release is controlled by controlling partitioning of drug out of oil into surrounding into aqueous medium
- For IM administration only
- No. of oils are limited.

Suspensions

Aqueous suspensions
- Given by IM or SC routes
- Conc. of solids should be 0.5 to 5%.
- Particle size should be <10 μm.
- Drug is continuously dissolving to replenish the lost.
- For oil soluble drugs
- Only crystalline and stable polymorphic drugs are given by this form.
- Viscosity builders can be used, e.g. crystalline zinc insulin.

Oil suspensions
- Given by IM route.
- Process of drug availability consists of dissolution of drug particles followed by partitioning of drug from oil solution to aqueous medium.
- More prolong drug action as compared to oil solution and aqueous suspension, e.g. penicillin G procaine in vegetable oil.

Emulsions

- Can be given by IM, SC, or IV routes.
- O/W systems are not used due to large interfacial area and rapid partitioning.
- W/O emulsions are used for water-soluble drugs.
- Multiple emulsions are used generally such as W/O/W and O/W/O since an additional reservoir is presented to the drug for partitioning which can effectively retard its release rate.
- Release of water-soluble drugs can be retarded by presenting it as oil suspension and vice versa. Water-soluble drug, e.g. 5-fluorouracil, oil soluble drug, e.g. lipidol.

Microsphere

- Each microsphere is basically a matrix of drug dispersed in a polymer from which release occurs by first order process.
- Polymers used are biocompatible and biodegradable.
- Polylactic acid, polylactide coglycolide, etc.
- Drug release is controlled by dissolution degradation of matrix.
- Small matrices release drug at a faster rate.
- For controlled release of peptide/protein drugs such as LHRH which have short half-lives.
- Magnetic microspheres are developed for promoting drug targeting which are infused into an artery.
- Magnet is placed over the area to localize it in that region.

Microcapsules

- Drug is centrally located within the polymeric shell.
- Release is controlled by dissolution, diffusion or both.
- For potent drugs such as steroids, peptides and antineoplastics.

Nanoparticles and Niosomes

- Nanoparticles are called nanospheres or nanocapsules depending upon the position of drugs.
- Polymers used are biodegradable ones, e.g. polyacrylic acid, polyglycolic acid.

- For selective targeting therapy.
- Nanosomes are closed vesicles formed in aqueous media from non-ionic surfactants with or without the presence of lipids.

Liposomes

- Spherule/vesicle of lipid bilayers enclosing an aqueous compartment.
- Lipid most commonly used is phospholipids, sphingolipids, glycolipids and sterols.
- Water-soluble drugs are trapped in aqueous compartment.
- Lipophilic ones are incorporated in the lipid phase of liposomes.
- Can be given by IM, SC, for controlled rate release.
- Can be given by IV for targeted delivery.

Resealed Erythrocytes

- Biodegradable, biocompatible, non-immunogenic.
- Can circulate intravascularly for days and allow large amounts of drug to be carried.
- Drug loading in erythrocytes is easy.
- Damaged erythrocytes are removed by liver and spleen.

Implant system

Implant systems are indicated in case of chronic therapy, such as hormone replacement therapy and chemical castration in the treatment of prostrate cancer. Parenteral implants can be highly viscous liquids or semisolid formulations both of which may be injected with a needle and implants may be in the form of tiny rods impregnated with a drug substance/a liquid which gel following administration. These parenteral implants are prepared from polymeric materials including—polysaccharides, polylactic acid coglycolic acid (no need for surgical removal of the implant after treatment) and non-degradable methacrylates. Various principles/mechanisms such as diffusion, dissolution, vapour-pressure, osmosis, and ion-exchange, etc. are exploited for implant system.

Implants can be further classified as:

1. **Solid implants:** Solid implants typically exhibit biphasic release kinetics, with initial burst of drug is usually due to the release of drug deposited on the surface of the implant although zero order kinetics may be achieved by coating the implant drug impermeable material.
2. ***In situ* forming implants:** Biodegradable injectable *in situ* forming drug delivery systems represent an attractive alternative to microspheres and implants as parenteral depot systems. The controlled release of bioactive macromolecules via (semi-) solid *in situ* forming systems has a number of advantages, such as:
   - Ease of administration,
   - Less complicated fabrication,
   - Less stressful manufacturing conditions for sensitive drug molecules.

Infusible Devices

- Osmotic pumps
- Vapour pressure
- Powered pumps
- Intraspinal infusion pumps
- Intrathecal infusion pumps

Polymers Used in Parenteral Controlled Drug Delivery System

Generally, biodegradable polymers are used for the preparation of parenteral controlled drug delivery system as they get degraded in the body and hence do not require removal from the body.

Classification of Biodegradable Polymers

Biodegradable polymer may be classified based on the mechanism of release of the drug entrapped in it:

Natural: Albumin starch, dextran, gelatin, fibrinogen, haemoglobin.

Synthetic: Aliphatic poly (esters), polyanhydrides, polyphosphazenes, polyamino acids poly-orthoesters, etc.

- Biodegradable polymers investigated for controlled drug delivery are polylactide/poly-glycolide polymers, polyanhydrides, polycaprolactone, polyorthoesters, pseudo-poly-amino acid, polyphosphazenes, natural polymers.

Desirable Characteristics of an Ideal Parenteral Drug Carrier

- Versatility in that carrier can deliver a variety of agents.
- High capacity to carry a sufficient quantity of drug per unit carrier to release therapeutic concentration to the target site without excessively loading host with the carrier.
- Restricting drug distribution to the desired target tissue.
- Uniform distribution within the capillary vasculature of the target tissue.
- Affording drug ready access to the parenchyma of target tissue.
- Restricting drug activity at the target site over a prolonged period.
- Minimizing systemic drug release during intravascular transit.
- Protecting drug from inactivation by plasma enzymes.
- Being biocompatible and minimally antigenic.
- Undergoing biologic degradation with prompt elimination and minimal toxicity of the breakdown products.

ADVANCES IN PUMP TECHNOLOGY: INSULIN PATCH PUMPS, COMBINED PUMPS AND GLUCOSE SENSORS, AND IMPLANTED PUMPS

In patients with type 1 diabetes, the benefits to glycaemic control and quality of life of external insulin pumps have been clearly established. The main indications for an external pump include persistently elevated HbA1c despite intensive multiple-injection insulin therapy, repeated hypoglycaemia and significant glycaemic variability. Other medical circumstances may also warrant pump treatment, such as pregnancy and type 2 diabetes that has failed to respond to intensified multiple-injection insulin therapy. Specific paediatric indications may also be seen in certain cases. Today's insulin pumps are the result of decades of design and engineering efforts towards the development of reliable, secure and user-friendly modern pumps. These pumps are small and light, and offer technical solutions that are suited to diabetic patients' needs. Their integrated software has also evolved, and can now keep track of the delivered insulin and blood glucose measurements, enable bolus calculation and permit link-ups with other compatible systems. The most recent pump-technology research concerns the development of insulin patch pumps and pumps coupled with glucose sensors.

Insulin Patch Pumps

Introduction

Although the benefits of external pump treatment have been clearly established, the treatment modality nonetheless requires strong patient motivation and involvement. However, certain features of the external pump could be improved to reduce treatment constraints and improve patients' quality of life. Indeed, the initial technical education on how to use the pump and insert the catheter takes time, some patients have the impression of being attached to an external object; equipment problems, such as catheter occlusion and bent cannulae, are common occurrences, disconnecting the pump is recommended before taking a shower, or engaging in water or other sports activities. Recent technological progress has resulted in the development of 'insulin patch pumps' that ought to simplify the technical aspects of treatment and improve patient comfort. The term 'patch', however, may be a misnomer. Although these new pumps are smaller and free of tubes, they often have subcutaneous cannulae through which insulin is injected. The patch pump is nevertheless an innovative system in the field of insulin pumps. The concept comprises an insulin reservoir, delivery system and cannula, all of which are integrated into a small, wearable, disposable or semidisposable device. The patch pump combines the functions of a conventional insulin pump with the following advantages: By eliminating the tubing, it is easy to use; to initiate pumping requires only simplified training; and it is discreet. The development of the patch pump has been initiated by a large number of companies ranging from start-ups to established firms. At present, a few of these pumps have been approved for marketing in the US by the Food and Drug Administration (FDA), while a wide range of other devices are also reported to be currently under development.

Currently Available Insulin Patch Pumps

Only the OmniPod® (Insulet Corp., Bedford, MA, USA) is currently available for use, and has been sold in the US for several years. The device, distributed by Ypsomed, will soon be available in whole world. The pump/reservoir unit (Pod) is a tube-free disposable device applied to the body with adhesive, and changed every 3 days. The Pod has an integrated infusion set and automated inserter, and communicates wirelessly with the personal data manager (PDM), a separate controller device that manages insulin delivery.

In addition, the PDM contains an integrated blood glucose meter and food database, and is waterproof, allowing it to be worn during showering or swimming. In one short-term study, type 1 diabetic patients preferred using the Pod to their conventional pump. Another prospective study demonstrated the safety and efficacy of 500 U of insulin delivered by OmniPod in type 2 diabetes insulin-resistant patients.

Approved Insulin Patch Pumps

Two patch pumps have been approved by the FDA.

1. The *Solo MicroPump Insulin Delivery System* (Medingo US, Inc., Tampa, FL, USA) has two parts: The micropump itself; and a remote device that programmes and directs the micropump. The micropump is small and slim, and consists of a 2 ml insulin reservoir, a cannula cradle infusion set and a pump base. The disposable insulin reservoir and cannula must be replaced every 2 to 3 days. The pump base includes a reusable 90-day unit that holds the electronics, memory, pump motor

and bolus buttons. The base must be clicked out of the cradle before swimming or engaging in contact sports. Boluses are delivered *via* the remote device or directly from the pump.

2. The Finesse patch pen (Calibra Medical, Inc., Redwood City, CA, USA) is a disposable and completely manual system that only delivers insulin boluses. As there are no electronics, the bolus is delivered by depressing bolus-release buttons.

Insulin Patch Pumps Under Development

There are numerous patch pumps currently being developed.

1. *The Cellnovo pump* (Cellnovo Ltd, London, United Kingdom) is a minipump that is programmable via a mobile handset based on the principles of Apple technology. It consists of a controller for the insulin pump and a blood glucose meter, and also contains a food library. The handset transmits data to a centralized server. The minipump's insulin reservoir has a capacity of either 0.5 ml or 1.5 ml, and is connected to a cannula and minitubing, each of which needs to be replaced every 3 days. The pump battery is rechargeable.

2. The *V-Go pump* (Valeritas, Inc., Bridgewater, NJ, USA) is a fully disposable transdermal device with a preset basal rate and on-demand bolus delivery. The device needs to be replaced daily. It has no programming, no electronics and no batteries.

3. The *Jewel PUMP* (Debiotech SA, Lausanne and ST Microelectronics, Geneva, Switzerland) is based on the MEMS Nanopump technology and comprises two parts: The reusable part contains the electronics and includes remote communication for distant programming; the other disposable parts include a reservoir, pumping mechanism and batteries. The insulin reservoir is refilled every 6 days.

4. The *CeQur pump* (Montreux, Switzerland) is intended for type 2 diabetes patients. The pump delivers a constant basal rate and on-demand bolus delivery at the push of a button.

5. The *PassPort Transdermal System* (Altea Therapeutics Corp., Atlanta, GA, USA), currently under phase-I clinical evaluation, dispenses only a basal rate of insulin. The system includes an applicator and a PassPort Patch, which contains a reservoir and a tiny metallic filament screen known as the "porator". The applicator delivers an electrical charge to the porator, thereby galvanizing the filaments and scattering the closest skin cells. Micropores are thus created on the surface of the skin, permitting transdermal passage of insulin. The delivery method can be configured to achieve either systemic or localized action of the therapeutic agent. The aqueous micropores allow the rapid and sustained flow not only of insulin, but also of proteins, peptides, carbohydrates and small molecules into the body without the use of needles or pumps.

6. *The Nilipatch disposable insulin pump system* (NiliMEDIX Ltd, Tirat-Carmel, Israel) delivers basal and bolus insulin. The pump uses a pressure-triggered release mechanism, and is controlled by a system of valves and sensors. The NiliPatch pump has been certified for marketing in the European Union and Israel.

7. *The Freehand system* (Medsolve Technologies, Inc., Manhattan Beach, CA, USA) is a remote-controlled basal and bolus insulin-delivery pump system with a 3-month lifetime. The system offers seven basal profiles. Basal delivery can be temporarily suspended, and boluses can be delivered either remotely or manually.

Little information is available at this time on the following models supposedly under development: The Medipacs patch pump (Medipacs, Inc., San Diego, CA, USA); the Medtronic patch delivery system (Medtronic, Inc., Minneapolis, MN, USA) and the SteadyMed patch pump (SteadyMed Ltd, Tel-Aviv, Israel).

There are many patch pumps at various stages of development, but a few are currently on the market or anticipated to soon be on the market. The very concept of a patch pump will improve patient comfort and eventually improve patient compliance with treatment. Moreover, it should reduce barriers to pump acceptance, particularly in type 2 diabetic patients.

Insulin Pumps Coupled with Glucose Sensors

The combined use of real-time continuous glucose monitoring (RT-CGM) and continuous subcutaneous insulin infusion (CSII) *via* an external pump is a logical development with a view towards an artificial pancreas for the optimal treatment of type 1 diabetes. The goal is to implement an automated system or 'closed loop' that permits the delivery of subcutaneous insulin adjusted to measured levels of subcutaneous glucose.

Non-Automated Coupling of Insulin Pumps and Glucose Sensors

While awaiting the development of an artificial pancreas, a preliminary step is the non-automated coupling of an insulin pump to a glucose sensor. The combined use of both systems appears consistent with the conceptual plan to optimize use of the pump. The patient can continuously adjust the delivery of insulin based on the values and trends indicated by real-time data from the glucose sensor. This is an example of an 'open-loop' device: The patient can maintain glucose control by interpreting the data from RT-CGM, and use it to modulate insulin basal rate, temporarily stop the pump and/or deliver additional insulin boluses. The theoretical value is such that systems incorporating insulin pumps and glucose sensors are already available to patients. These sensor-augmented pump devices include a subcutaneous glucose sensor with a 6 to 7 days lifetime that communicates via telemetry with an external insulin pump. The pump's screen displays glucose sensor data and emits an audible alarm whenever high or low values are detected. The first such system, sold in 2006, was the MiniMed Paradigm REAL-Time System® (Medtronic, Inc.). Another system soon to appear on the market is the Animas® VibeTM (Animas Corp., West Chester, PA, USA). Self-monitoring of blood glucose (SMBG), in its common clinical use, only reports glycaemia levels at a precise point in time, generally before meals and at bedtime. It has been shown that the frequency of SMBG is inversely correlated to the value of HbA1c. In practice, most patients rarely take more than four to six blood glucose measurements per day. On the other hand, even if sustained, the SMBG provides glucose information for only one point in time, with no information on the kinetics of blood glucose and/or its rate of change. For these reasons, RT-CGM from the start appears to have added value when combined with CSII. This added value can be examined in recent randomized studies evaluating the effectiveness of sensor-augmented pumps.

Implanted Pumps

The use of implanted insulin pumps began enthusiastically a little over 20 years ago. The objective was to free the patient from the constraints of injections as well as to develop the components for an implantable artificial pancreas by taking advantage of the benefits derived from the use of intraperitoneal insulin delivery.

Intraperitoneal Route

Subcutaneous (SC) insulin absorption is slow, variable and induces secondary hyperinsulinaemia. These limitations have led to alternative routes being sought for continuous ambulatory infusion of insulin. Studies in animals have shown the benefits of the intraperitoneal (IP) route, which has pharmacokinetics that are closer to physiological than the SC route. After delivery into the peritoneal cavity, insulin is primarily resorbed in the portal vein. There is an approximately 50% degradation during the first hepatic passage, thereby recreating a physiological insulin gradient between the portal vein and systemic circulation. Compared with the SC route, the IP route induces lower peripheral insulinaemia while allowing resorption and a faster return to baseline plasma levels. This insulin kinetics is more physiological, maintaining reproducibility of insulin profiles in the long term and resulting in an improved glucagon response to hypoglycaemia. The use of the IP route for type 1 diabetes treatment was made possible by the development of programmable implantable pumps that deliver insulin through an IP catheter. Pilot trials conducted in the 1980s, demonstrated the feasibility, efficacy and safety of this therapeutic approach. Insulin therapy via an implanted pump began in 1989 with its primary development in France. As a result, the French data are foremost in the world. There are 15 centres in France included in the association EVADIAC (evaluation dans le diabete du traitement par implants actifs; evaluation of treatment with active implants in diabetes). EVADIAC monitors and gathers information into a computerized central registry. The current implant, the MIP 2007 model (Medtronic-MiniMed, Northridge, CA, USA), underwent improvements to the electronic and battery components of the previous model. It has been in use since 2000 and has a 7- to 10-year battery life. Insulin delivery options are similar to those of the most up-to-date external pumps, and are programmable through a personal pump communicator (PPC). The catheter is inserted into the peritoneal cavity, while the pump itself is implanted in the abdominal wall. In 2007, the MIP 2007 device and Insuplant® 400 IU/ml (Aventis Pharma, Frankfurt, Germany), a semi-synthetic insulin used in implanted pumps, received marketing approval from the French regulatory agency. However, currently, Insuplant 400 IU/ml has been replaced by Insuman Implantable 400 IU/ml (Aventis Pharma), an ordinary recombinant insulin. As with Insuplant, this new insulin has been stabilized to prevent denaturation and precipitation in the implanted pump reservoir. The AMM is pending.

The current indications for an implanted pump are related to user experience and the metabolic benefits observed, and were presented in an EVADIAC 'position statement' that has since been recently updated. Treatment with an implanted insulin pump is indicated for type 1 diabetic patients with an HbA1c >7% and/or presenting with large blood glucose fluctuations, including moderate and/or severe recurrent hypoglycaemic events despite intensified treatment with SC insulin. At this time, implanted insulin pump therapy is limited to a minority of selected patients based on who is likely to obtain the most benefit. There are currently 458 diabetic patients with an implantable pump: 370 in France, 3 in Belgium, 63 in the Netherlands and 22 in Sweden. The limitations of this treatment mode are the result of its technically specialized medical requirements, significant cost and reimbursement guidelines, as well as its limited manufacturing. Despite these limitations, however, the benefits provided to patients requiring this form of insulin therapy should be borne in mind. The need to improve diabetes management to reduce the frequency, severity and consequences of hypoglycaemic events and degenerative complications constitutes a major public-health issue. Considering the health costs generated by the management of diabetes complications (such as hospitalization, work absences, medical transports, dialysis, retinal laser treatment, vascular bypasses and amputations), treatment with an implanted insulin pump should certainly constitute an acceptable cost and remain available when validly indicated. Moreover, as regards implanted pumps coupled with glucose sensors, the implanted insulin pump is part of an innovative technology for diabetes and an important step towards the development of an artificial pancreas. Indeed, the pharmacokinetic properties of IP-administered insulin give it a high reactivity that is of particular interest for use in a closed-loop system. Pilot studies have also shown encouraging results with implanted pumps coupled with intravenous and SC glucose sensors. Thus, important advances have been made in the technology of insulin pumps, and the research is ongoing. The immediate expected patients' benefits are accurate data, ease of use, and improvements in metabolic control, quality of life and compliance. The benefits to come are related to its implementation as a component of an artificial pancreas.

QUESTIONS

A. Short Answer Type Questions

1. Give a short note on emulsion for parenteral controlled drug delivery system.
2. Write a short note on insulin pump.
3. Write the desirable characteristics for an ideal parenteral drug carrier.
4. What are resealed erythrocytes?
5. Write the different approaches for parenteral formulation.
6. Mention different additive for parenteral formulation.
7. What are implanted pumps?

B. Long Answer Type Questions

1. Discuss about parenteral controlled drug delivery system in detail.
2. Describe advantages and disadvantages for parenteral controlled drug delivery system in detail.
3. Write different approved insulin patch pump by FDA.
4. Write about phytophospholipid interactions in detail.
5. Give a detail note on intraperitoneal rout.

Novel Drug Delivery Systems for Phytoconstituents and Phospholipids as Carrier for Herbal Drugs

INTRODUCTION

Natural resources continue to be an invaluable source of new, novel chemical entities of therapeutic utility due to the vast structural diversity observed in them. The quest for new and better drugs has witnessed an upsurge in exploring and harnessing nature especially for discovery of antimicrobial, antidiabetic, and anticancer agents. The imbalance of hydrophilicity and lipophilicity along with a large molecular size (due to a unique chemical structure) of natural compounds or plant actives poses a significant challenge for their absorption through a biological membrane and thus, alters the therapeutic efficacy. Therefore, it is desirable to have a novel approach for such formulation in order to improve the solubility and bioavailability of these phytoconstituents as a phospholipid complexation. Herbal drugs are precisely, embedded and bound by phospholipids to form vesicular structures which are amphoteric in nature. Thus, the phytolipid complex technology is unique, in the respect that it has a higher stability profile owing to its amphoteric nature or owing to its solubility in aqueous as well as oil media. It also exhibits a greater absorption and bioavailability, as the drug molecules are embedded in the pockets of the phytosomal assembly, therefore, with more drug loading capability, protection from the gastric environment, and subsequently inactivation in gastrointestinal tract (GIT). Phytolipid complexes have a great potential in the field of medicine, pharmaceuticals and cosmetics due to improved pharmacokinetics and pharmacological attributes.

IMPORTANCE OF NOVEL HERBAL DRUG DELIVERY SYSTEM

Most of the active constituents present in the herbal drugs are flavonoids, glycosides, etc. These are mainly hydrophilic molecules due to that they are limited in their effectiveness and are poorly absorbed when they are taken internally and when applied topically. Apart from that due to its larger molecular size which cannot be absorbed by passive diffusion and due to their poor lipid solubility limiting its ability to pass across the lipid-rich outer membranes of the enterocytes (the cells that line the small intestine) resulting poor bioavailability of drugs. Therefore, a larger dose is usually required for dosage regimens. These aspects constitute a drawback against the widespread usage of phytomedicines in the pharmaceutical field. The effectiveness of many herbal drugs is mainly based upon delivering an effective level of the active phytoconstituents present in it. These can be overcome by suitable incorporation of the novel drug delivery technology to herbal extracts minimizes the drug degradation or pre-systemic metabolism and serious side effects by accumulation of drugs to the non-targeted areas and improves the ease of administration in patients. Various phytochemical and phyto-pharmacological studies prove that the compositions, therapeutics and overall health enhancing capacities of various plant extracts but there is a great interest and medical need for the improvement of bioavailability of large number of herbal drugs and plant extracts which is having poor lipid solubility and poor bioavailability. Many herbal drugs unlike their extraordinary potential *in vitro* finding show less or no *in vivo* actions as a reason of their poor lipid solubility and larger molecular size finally resulting poor absorption and bioavailability of the drug. Numerous phytoconstituents present in it may produce a combined action of the phytoconstituents and various methods like purification and separation of the plant parts lead to a partial loss of specific activity due to the removal of chemically related substances contributing the activity of the main components present in it. Very often the chemical complexity of the extract is important for the bioavailability of then active components. Most of the plant constituents specifically phenolics are water soluble and so the major problem for less bioavailability is the inability to cross the lipid-rich biological membranes. Novel drug delivery system is useful in delivering the herbal drug at a predetermined rate and delivery of drug at the site of action which reduces the side effects with increase in bioavailability of drugs. In novel drug delivery technology, control of the distribution of drugs is obtained by incorporating the drug in suitable carrier system or by converting the structure of the drug at molecular level. Incorporation of herbal drugs in the delivery system also aids to increase its solubility, enhanced stability, protection from toxicity, enhanced pharmacological activity, improved tissue macrophage distribution, sustained delivery and protection from physical and chemical degradation. For good bioavailability, natural products must have a good balance between hydrophilicity and lipophilicity to cross lipid biological membranes. The novel carrier should ideally fulfill to requirements such as it should deliver the drug at the rate directed by the needs of the body and over the period of treatment; secondly it should be a channel for the active entry of herbal drug to the site of action. Incorporating the herbal drugs into the novel drug delivery system reduces the repeated administration of drug to overcome non-compliance which helps to increase the therapeutic value by reducing toxicity and increases the bioavailability. Novel drug delivery admits to either prolonged drug action at a predetermined rate or by maintaining the relatively constant active drug level in the body with minimization of undesirable toxic effects.

Advantages of Novel Herbal Drug Delivery System

- Help to increase the efficacy and reduce the side effect of various herbal compounds.
- Quantity of component becomes less with improving quality of drug effect.
- Fewer raw materials are required to achieve the desire effect and control drug delivery to provide exact specification regarding drug dose form.
- Ready to use devices are acceptable in today's fast lifestyle where time is important.
- Carry maximum amount of drug to the site of action by passing all barriers such as acidic pH of stomach.
- Increases prolong circulation of drug into blood due to their small particle size.
- Reduce repeat dose administration.

RECENT ADVANCES IN NOVEL HERBAL DRUG DELIVERY SYSTEMS

Various approaches in case of novel herbal drug delivery include different types of formulation such as liposomes, phytosomes, niosomes, nanoparticles, microspheres, transferosomes, ethosomes, herbal transdermal patches and proniosomes, etc. These are discussed below.

Nanoparticles

The past two decades have witnessed that many therapeutics based on nanoparticles (NPs) have been introduced in the market for therapeutic management of cancer. Advances in nanotechnology and an increased understanding of the importance of nanoparticle characteristics (size, shape, and surface properties) for biological interactions at the molecular level have created novel opportunities for development of NPs for versatile therapeutic applications.

Magnetic Nanoparticles

Magnetic nanoparticles (MNPs), in particular iron oxide (also called magnetite or Fe_3O_4) NPs and their multifunctionalized counterparts are an important class of nanoscale materials that have attracted great interest for their potential applications in drug delivery and disease diagnosis. Owing to the recent advances in synthesis and surface modification technologies, a variety of new potential applications have become feasible for this class of nanomaterials that may revolutionize current clinical diagnostic and therapeutic techniques. The well-developed surface chemistry of Fe_3O_4 MNPs allows loading of a wide range of functionalities, such as targeting ligands, imaging, and therapeutic features onto their surfaces. It is now possible to fine-tune the physical parameters of MNPs, such as size, shape, crystallinity, and magnetism. Furthermore, MNPs have the potential for replacement or modification of the coating materials post-synthesis allowing tailoring of the nanoparticle's surface charge, chemical groups, and overall size. Due to their unique physicochemical properties and ability to function at the cellular and molecular level of biological systems, MNPs are being actively investigated as the next generation of targeted drug delivery vehicle. The design of such drug delivery systems requires that the carriers be capable of selectively releasing their payloads at specific sites in the body and thereby treat disease deliberately without any harmful effect on the healthy tissues. In this regard, MNPs represent a promising option for selective drug targeting as they can be concentrated and held in position by means of an external magnetic field. This allows high dose drug loads to be delivered to a desired target tissue while minimizing the exposure of healthy tissues to the side effects from highly toxic drugs, e.g. chemotherapeutic agents. In addition, preclinical and clinical studies have proven them to be safe and some formulations are now FDA approved for clinical imaging and drug delivery. Thus, fabrication of MNPs as drug conjugates has the potential to greatly benefit inflammatory disease and cancer treatments, and diagnostics.

Liposomes

Liposomes are nanosized lipid carriers formed by the self-assembling phospholipid molecules in an aqueous environment. As liposomes are made up of lipids, they are rapidly absorbed in liver and taken up by macrophages thus decreasing their efficacy. This can be avoided by coating liposome lipid surface with ligands such as monosialoganglioside or by incorporating cholesterol, polyvinylpyrrolidone polyacrylamide lipids, glucuronic acid lipids, or phospholipid distearoylphosphatidylcholine (DSPC) into liposomes that increases their circulating time in body. When the liposomes are coated with monosialoganglioside they are called stealth liposomes. The size of these liposomes is about 100 nm. The other type of liposomes, i.e. non-stealth liposomes, prepared from high phase transition temperature phospholipids help in increasing circulation times and also accumulate within tumour tissue despite high levels of liver uptake. This surface modification of liposomes improves duration of drug release and also improves targeting of the drug to its site of action along with increased circulation time. Stability of the liposomes can be increased by incorporating cholesterol into it. The concentration of cholesterol is a crucial factor as it regulates the membrane properties. The advantages of using liposomal drugs as opposed to free drugs are well-documented in the literature and include the ability to selectively deliver liposomes to the desired site in the body.

Carbon Nanotubes

Carbon nanotubes are long, thin cylinders made up of carbon. These are synthetic rods that are only half the width of DNA. These are large macromolecules that are unique for their size, shape, and remarkable physical properties. The carbon nanotubes are derived from Graphene. As in grapheme, carbon atoms, arranged in sp2 bonded structure, form honeycomb-like patterns. They are of two types: Single-wall carbon nanotubes (SWCNTs) that have single layer of graphene and multi-wall carbon nanotubes (MWCNTs) that have more than one well of graphene. MWCNTs consist of concentric cylinders with the regular periodic interlayer spacing with a hollow centre. This central core has a spacing of around 0.34–0.39 nm. This inner diameter differs depending on the number of layers. The outer diameter of these nanotubes ranges from 20 to 30 nm. The tips of MWCNTs are usually closed and their ends are capped. A property of carbon nanotubes is that they absorb near-infrared light waves and pass harmlessly through cells. However, when a beam of near-infrared light falls on carbon nanotubes, the excitation of electrons in the nanotubes occurs as a result the excess energy is produced in the form of heat that leads to the thermal destruction of cancer cells *in vivo*. The surface of cancer cells contains numerous receptors for vitamins known as folate, thus the nanotubes coated with the folate molecules would be attracted to folate receptors of diseased cells. This treatment induces coagulative necrosis, a form of cell death that involves protein denaturation and membrane lysis. Use of MWCNTs enables ablation of tumours with low laser power (3 W/cm^2) and very short treatment time with minimal local toxicity and no evidence of systemic toxicity.

Dendrimers

Dendrimers are spherical macromolecules having highly branched structure of large number of peripheral groups that aid in encapsulation of hydrophobic drug compounds. They consist of a central core, branching units and terminal functional groups. The environment of the nanocavities and solubilizing properties of these cavities depend on the central core. Liquid crystals show the combined properties of both liquid and solid states. They can be made to form different sizes and shapes, with alternative polar and non-polar layers which include aqueous drug solutions. Because of their unique physical properties (like monodispersity, water solubility and encapsulation ability), these macromolecules are very helpful in production of drug delivery vehicles. The properties of dendrimers are dominated by the functional groups on the molecular surface; however, there are examples of dendrimers with internal functionality. Dendrimers have a well-defined nanoscale architecture and large internal volume make them an attractive option for drug delivery and other biomedical applications. Their systematic structural architecture, the unique properties of dendrimers, as compared to linear polymers, renders them of interest for intracellular drug delivery system for cancer therapy. Dendritic encapsulation of functional molecules allows for the isolation of the active site, a structure which mimics that of active sites in biomaterials. Also, it is possible to make water-soluble dendrimers, unlike most polymers, by functionalizing their outer shell with charged species or other hydrophilic groups.

Micelles

Micelles are collection of amphiphilic surfactant molecule that spontaneously aggregate and forms a spherical vesicle in water (size range of several tens of nanometers). The inner core of micelle is hydrophobic, thus can help in incorporation of hydrophobic drugs which are then released by some drug delivery mechanisms. Conventional micelles consist of hydrophilic head and a hydrophobic tail made of small molecules consisting of the hydrocarbon portion of long fatty acids. They are most of the times used as carriers for hydrophobic drugs and can be administered directly into the circulation. The molecular weight of polymer micelles is often high thus enabling maximum storage in the tissue of solid cancers. Micelles enter the tumour tissue easily as compared to other tissues. The concentration of micelles is often one order higher than in the surrounding area. The drug can be dissolved in the hydrophobic micelle core, or are bound chemically on the biodegradable polymer carrier. The preparation of polymeric micelles is simple but controlling the rate of drug release from these polymeric micelles is a tedious job. So, the surface modified micelles are prepared, the chemical bond on the surface helps to control drug release. The activation of the micelles occurs in the tumour tissue environment thus preventing the drug release in the blood while circulation thus decreasing the toxicity of drug to normal cells.

Solid Lipid Nanoparticles

Solid lipid nanoparticles (SLNPs) are widely used as a nanocarrier system for many drugs. These particles have size ranging from 50 to 1,000 nm and are made up of lipids which are stable at room temperature and body temperature. The lipids used in preparation of SLNPs include lipid acids, mono-, di-, or triglycerides, glyceride mixtures, or waxes that are stabilized using biocompatible surfactants. Over other drug deliveries, the SLNPs have advantages of physical stability, protection of labile drugs from degradation, controlled release and ease of preparation. Production of SLNPs is relatively cost efficient and amenable to large scale production. The storage and drug leakage problems are very less in SLNPs than in liposomes.

Glycerosomes

Topical drug delivery, compared to conventional routes of administration such as oral or parenteral delivery, is both potentially advantageous since it avoids active principle degradation in gastrointestinal tract and first pass hepatic metabolism and it is more acceptable by patients. However, the skin, which consists of two layers, the deeper one or dermis and the external layer or epidermis, behaves as a difficult to permeate barrier for most drug substances. The deeper layer or dermis, whose thickness is between 0.3 and 4 mm, consists of connective tissue embedded with blood vessels, pilosebaceous units (hair follicles and sebaceous glands) as well as nerve endings which make skin a true sense organ. At dermis level, active principles can cross the capillary walls to enter into the circulatory system and reach different tissues. The outermost layer of the skin or epidermis, whose thickness is between 50 and 150 μm, is covered by a hydrolipidic film and performs a barrier function against microorganisms and other exogenous molecules from the surrounding environment. Keratinocytes are the typical epidermis cells that originate at the innermost layer close to dermis and undergo a gradual differentiation process called keratinization ending with migration to surface to form a horny layer of dead cells (statum corneum) with thickness between 10 and 30 μm. The horny layer acts as an effective barrier limiting the passage of active principles whose rate of transdermal absorption correlates with the generally very low rate of their penetration through the horny layer. Due to this barrier effect, the topical administration of drugs normally results in a reduced bioavailability. Different approaches have been investigated to improve the diffusion of drugs through the skin including physicochemical methods based on the use of penetration enhancers such as dimethylsulphoxide, fatty acids, propylene glycol and urea as well as physical methods including, among others, iontophoresis, electroporation and low-frequency ultrasound or a combined application of both physical methods and chemical enhancers. A different approach to improve the transdermal diffusion of drugs is based on the carrier properties of vesicular structures generally indicated as liposomes and nanovesicular carriers.

The skin acts as the main target as well as a principal barrier for dermal and transdermal drug delivery. It also represents an ideal route of drug administration in terms of accessibility and ease of application. Indeed, topical drug delivery has several advantages over other routes of administration including improved bioavailability for drugs that suffer the gastrointestinal environment and/or hepatic first effects. Moreover, topical application can give both a constant, continuous drug delivery and/ or a targeting of the active with consequent fewer side effects and improved patient compliance. However, the barrier nature of the skin represents a significant obstacle for most drugs to be delivered into and through it. In order to overcome the barrier properties of the stratum corneum (SC) and to enhance drug transport across intact skin, several techniques have been developed. They include chemical methods based on the use of different penetration enhancers as well as physical methods (ionophoresis, electroporation and low-frequency ultrasound). One of the most controversial methods is the use of vesicular formulations as drug skin delivery systems. Over the last two decades, the lack of ability of conventional liposomes to efficiently deliver drugs across the skin has led to intensive research in the field, with the introduction and development of new classes of lipid vesicles. Recently, it has become evident that vesicle composition plays a significant role in vesicles as skin delivery systems and many authors have reported that specially designed vesicular carriers can be used to increase penetration and permeation through the SC for systemic delivery, but they can also be employed to localize the drug in the skin layers and deeper soft tissues (subcutaneous adipose and skeletal muscle tissue) for local treatment in the context of various diseases.

Therefore, new, modified formulations have been tested and the so-called deformable/ elastic liposomes, niosomes as well as ethosomes are introduced. Recently, different authors have tested various penetration enhancers as 'edge activator' in the formulation of new phospholipid vesicles such as propylene glycol-liposomes, invasomes, and PEVs (penetration enhancer containing vesicles). A new approach to increase liposome properties as dermal and transdermal drug delivery systems by modifying liposomal bilayer fluidity is represented by glycerosomes, which are obtained from different phospholipids and high concentrations of glycerol (10–30%, v/v), a harmless and fully accepted compound for topical administration. Glycerosomes are versatile vesicular carriers that might contain one or more of the additives commonly used in the composition of conventional liposomes such as cholesterol. Moreover, they can be obtained by any of the different techniques commonly used for the preparation of conventional liposomes.

Glycerosomes are firstly designed in 2012 using DPPC and high concentrations of glycerol (10–30%) in the water phase. Glycerosomes containing 20 and 30% glycerol are able to ameliorate both accumulation and transdermal delivery of diclofenac sodium salt, one of the most potent non-steroidal anti-inflammatory compounds, in comparison with basic liposomes. Glycerosomes are phospholipid vesicles containing glycerol (10–30%) in the water phase. Glycerosomes are obtained from dipalmitoylglycero-phosphatidylcholine cholesterol, and different amounts of glycerol. Formulations are prepared, characterized, and tested as carriers of diclofenac, one of the most potent and commercially successful non-steroidal anti-inflammatory drugs (NSAIDs), which has been very often used as a model drug in (*trans*) dermal drug delivery by using different vesicular carriers. Diclofenac is encapsulated into glycerosomes as sodium salt and formulations are fully characterized by using different methods, transmission electron microscopy; photon correlation spectroscopy, differential scanning calorimetry, to obtain more information regarding glycerosomes' structure and properties and go deeply into the role of glycerol in affecting their features as (*trans*) dermal drug delivery system (Figs 11.1 and 11.2).

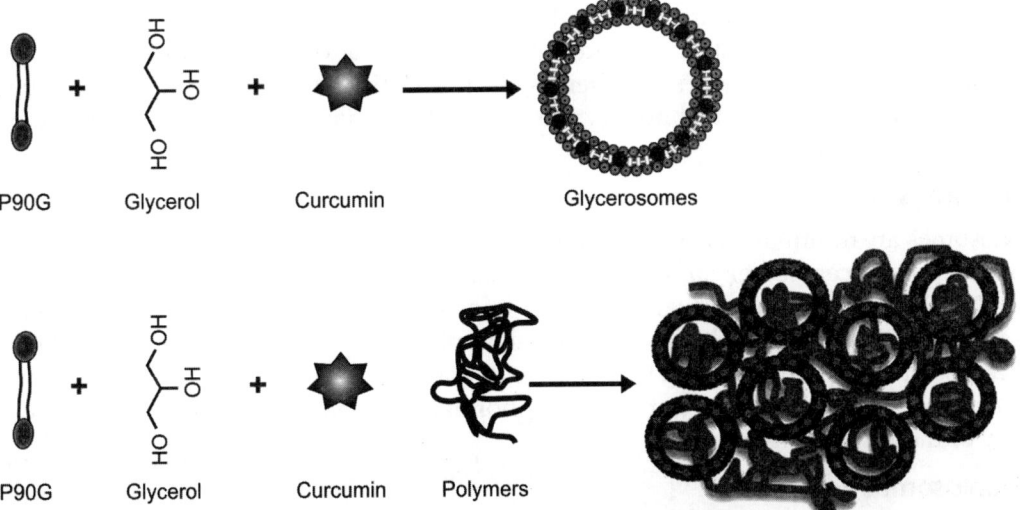

Fig 11.1: Curcumin encapsulated glycerosomes

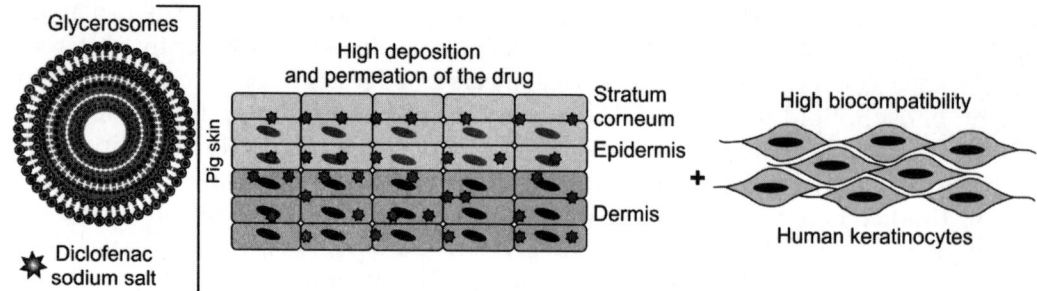

Fig 11.2: Diclofenac encapsulated glycerosomes

Glycethosomes (Glycerol-Ethanol Phospholipid Vesicles)

Lipids, surfactant and payload are mixed and hydrate with water to obtain liposomes; water and glycerol (50:50 v/v) to obtain glycerosomes; water and ethanol (50:50 v/v) to obtain ethosomes; glycerol, ethanol and water (50:25:25 v/v) to obtain glycethosomes. Glycethosome is the smallest vesicles (~140 nm), most homogeneously dispersed (PI 0.32) and highly negatively charged (–42 mV). The mean diameter of other vesicles is 2–3 times higher. Additionally, the dispersion is very instable and after a few days formed two phases.

Phytosomes

Most of the bioactive constituents of phytomedicines are flavonoids, which are poorly bioavailable when taken orally. Water-soluble phytoconstituent molecules (mainly polyphenols) can be converted into lipid compatible molecular complexes, which are called phytosomes. Phytosomes are more bioavailable as compared to simple herbal extracts owing to their enhanced mental ability to skip through the lipid rich biomembranes and finally arriving to the origin. The lipid phase substances employed to make phytoconstituents lipid compatible are phospholipids from soy, mainly phosphatidylcholine. Phytosomal complexes are first investigated for cosmetic applications, but mounting evidence of potential for drug delivery has been amassed over the past few years, with beneficial activity in the realms of cardiovascular, anti-inflammatory, hepatoprotective, and anticancer applications. Phytosome complexes show better pharmacokinetics and therapeutic profile than their non-complexed herbal extract. The phytosome technology has markedly enhanced the bioavailability of selected phytochemicals.

Niosomes

Niosomes are multilamellar vesicles formed from non-ionic surfactants of the alkyl or dialkylpolyglycerol ether class and cholesterol. Niosomes are different from liposomes in that they offer certain advantages over liposomes. Liposomes face problems such as they are expensive, their ingredients such as phospholipids are chemically unstable because of their predisposition to oxidative degradation, they require special memory and handling, and purity of natural phospholipids is variable. Niosomes do not have any of these problems.

Proniosomes

Proniosome gel system is step forward to niosome, which can be utilized for various applications in delivery of actives at desired site. Proniosomal gels are the formulations, which on *in situ* hydration with water from the skin are converted into niosomes. Proniosomes are water soluble carrier particles that are coated with surfactant and can be hydrated to form niosomal dispersion immediately before use on brief agitation in hot aqueous media.

Microspheres

Microspheres are discrete spherical particles ranging in average particle size from 1 to 50 μ. Microparticulate drug delivery systems are studied and taken on as a reliable one to rescue the drug to the target site with specificity, to assert the desired concentration at the situation of interest without untoward effects. Microencapsulation is a useful method which extends the duration of drug effect significantly and improves patient compliance. Finally, the entire dose and a few adverse reactions may be thinned out since a steady plasma concentration is kept. So far, a series of active ingredients of plants, such as rutin, camptothecin, zedoary oil, tetrandrine, quercetine, and *Cynara scolymus* extract, has been made into microspheres. In addition, reports on immune microsphere and magnetic microsphere are also usual in recent years. Immune microsphere possesses the immune competence as a consequence of the antibody, and antigen is coated or adsorbed on the polymer microspheres.

Herbal Transdermal Patches

Transdermal drug delivery systems facilitate the passage of therapeutic quantities of drug substances through the skin and into the general circulation for their systemic effects. Herbal transdermal patches are medicated adhesive pad designed to release active ingredients at a constant rate over a period of several hours or days after application to skin. Herbal penetration enhancers like some terpenes are found to be potential enough to replace the conventionally available penetration enhancers.

Emulsions

Emulsion refers to a non-homogeneous dispersion system that is composed of two kinds of liquids unable to dissolve each other, and one of which disperses in the other one in a form of droplets. Broadly speaking, the emulsion is composed of the oil phase, water phase, surfactant, and subsurfactant. Its appearance is translucent to transparent liquid. Emulsion can be split up into ordinary emulsion (0.1–100 μm), microemulsion (10–100 nm), sub-microemulsion (100–600 nm), etc. Among them, the microemulsion is also called nanoemulsions, and the sub microemulsion is also called lipid emulsion. As a drug delivery system, emulsion gets distributed *in vivo* in the targeted areas due to its affinity towards lymphatic fluids. In addition, the drug can be a sustained release in a long time because the drug is packaged in the inner phase and kept off direct touch with the body and tissue fluid. Afterward, along the oily drugs or lipophilic drugs being made into O/W or O/W/O emulsion, the oil droplets are phagocytozed by the macrophage and get a high concentration in the liver, spleen, and kidney in which the quantity of the dissolved drug is truly heavy. While water soluble drug is produced into W/O or W/O/W emulsion, it can be well contracted in the lymphatic system by intramuscular or subcutaneous injection. The size of the emulsion particle has an impact on its target distribution. Aside from its targeted sustained release, producing the herbal drug into emulsion will also beef up the stability of the hydrolyzed materials, improve the penetrability of drugs to the skin and mucous, and reduce the drugs' stimulus to the tissues. So far, some kinds of herbal drugs, such as camptothecin, Brucea javanica oil, coixenolide oil, and zedoary oil, have been made into emulsion.

Ethosomes

Newer advancements in the patch technology have led to the development of ethosomal patch, which consists of drug in ethosomes. Ethosomal systems are made up of soya phosphatidylcholine, ethanol and water. They may form multilamellar vesicles and have a high entrapment capacity for particles of various lipophilicities. The elastic vesicles and transfersomes have also been used as drug carriers for a range of small molecules, peptides, proteins and vaccines. Ethosome has a high deformability and entrapment efficiency and can penetrate through the skin completely and improve drug delivery through the skin. Likened to other liposomes, the physical and chemical properties of ethosomes make the legal transfer of the drug through the stratum corneum into a deeper skin layer efficiently or even into the blood circulation. This property is very important as the topical drug carrier and transdermal delivery system. Moreover, the ethosomes carrier also can provide an efficient intracellular delivery for both hydrophilic and lipophilic drugs, percutaneous absorption of matrine an anti-inflammatory herbal drug is increased, it also permits the antibacterial peptide to penetrate into the fibrocyte easily.

Transfersomes

Transfersomes are specially optimized particles or vesicles that can respond to an external stress by rapid and energetically inexpensive, shape transformations. The development of novel approaches such as transfersomes have immensely contributed in overcoming problem faced by transdermal drug delivery such as unable to transport larger molecules, penetration through the stratum corneum is the rate-limiting step, physicochemical properties of drugs hinder their own transport through skin. These elastic vesicles can squeeze themselves through skin pores many times smaller than their own size and can transport larger molecules. Transfersomes are applied in a non-occluded method to the skin, which permeate through the stratum corneum lipid lamellar regions as a result of the hydration or osmotic force in the skin. It can be applicable as drug carriers for an orbit of small molecules, peptides, proteins and herbal elements. Transfersomes can penetrate the stratum corneum and supply the nutrients, locally to maintain its functions resulting maintenance of skin. Transfersomes are a form of elastic or deformable vesicle, which are first introduced in the early 1990s and their elasticity is generated by incorporation of an edge activator in the lipid bilayer structure.

PHOSPHOLIPIDS: A NOVEL ADJUVANT IN HERBAL DRUG DELIVERY SYSTEMS

Introduction

Phytoconstituents have been used extensively in modern science because of their various pharmacological actions with a few side effects. Regardless of their excellent therapeutic activity, several phytoconstituents have shown poor bioavailability *in vivo*. Phytoconstituents possess properties such as poor lipid solubility, large molecular size, and degradation in the gut due to the acidic environment. Gastric enzymes always limit their use. Phospholipids seem to be a major carrier for plant active molecules, which not only interact with the plant constituents on a molecular level but also protect the active components of the plant from degradation and increase the bioavailability of the active components by imparting lipid solubility to them. Complexation techniques enable researchers to convert the phytophospholipids into various dosage forms, including tablets and capsules. In the cosmetic industry, however, these complexes have acquired wider applicability in the form of gels and emulsions. Complexation of phospholipids with active components of plants improves their bioavailability and is being extensively studied by researchers, and further research in this regard is expected in the future.

All biological membranes consist of a mixture of different classes of phospholipids, such as phosphatidylcholine (PC), phosphatidylethanolamine (PE), phosphatidylinositol (PI), phosphatidic acid (PA), and phosphatidylserine (PS). Phospholipids are amphipathic and are composed of a hydrophilic portion (the head group; negatively charged phosphates) and a hydrophobic portion (the tail group; long fatty acid hydrocarbon chains), thus forming lipid bilayers. Structural differences among phospholipids depend on the variability of the head group, variation of the chain length, and degree of saturation of the fatty acid ester groups. Phospholipids containing glycerols are called glycerophospholipids. Plant-derived active components have recently gained wide importance in the therapeutic field and are part of remarkable breakthrough in therapeutic drug delivery.

Traditional systems using crude plant extracts may at times be harmful because they contain different ingredients along with the active constituents; these traditional systems have been replaced with modern analytics of plant active components, both quantitatively and qualitatively. Advances in modern science allow researchers to extract and isolate specific active constituents for specific medical applications. More standardized herbal extracts are prepared in herbal medicine systems that exhibit beneficial therapeutic effects. However, because of poor solubility, extensive research has been done to enhance the solubility and bioavailability of herbal extracts and their constituents. Modern drug delivery helps researchers to formulate various formulations of these plant active components, thus improving their bioavailability. When combined with phospholipids, phytoconstituents offer plenty of advantages, such as enhanced permeation of the drug through the skin, which is advantageous for herbal active components. Several herbal active components with low bioavailability can be delivered effectively when complexed with phospholipids and offer a low toxicity profile. Phospholipids recently emerged as a potential carrier for complexing with plant active components to increase their bioavailability. These techniques are widely used now and have proved efficient in enhancing the bioavailability of poorly absorbed plant constituents. Complexing PC with plant active components (standardized herbal extracts) also improves the membrane permeability, water–oil partition coefficient, and hence the systemic bioavailability of the plant active components. Complexation of water-soluble drugs with phospholipids enhances bioavailability by increasing the penetration of complex-containing active components through lipoidal plasma membrane, whereas increased bioavailability of phospholipid complexes of poorly water-soluble drugs is attributed to an increase in the solubility of the complex in gastric fluids (Fig. 11.3).

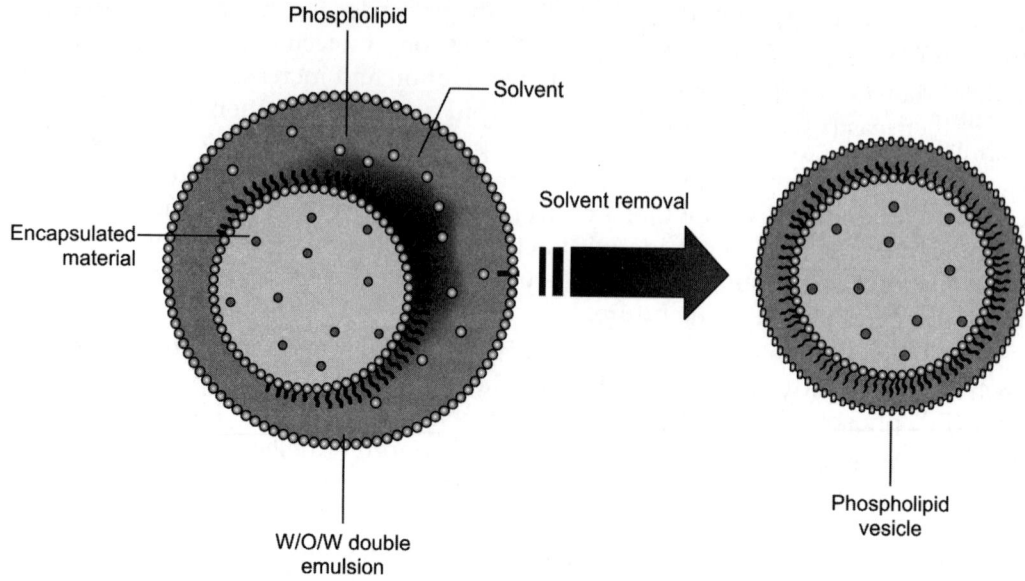

Fig 11.3: Phospholipid vesicles

Phospholipids in Human/Animal Tissues and Natural Sources

Phospholipids are found in every part of the body and, as an essential component of membranes, serve a structural as well as functional purpose in the body. Phospholipids are present in eggs, particularly in the yellow yolk, in addition to protein and carbohydrates. Egg yolk contains major lipids as phospholipids (12% by weight of wet tissue) and triglycerides (24% by weight of wet tissue). Milk is another important source of phospholipids. It contains glycerophospholipids and sphingolipids that are usually present in the milk fat globule membrane and in other membranous materials of the skim milk phase. Principally, PC, PE, PI, and PS come under glycerophospholipids, whereas sphingomyelin is the dominant species of sphingolipids. The milk fat globule membrane is a triple-layer lamina; an initial surface-active layer composed of proteins completely surrounds the intracellularly present neutral lipids. The inner part of the membrane is covered with a bilayer membrane that is derived from the secretory cell apical plasma membrane. Phospholipids are mainly located on the outer leaflet and are arranged as a free liquid phase co-organized with a lipid phase; the latter is rich in sphingomyelin and cholesterol. Vegetable materials normally contain very low quantities of phospholipids, ranging from 0.3 to 2.5 w/w (PC, PE, and PI). Rice bran, papaya, cucurbit, corn, and castor bean are some plant sources of phospholipids. Phospholipids constitute 0.3–0.6% of soybean seed (1.5–3.0% of crude soybean oil). Other minor constituents of soybean phospholipids are water, pigment, galactosyl glyceride, glycolipids, carbohydrates, sterols, and tocopherol. Soybean phospholipids are the byproducts of the soybean oil refining process; hence phospholipid composition may vary each time the process is done. Soybean phospholipids are soluble in aliphatic, aromatic, and halogenated hydrocarbon solvents, such as ether, benzene, chloroform, and petroleum ether, and in aliphatic alcohol, in particular ethanol. Like other non-polar surfactants, soybean phospholipids are insoluble in polar solvents. Soybean phospholipids are soluble in animal fats and vegetable oils, mineral oils, and fatty acids; however, they are insoluble in cold conditions. Because of the presence of a hydrophilic phosphate group and hydrophobic hydrocarbon keys, phospholipid molecules possess a hydrophilic colloid property that makes them easily form an interface between water and oil, which lowers the interfacial tension between water and oil and makes them colloidally stable molecules. When a phospholipid molecule comes in contact with hot water, it absorbs water and expands, forming a stable colloidal solution.

Digestion of Phospholipid

Researchers have been exploring several issues involving lipid digestion in the body. Understanding lipid pharmacokinetics will help the researchers in developing pathways that may reduce the risk of lipid-associated disorders. Lipid digestion starts as soon as it enters the oral cavity, when it is exposed to lingual lipases secreted by glands in the tongue, which are mainly responsible for the digestion of triglycerides. Digestion continues in the stomach through enzymes (lingual and gastric). Emulsification of dietary fat and fat-soluble vitamins also occurs in the stomach. The emulsion of dietary fat enters the duodenum as fine lipid droplets and mixes with the bile and pancreatic juices that provide pancreatic lipase and bile salts to the body, which function synergistically to ensure lipid digestion and absorption. The digestion of PC, in particular phospholipids found in lumen of the small intestine, primarily occurs by pancreatic phospholipase A2 and other lipases secreted by the pancreas. Luminal PC is cleaved by the enzyme phospholipase A2 from the pancreatic juice into fatty acids and lysophosphatidylcholine. These two breakdown products are further absorbed and cross the intestinal mucosa. Researchers studied the mechanism of intestinal absorption of polyunsaturated PC in an oil medium. They found that the absorption rate, as measured by disappearance from the gastrointestinal tract, is relatively rapid in the first 6–8 hours. The study results revealed that one part of the absorbed polyunsaturated PC is hydrolyzed to 1-acyl-lysophosphatidylcholine during the absorption process and reacylated again to PC upon entering the mucosa cell, whereas the other part is completely hydrolyzed to free fatty acids and glycerophosphocholine.

Phytophospholipid Interactions

M/s Indena, an Italian pharmaceutical and neutraceutical company, has patented the first phospholipid complexation technique in the name of Phytosome (a combination of soy lecithin with any standardized extracts containing polyphenolic compounds). Phytosomes have been developed using boswellic acids, selected triterpenes from the leaves of *Centella asiatica*, ginkgo flavonglycosides, ginkgo terpenes, bilobalide and ginkgolides from the leaves of *Ginkgo biloba,* typical ginseng constituents from the roots of Panax ginseng, polyphenols from young leaves of *Camelia sinensis*, proanthocyanidins from the seeds of *Vitis vinifera,* silybin-like substances from the fruit of *Silybum marianum,* and curcuminoids from *Curcuma longa.* PC comprises two major parts, namely the phosphatidyl moiety (lipophilic) and the choline moiety (hydrophilic). Choline binds to the respective active compounds/extracts and the phosphatidyl portion encloses the choline-bound structure as an envelope. The shape and integrity of the phytophospholipid plant active component complex contributes to easy diffusion across the cell barrier because phosphatidyl choline is a major molecular building block of the cell membrane and is easily solubilized in water; in addition, the oil/lipid environment acts as convoy for phytoconstituents that allows them to pass through biological membranes. Plant active components, particularly polyphenolic compounds, interact with the phospholipid molecules by forming chemical bonds (complexes) between them. Many researchers have prepared these complexes and characterized them with the help of fourier transform infrared (FTIR) spectroscopy, nuclear magnetic resonance (NMR) spectroscopy, and differential scanning calorimetry (DSC) analysis (Fig. 11.4).

Beneficial Effects of Phospholipids

Inflammation is a complex biological response to harmful stimuli such as pathogens or irritants, leading to a biochemical cascade that releases inflammatory mediators such as cytokines, chemokines, and eicosanoids. Many researchers investigated the effects of exogenous PC with nonsteroidal diclofenac supplementation on polymorphonuclear cell influx in Wistar rats with carrageenan-induced arthritis. A mixture of 2% carrageenan and 4% kaolin is injected intramuscularly into animal knee joints to induce arthritis. They found that the development of arthritis is accompanied by a significant increase in the number of adherent leucocytes, but this increment is drastically controlled (by approximately 40%) by PC. The treatment of arthritis with PC greatly reduced perivascular infiltration of the neutrophil leucocytes and the expression of intercellular adhesion molecule-1. This study of arthritis clearly indicates

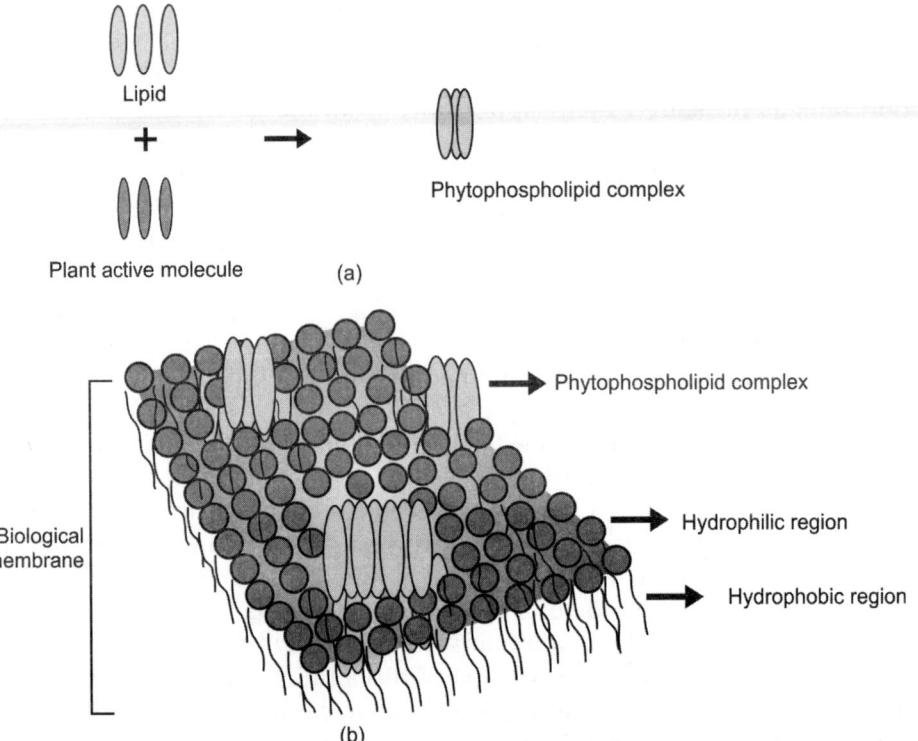

Fig. 11.4: (a) Schematic representation of phospholipid complexation with active plant components. (b) Interaction of a phytophospholipid complex with the biological membrane.

the potential anti-inflammatory effects of PC, which are attributed to the reduction of neutrophil leucocyte-mediated microcirculatory inflammatory reactions. The potential use of dietary PC as an anti-inflammatory substance in a murine model of chronic rheumatoid arthritis has been studied. PC pretreatment reduced the hypersensitivity of collagen-induced arthritis and produced a remarkable decrease in the number of leucocyte endothelial cell interactions. The results of the study suggested the use of PC pretreatment for rheumatoid arthritis seemed to exert beneficial effects on the morphological, functional, and microcirculatory characteristics of chronic arthritis. The authors reported the use of oral PC as a preventive approach in ameliorating experimental rheumatoid arthritis-induced joint damage.

Researchers investigated the use of PC-derived choline for anti-inflammatory action in stress conditions. PE and N-acyl PEs, which are endogenous bioactive phospholipids linked to PC, also are investigated for anti-inflammatory responses. The treatment of mice with dietary PC + PE + N-acyl PE supplementation significantly decreased the leucocyte reaction and suppressed the activity of pulmonary proinflammatory enzymes. The study results reported that PC-derived choline can be used as a novel preventive or pharmacotherapeutic option in inflammatory pathologies. Researchers investigated the possible use of PCs in the treatment of ulcerative colitis. PCs with different fatty acid side chains are applied on differentiated and non-differentiated Caco-2 cells treated with tumour necrosis factor (TNF)-α to induce a proinflammatory response that is detected with the help of a quantitative real-time polymerase chain reaction analysis. Prolonged inhibition of TNF-α-induced proinflammatory signaling is reported after application of PC; this is attributed to a shift of the TNF-α receptors at the surface of lipid rafts. The study results may offer a potential treatment of ulcerative colitis.

Researchers investigated the capacity of phospholipids to reduce adhesions of gastric cancer cells in extracellular matrix components. Human gastric cancer cells from NUGC-4 (Japanese Cancer Research Resources Bank, Tokyo, Japan) are used in the investigation. Phospholipids are added in concentrations of 0.05, 0.1, 0.5, 0.75, and 1.0/100 µl medium to a precoated plate of collagen IV, laminin, and fibronectin. Phospholipid concentrations of 0.5 mg/100 µl or higher can significantly reduce the attachment of gastric cancer cells to collagen IV, laminin, and fibronectin. Researchers investigated the effect of n-3 polyunsaturated fatty acids (PUFAs) as a growth inhibitor on chemically induced (1, 2-dimethylhydrazine) colon cancer in rats. They found that PC potently inhibited the growth of Caco-2 cells, and experimental diets containing n-3 PUFAs suppressed colon cancer in rats. The study reported the use of marine-derived diets containing PC that may prove to be a valuable dietary protective factor against colon cancer.

Researchers investigated the effect of PUFAs, docosahexaenoic acid (DHA), and eicosapentaenoic acid on carcinogenic processes. The effect of PUFAs on 3 colon cancer cell lines (HT-29, Caco-2, and DLD-1) is examined. PUFAs have the strongest growth-inhibitory effect on HT-29 cells than Caco-2 and DLD-1 cells. Another study done by researcher investigated the effect of two phospholipids, polyunsaturated PC and PS, on butyrate-induced growth inhibition, differentiation, and apoptosis using Caco-2 cells. The addition of PC inhibited the growth of cancer in 24 hours in Caco-2 cells, whereas PS took 48 hours to inhibit growth. The study suggests the potential use of marine PC and PS as a promising active component against colon cancer chemotherapy with high bioavailability. Age-related memory impairment now affects a vast group of the population worldwide. As aging progresses, the lipid composition of the brain cells also changes. The amount of 3-PUFAs in the brain correspondingly decreases as aging progresses; thus, a decrease in membrane fluidity and other related activities such as cholinergic pathways seem to be affected because they require PC and PUFAs for proper functioning and release of neurotransmitters. Researchers demonstrated the effective use of phospholipids as a potential carrier of PUFAs (e.g. DHA) to the brain. Kinetics and tissue distribution of ingested 13C-labelled DHA and radio-labelled DHA is analyzed after being injected in a non-esterified form compared with the fatty acid esterified in lyso-PC. The capacity of the 2 latter forms to cross a reconstituted blood–brain barrier consisting of co-cultures of brain capillary endothelial cells and astrocytes is examined. On the whole, the study suggests phospholipids as the preferred carrier of DHA in the brain.

Researchers investigated and summarized important clinical findings that emphasized the intake of essential phospholipids (EPLs) from soybean in liver diseases. These EPLs contain a highly purified extract of polyenyl PC molecules from soybean. Regarding *in vitro* analysis done on animals, EPLs performed several functions, such as antioxidant, anti-inflammatory, antifibrotic, apoptosis-modulating, regenerative, membrane-repairing and -protective, cell-signaling and receptor-influencing, as well as lipid-regulating effects in models of intoxication with chemicals or drugs. Clinical data from European and Asian countries also reported that remarkable improvement in subjective symptoms; clinical, biochemical, and imaging findings; and histology in liver indications such as fatty liver of different origins, drug hepatotoxicity, and adjuvants in chronic viral hepatitis and hepatic coma. On the whole, the clinical data suggest the potential use of EPLs as evidence-based medicine in the treatment of liver disorders.

QUESTIONS

A. Short Answer Type Questions

1. Give a short note on glycethosomes.
2. Write a short note on liposomes.
3. What do you mean by glycerosomes?
4. What is phospholipid?
5. Write the significance of phospholipid in herbal drug delivery system.
6. Mention the application of nanoparticles.
7. What are the differences between niosomes and proniosomes?

B. Long Answer Type Questions

1. Discuss about novel drug delivery systems for phytoconstituents.
2. Describe importance of novel herbal drug delivery system.
3. Write beneficial effect of phospholipid in herbal drug delivery system.
4. Write about phytophospholipid interactions in detail.
5. Give the advantages of phytosomes.

Index